Medical Radiology

Diagnostic Imaging

For further volumes:
http://www.springer.com/series/4354

Sabine Weckbach
Editor

Incidental Radiological Findings

Springer

Editor
Prof. Dr. Sabine Weckbach
Diagnostic and Interventional Radiology
University Hospital Heidelberg
Heidelberg
Germany

ISSN 0942-5373 ISSN 2197-4187 (electronic)
Medical Radiology
ISBN 978-3-319-42579-5 ISBN 978-3-319-42581-8 (eBook)
DOI 10.1007/978-3-319-42581-8

Library of Congress Control Number: 2017937774

Printed on acid-free paper

This Springer imprint is published by Springer Nature
The registered company is Springer International Publishing AG
The registered company address is: Gewerbestrasse 11, 6330 Cham, Switzerland

Contents

Part I: Introduction

Incidental Findings: Definition of the Concept 3
Reinold Schmücker

Incidental Findings – Ethical Aspects 9
Pia Erdmann

Medicolegal Aspects and Informed Consent 25
Leonard Berlin

Part II: IFs in Population Based Imaging/Research Setting

Technical Prerequisites of Population-Based Imaging 37
Sergios Gatidis and Fabian Bamberg

Part III: Handling / Management of IFs in Different Countries/ Population Based Studies

Management of Incidental Findings in the Study of Health in Pomerania 45
Carsten-Oliver Schmidt and Katrin Hegenscheid

Management of Incidental Findings in the German National Cohort 57
Robert C. Bertheau, Oyunbileg von Stackelberg, Sabine Weckbach, Hans-Ulrich Kauczor, and Christopher L. Schlett

Management of Incidental Findings on Multimodal Imaging in UK Biobank 71
Lorna M. Gibson, Jonathan Sellors, and Cathie L.M. Sudlow

Management of Incidental Findings on Neuroimaging in the Rotterdam Study 79
Daniel Bos and Meike W. Vernooij

Incidental Findings in a Population Based Study Using Cardiac CT: Experience from the Multi-Ethnic Study of Atherosclerosis (MESA) 87
Sina Rahmani and Matthew J. Budoff

Incidental Findings and Their Handling in the Swedish CArdioPulmonary bioImage Study (SCAPIS) 91
Åse Johnsson, Oskar Angerås, Anders Blomberg, David Erlinge, Agneta Flinck, Christer Janson, Hanna Markstad, Jonas Persson, Lennart Persson, Eva Swahn, Kjell Toren, Jenny Vikgren, Mats G. Hansson, and Göran Bergström

Part IV: Differences Between IF in Population Based Imaging and Patients

Management of Incidental Findings in Patients 105
Katharina Müller-Peltzer, Melvin D' Anastasi, and Wieland Sommer

Classification of Incidental Findings 113
Lale Umutlu

Incidental Findings on Abdominal CT 127
Mikael Hellström

Incidental Findings in ^{18}F-FDG PET/CT and PET/MR 169
Benedikt M. Schaarschmidt and Christian Buchbender

Incidental Findings in Ultrasound 197
J. Rübenthaler and D.-A. Clevert

Index 205

Contributors

Oskar Angerås Department of Molecular and Clinical Medicine, University of Gothenburg, Gothenburg, Sweden

Department of Cardiology, Sahlgrenska University Hospital, Gothenburg, Sweden

Fabian Bamberg Department of Diagnostic and Interventional Radiology, University of Tuebingen, Tübingen, Germany

Göran Bergström Department of Radiology, Sahlgrenska University Hospital, Gothenburg, Sweden

Department of Clinical Physiology Sahlgrenska University Hospital Gothenburg, Sweden

The Wallenberg Laboratory for Cardiovascular and Metabolic Research, Sahlgrenska University Hospital, Gothenburg, Sweden

Leonard Berlin Radiology Department, Skokie Hospital, Skokie, IL, USA
Rush University, Chicago, IL, USA
University of Illinois, Chicago, IL, USA

Robert C. Bertheau Department of Diagnostic and Interventional Radiology, University Hospital Heidelberg, Heidelberg, Germany

Anders Blomberg Department of Public Health and Clinical Medicine, Division of Medicine/Respiratory Medicine, Umeå University, Umea, Sweden

Daniel Bos Departments of Radiology and Epidemiology, Erasmus MC, University Medical Centre Rotterdam, Rotterdam, The Netherlands

Christian Buchbender Medical Faculty, Department of Diagnostic and Interventional Radiology, University Dusseldorf, Dusseldorf, Germany

Matthew J. Budoff Division of Cardiology, Los Angeles Biomedical Research Institute at Harbor-UCLA, Torrance, CA, USA

D.-A. Clevert Department of Clinical Radiology, Interdisciplinary Ultrasound Center, Ludwig-Maximilians-University of Munich-Grosshadern Campus, Munich, Germany

Pia Erdmann Ernst-Moritz-Arndt-Universität Greifswald, Theologische Fakultät, Lehrstuhl für Systematische Theologie, Greifswald, Germany

David Erlinge Department of Cardiology, Clinical Sciences, Lund University, Lund, Sweden

Agneta Flinck Department of Radiology, Sahlgrenska University Hospital, Gothenburg Sweden

Department of Radiology, University of Gothenburg, Gothenburg, Sweden

Lorna M. Gibson University of Edinburgh, Centre for Clinical Brain Sciences, Edinburgh, UK

Mats G. Hansson Department of Public Health and Caring Sciences, Centre for Research Ethics and Bioethics, Uppsala University, Uppsala, Sweden

Katrin Hegenscheid Institut für Community Medicine – SHIP-KEF, Universitätsmedizin Greifswald, Greifswald, Germany

Christer Janson Department of Medical Sciences: Respiratory, Allergy and Sleep Research, Uppsala University, Uppsala, Sweden

Åse Johnsson Department of Radiology, Sahlgrenska University Hospital, Gothenburg, Sweden

Department of Radiology, University of Gothenburg, Gothenburg, Sweden

Hans-Ulrich Kauczor Department of Diagnostic and Interventional Radiology, University Hospital Heidelberg, Heidelberg, Germany

Hanna Markstad Department of Diagnostic Radiology, Lund University and Skåne University Hospital, Lund, Sweden

Jonas Persson Division of Cardiovascular Medicine, Department of Clinical Sciences, Danderyd Hospital, Karolinska Institutet, Stockholm, Sweden

Lennart Persson Department of Medical and Health Sciences, Linköping University, Linkoping, Sweden

Sina Rahmani Division of Cardiology, Los Angeles Biomedical Research Institute at Harbor-UCLA, Torrance, CA, USA

J. Rübenthaler Department of Clinical Radiology, Interdisciplinary Ultrasound Center, Ludwig-Maximilians-University of Munich-Grosshadern Campus, Munich, Germany

Benedikt M. Schaarschmidt Medical Faculty, Department of Diagnostic and Interventional Radiology, University Dusseldorf, Dusseldorf, Germany

Christopher L. Schlett Department of Diagnostic and Interventional Radiology, University Hospital Heidelberg, Heidelberg, Germany

Carsten Oliver Schmidt Institut für Community Medicine – SHIP-KEF, Universitätsmedizin Greifswald, Greifswald, Germany

Reinold Schmücker Westfälische Wilhelms-Universität Münster, Münster, Germany

Jonathan Sellors University of Oxford, Clinical Trial Service Unit and Epidemiological Studies Unit, Nuffield Department of Population Health, Oxford, UK

UK Biobank Coordinating Centre, Adswood, Stockport, UK

Cathie L. M. Sudlow University of Edinburgh, Centre for Clinical Brain Sciences, Edinburgh, UK

UK Biobank Coordinating Centre, Adswood, Stockport, UK

Eva Swahn Department of Medical and Health Sciences, Linköping University, Linkoping, Sweden

Kjell Toren Section of Occupational and Environmental Medicine, Institute of Medicine, University of Gothenburg, Gothenburg, Sweden

Gatidis Tübingen Department of Diagnostic and Interventional Radiology, University of Tuebingen, Tübingen, Germany

Lale Umutlu University Hospital Essen, Department of Diagnostic and Interventional Radiology and Neuroradiology, Essen, Germany

Meike W. Vernooij Departments of Radiology and Epidemiology, Erasmus MC, University Medical Centre Rotterdam, Rotterdam, The Netherlands

Jenny Vikgren Department of Radiology, Sahlgrenska University Hospital, Gothenburg, Sweden

Department of Radiology, University of Gothenburg, Gothenburg, Sweden

Oyunbileg von Stackelberg Department of Diagnostic and Interventional Radiology, University Hospital Heidelberg, Heidelberg, Germany

Sabine Weckbach Department of Diagnostic and Interventional Radiology, University Hospital Heidelberg, Heidelberg, Germany

Part I

Introduction

Incidental Findings: Definition of the Concept

Reinold Schmücker

Contents

1 **Incidental Findings in a Broad Sense** 4

2 **Incidental Findings in a Narrow Sense** 5

3 **Incidental Finding or Signal Abnormality?** 5

4 **The Differing Indicative Dignity of Incidental Findings** 6

5 **The Context of the Occurrence of Incidental Findings** 6

References 7

Abstract

In a broad sense, any findings can be called incidental that occur in the context of medical diagnostics and that potentially affect the health (including the reproductive capacities) of a living being – if the diagnostic means were not intended to produce such findings. It would be wrong to only talk about an incidental finding once the relevance for the health or reproductive capacity of the concerned individual has been established. The concept of an incidental finding rather includes – in its broad as well as narrow sense, which will be explained in the next paragraph – both marginal findings with no clinical relevance and false positive findings. This use of the concept makes sense, because the artefactual character of false positive findings in particular usually only becomes clear after further evaluation. Since this evaluation would not take place without the misleading primary finding, the concept of a finding cannot plausibly depend on the factual correctness or clinical relevance of diagnostic discoveries.

This chapter is derived from my handbook entry Schmücker (2013).

R. Schmücker
Westfälische Wilhelms-Universität Münster, Münster, Germany
e-mail: schmuecker@uni-muenster.de

Med Radiol Diagn Imaging (2016)
DOI 10.1007/174_2016_96, © Springer International Publishing Switzerland
Published Online: 17 Dec 2016

1 Incidental Findings in a Broad Sense

In a broad sense, any findings can be called incidental that occur in the context of medical diagnostics and that potentially affect the health (including the reproductive capacities) of a living being – if the diagnostic means were not intended to produce such findings. It would be wrong to only talk about an incidental finding once the relevance for the health or reproductive capacity of the concerned individual has been established. The concept of an incidental finding rather includes – in its broad as well as narrow sense, which will be explained in the next paragraph – both marginal findings with no clinical relevance and false positive findings. This use of the concept makes sense, because the artefactual character of false positive findings in particular usually only becomes clear after further evaluation. Since this evaluation would not take place without the misleading primary finding, the concept of a finding cannot plausibly depend on the factual correctness or clinical relevance of diagnostic discoveries.

Incidental findings understood in this sense can occur in the context of research in life sciences or while diagnostic means are employed to confirm the presence of a certain disease. They can also occur when magnetic resonance images are taken for an anatomical atlas or when a follow-up examination for a cured disease shows indications of a different disease.

Diagnostic findings that occur in the context of the doctor-patient relationship while searching for the cause of certain symptoms, but that do not comply with the doctor's expectations concerning this cause, are not incidental findings – not even according to the broad concept of incidental findings. The examination is aimed at establishing findings that would explain the reported symptoms, even if those findings do not comply with the physician's expectations. Diagnostic findings that occur in the context of *direct-to-consumer* genetic analyses or *direct-to-consumer* whole-body MRI examinations that are offered by commercial companies as individual check-ups also do not count as incidental findings. For there is, although no treatment contract is involved here, a contractual relationship between the subject of the preventive examination and the provider of the latter that resembles the relationship between doctor and patient in at least one respect, due to the preventive aim it is based on: the purpose of the contract and the examination is to collect information relevant for the subject's health. This information can help the subject make an informed decision about measures that will serve sustain her health for as long as possible. Even in the broad sense of the concept, it is *not* an instance of incidental findings if (a) a diagnosis is carried out, because the examined person demanded it – even without presenting any symptoms – in order to find out about a potential need for medical intervention or (b) a cause of the patient's symptoms is found that differs from what is expected by the physician who is responsible for the diagnosis. In the latter case, the findings differ from what is expected or considered likely by the physician. So the findings are unexpected, but not incidental. It is not the case that the use of the diagnostic means did not intend to produce the findings. This becomes clear once we consider the intention of the physician when employing diagnostic means. The physician does not primarily examine the patient with the aim of finding the cause of a symptom or confirming the presence of a certain disease. She rather wants to find out which therapeutic measures should be undertaken for the patient's benefit. The physician's intention is not primarily to confirm her own suspicion concerning the cause of the symptoms. The aim is usually rather to cure the patient as soon as possible. This can also be seen in the fact that an experienced physician will abstain from any further diagnostic procedures if she is confident that further differential diagnostics will be irrelevant for the indication of adequate therapeutic measures. In this case, any further examination would be unnecessary for the treatment of the patient and would only be carried out for the sake of confirming the physician's hypothesis. Since the latter is not the aim of the physician's conduct, no further examinations are required.

The occurrence of an incidental finding can nowadays not be regarded as unexpected. It has become evident – and is a matter of basic knowledge in modern research – that the use of high-resolution imaging diagnoses in medical studies yields a relatively high number of findings that the study was not aimed at detecting (Rangel 2010, 124). In brain MRI scans, 1–8% of subjects featured incidental findings that were considered in need of further examination (Katzman et al. 1999; Alphs et al. 2006; Weber and Knopf 2006; Vernooij et al. 2007; Schleim et al. 2007; Gupta and Belay 2008). In cohort studies employing whole-body MRI, the number of incidental findings is even higher (Langanke and Erdmann 2011, 206). Unexpected findings neither are always incidental nor are incidentally discovered findings always unexpected. Therefore it would be inadequate to characterize incidental findings as unexpected findings (pace, e.g. Illes et al. 2006, 783; Heinemann et al. 2007, A1982). Incidental findings should rather be characterized as unintended findings whose discovery was not intended by a treating physician or medical researcher. Their discovery was not intended, because the intention of a treating physician is not – in contrast to, e.g. the provider of direct-to-consumer whole-body MRI examinations – to discover a clinically not (yet) manifested disease, and the intention of the researcher in life sciences is not to provide a diagnosis for the subject's disease.

2 Incidental Findings in a Narrow Sense

In the relevant literature, the concept of incidental findings is, however, often used in a different, narrower, sense than the one described above. According to this narrow understanding, incidental findings are characterized by three features:

1. They occur in participants during a scientific study.
2. They potentially affect the health or reproductive capacities of the concerned participant.
3. They are findings, the discovery of which was not intended in the context of the study's aim.

Incidental findings in this narrower sense – based on a suggestion by Wolf et al. (2008: 219) – are only those unintended findings that occur in the context of scientific research. Incidental findings in this narrow sense raise ethical problems. These problems are not raised by the broad sense according to which such findings can also occur in the context of the doctor-patient relationship. If there is a doctor-patient relationship, it is clear that strategies for avoiding the discovery of any incidental findings are illegitimate. The aim of gaining information about therapeutic measures that should be taken for the patient's benefit does not allow for avoiding certain findings. The existence of a doctor-patient relationship also means that the non-disclosure of an incidental finding cannot be justified but for it is in the immediate interest of the patient. If there is no doctor-patient relationship, however, avoiding findings and non-disclosure may not always be illegitimate.

3 Incidental Finding or Signal Abnormality?

Independently of the diagnostic methods that are employed, specific data can only be called incidental findings if they are registered as a deviation from the norm, an abnormality and hence a potential symptom. Incidental findings do not occur independently of their interpretation as *potential* symptoms. They are always the result of an at least rudimentary assessment, because they are categorized based on the comparison with an expectation that is derived from other data, or with the norm.

Heinemann et al. (2009: 2–3) distinguish between a "signal abnormality […] in the collected image data that is detected by the researcher while inspecting and analysing the data with respect to their usability for the collective scientific evaluation of the research study" and a "signal abnormality with respect to a potential clinical relevance for the individual study participant." This distinction is, however, artificial. It presupposes that it is, in principle, possible for the researcher to observe a signal abnormality as such without, at the same time, seeing it as a potential indication of a disease. Even if this is theoretically conceivable, it is practically impossible for a trained doctor or a similarly competent researcher. A researcher could deliberately *ignore* the indicative character of an abnormality and the clinical relevance for the participant. She cannot, however, evaluate (imaging) data without referring to her specific knowledge about the subject nor can she only refer to that knowledge to the extent required for the aim of the study *without intending such a limitation of the use of her knowledge*. Brain researchers cannot, as Schleim et al. (2007: 1044) concede, "take their entire measurements with closed eyes." The possibility of incidental findings therefore raises an important normative question: is it legitimate to evaluate the data collected in research with human subjects by only partially making use of the available knowledge about the analysis of data? The question is, in particular, whether it is legitimate to abstain from the use of such knowledge in research with human subjects, if using that knowledge could lead to a discovery that is potentially clinically relevant for the subject. This normative question requires a convincing normative answer. It should not be covered up by conceptual distinctions suggesting that discovering abnormalities in study participants could not only be separated from discovering potential disease symptoms analytically but also in research practice.

4 The Differing Indicative Dignity of Incidental Findings

Incidental findings do not always have the same indicative dignity. Three different classes of dignity can be distinguished from each other here. The first class contains those incidental findings whose clinical relevance is evident. These could be abnormalities or changes that evidently indicate, for example, a renal tumour. The second class contains incidental findings that – according to the current state of medical knowledge – are not clinically significant. One example would be an arachnoid cyst found during a brain MRI examination. The third class contains abnormalities whose clinical relevance is unclear, such as an intervertebral disc degeneration that is only clinically relevant if the anamnesis or examination of the person concerned yields indications of complaints or failure of the nerves. Findings of this type are more common in research contexts than in clinical contexts, because in research, a very high number of subjects is examined – and not only in one but in many respects. For this class, it might be thought maintainable to merely speak of signal abnormalities, because there is no (sufficient) evidence that the abnormality is indicating a disease. However, assigning an abnormality to this class always presupposes an evaluation by the researcher and thus her use of her knowledge about analysing the relevant data. Therefore the possibility of abnormalities belonging to this class does not contradict the above statement that the evaluator's knowledge about analysing the relevant data always influences the evaluation of the participants' data. This suggests that abnormalities of this class should also be characterized as incidental findings, if necessary.

Further distinctions can be made within the three classes of dignity. In particular, it would be appropriate to differentiate between clinically relevant incidental findings where a medical intervention is required and those where a risk assessment suggests the contrary. For these distinctions, knowledge about the natural history of the disease in question is required, and for many incidental findings, this is still missing.

5 The Context of the Occurrence of Incidental Findings

Incidental findings (in the narrow sense) concern diseases for which the participant showed no symptoms prior to the study. Findings of this kind occur in different research contexts. Currently they mostly occur (a) in the context of clinical studies with the aim of reviewing the therapeutic efficacy of a drug or a certain medical intervention and of reviewing their potential adverse effects in order to judge whether the latter are acceptable; (b) in the context of fundamental research in life sciences with the aim of deepening the scientific understanding of human beings or the interaction between human beings and their environment by examining, e.g. the function of certain brain regions or the reactions of the brain to specific external stimuli; (c) in medical fundamental research with the aim of benefitting the health care of future patient generations. The currently most prominent field of fundamental research in life sciences, where a large number of incidental findings occur, is the neuroscientific localization of specific functions in the human brain. In medical fundamental research, a large number of incidental findings occur in epidemiological cohort studies, which include MRI scans in most cases. Clinical studies include medical interventions; fundamental research does not (besides interventions that are necessary for a diagnosis such as the infusion of a contrast medium, the application of stimuli and the like). These three types of research contexts also differ from each other in their respective type of study participant. Clinical studies are mostly carried out with "patient subjects" (Heinemann et al. 2009: 3), i.e. with participants who already show a clinically manifest disease and hope for a (higher) chance of a cure by participating in the study. Neuroscientific fundamental research is often carried out with young, healthy subjects, where the chances of a disease-related partial dysfunction of the brain are relatively low. Neuroscientific studies also include patients who had a stroke, however, in order to investigate neuroplasticity. Population-based epidemiological studies require representative random samples from the general public.

References

Alphs HH, Schwartz BS et al (2006) Findings on brain MRI from research studies of occupational exposure to known neurotoxicants. Am J Roentgenol 187: 1043–1047

Gupta SN, Belay B (2008) Intracranial incidental findings on brain MR images in a pediatric neurology practice: a retrospective study. J Neurol Sci 264:34–37

Heinemann T, Hoppe C et al (2007) Zufallsbefunde bei bildgebenden Verfahren in der Hirnforschung: Ethische Überlegungen und Lösungsvorschläge. Deutsches Ärzteblatt 104:A-1982/B-1748/C-1684

Heinemann T, Hoppe C et al (2009) Ethisch angemessener Umgang mit Zufallsfunden bei bildgebenden Verfahren in der Hirnforschung. – Leitlinienvorschlag – (19. Juni 2009) http://www.psychologie.hu-berlin.de/institut/intra/ethik/Leitlinie%20Zufallsfunde

Illes J, Kirschen MP et al (2006) Incidental findings in brain imaging research. Science 311:783–784

Katzman GL, Dagher AP, Patronas NJ (1999) Incidental findings on brain magnetic resonance imaging from 1000 asymptomatic volunteers. J Am Med Assoc 282:36–39

Langanke M, Erdmann P (2011) Die MRT als wissenschaftliche Studienuntersuchung und das Problem der Mitteilung von Zufallsbefunden. Probandenethische Herausforderungen. In: Theißen H, Langanke M (eds) Tragfähige Rede von Gott. Festgabe für Heinrich Assel zum 50. Geburtstag. Dr Kovac, Hamburg, pp 197–240

Rangel EK (2010) The Management of Incidental Findings in Neuro-Imaging Research: Framework and Recommendations. J Law Med Ethics 38:117–126

Schleim S, Spranger TM et al (2007) Zufallsfunde in der bildgebenden Hirnforschung. Empirische, rechtliche und ethische Aspekte. Nervenheilkunde 26:1041–1045

Schmücker R (2013) Zufallsbefunde – was gebietet die Menschenwürde? In: Joerden JC, Hilgendorf E, Thiele F (2013) Menschenwürde und Medizin. Duncker & Humblot, Berlin, pp 949–981

Vernooij MW, Ikram MA et al (2007) Incidental findings on brain MRI in the general population. N Engl J Med 357:1821–1828

Weber F, Knopf H (2006) Incidental findings in magnetic resonance imaging of the brains of healthy young men. J Neurol Sci 240:81–84

Wolf SM, Lawrenz FP et al (2008) Managing Incidental Findings in Human Subjects Research: Analysis and Recommendations. J Law Med Ethics 36:219–248

Incidental Findings – Ethical Aspects

Pia Erdmann

Contents

1 **Introduction** 9
1.1 Frequency of Occurrence 10
1.2 Typical Fields of Ethical Challenges 11
1.3 Potential Outcome Resulting from the Question "Who Should Interpret the Images?" 11
1.4 Disclosure and Non-disclosure of IFs in the Research Context and Communication of Suspicious Findings in the Clinical Context 12
1.5 Positive and Negative Effects That May Arise from Decision About Which IFs Will Be Disclosed 13
1.6 The Approach to Disclosing IFs and Possible Consequences 14

2 **Ethical Prerequisites and Principles** 14

3 **Recommendations** 17
3.1 Disclosure Algorithms 18
3.2 Disclosure or Non-disclosure of IFs in the Research Context or the Communication of Suspicious Findings in the Clinical Context 18
3.3 Who Should Interpret the Images and Decide About the Disclosure of IFs? 20
3.4 Informing About the Handling of IFs/Consent Processes 21
3.5 Designing a Study Protocol in Research 21

Final Considerations 22

References 23

P. Erdmann, MA
Ernst-Moritz-Arndt-Universität Greifswald, Theologische Fakultät, Lehrstuhl für Systematische Theologie, Am Rubenowplatz 2–3, Greifswald 17487, Germany
e-mail: perdmann@uni-greifswald.de

Abstract

This article deals with ethical aspects of incidental/secondary resp. discovery findings (IFs) from imaging techniques that are generated in clinical care, medical research or the context of direct-to-consumer services. After the questions and challenges, typically raised by IFs are introduced, the second part focusses on ethical prerequisites and reflects principles that are capable of providing a normative foundation in dealing with IFs. The final part presents recommendations on the basis of these principles as a guideline to ensure responsible planning as well as to take suitable measures, to avoid (or at least mitigate) the hazards of IFs.

1 Introduction

Incidental findings (IFs) regularly evoke a discussion about ethical challenges that accompany them. The corresponding dispute started about one decade ago (Wolf et al. 2008) and the handling of those "incidentalomas" (abnormalities revealed during imaging, which were not accompanied by any symptoms) (Kohane et al. 2006; Salman et al. 2007; Brothers et al. 2013) has been lively debated since then. The present chapter tries to demonstrate that IFs indeed pose ethical challenges, but in the majority of cases, the investment of careful and responsible planning and suitable measures once IFs are revealed

Med Radiol Diagn Imaging (2016)
DOI 10.1007/174_2016_69, © Springer International Publishing Switzerland
Published Online: 22 Oct 2016

can succeed: either the total number of IFs, particularly of false-positives and false-negatives, can be reduced or, in case of exposure, appropriate measures can at least mitigate potential adverse effects.

Due to the radiological setting of this book, the following considerations focus on IFs arising in the context of medical imaging, even though IFs can certainly arise in other contexts. Instead of expanding this discussion to include IFs from other modalities, such as large-scale genomic sequencing, we will instead expand this examining in another interesting direction: We will address not only incidental or secondary findings, but also *discovery findings*. The outstanding report "Anticipate and Communicate. Ethical Management of Incidental and Secondary Findings in the Clinical, Research, and Direct-to-Consumer Context" published by the Presidential Commission for the Study of Bioethical Issues (Presidential Commission for the Study of Bioethical Issues 2013) treats only incidental and secondary findings, whereas so-called discovery findings are deliberately ignored. Discovery findings, in contrast with incidental and secondary findings, occur in their definition primarily in examinations or tests intended to detect diseases in a presymptomatic stage (Presidential Commission for the Study of Bioethical Issues 2013). As an example for a modality typical for discovery findings, the Commission quotes the "wellness scan" which is conducted to search for anything abnormal throughout the body (Presidential Commission for the Study of Bioethical Issues 2013). Interestingly the Commission only refers to discovery findings in the direct-to-consumer [hereafter: DTC] testing, although hospitals and other institutions sometimes offer it. Whole-body scans, which are conducted within the research context, e.g., whole-body MRIs (WB-MRI) in SHIP (see Chap. 5 Ship) or the National Cohort in Germany (see Chap. 6 Nako), are not mentioned. It can only be speculated why the deliberations of the Commission did not explicitly include examinations of this kind. The fact is that findings in this research field, regardless of whether you name them incidental or discovery, regularly pose problems, including the question of whether to disclose them. We will therefore include discovery findings in the following considerations. To simplify matters, the generic term incidental finding (IF) will be used to refer to all three classes of findings, even discovery findings, since this is the most commonly used term, thereby taking the risk of occasional slight inaccuracies.

1.1 Frequency of Occurrence

Generally IFs can occur as well in clinical research as in DTC contexts. The frequency with which they occur naturally differs depending on the application of technique, the defined field of view, and the purpose of the examination as well as the expertise of the person who interprets the images. For instance, a WB-MRI in the field of research will generate more IFs than an ultrasound of the kidney carried out in a hospital with the target of clarification (Presidential Commission for the Study of Bioethical Issues 2013; The Royal College of Radiologists 2011). But even in the clinical context, the frequency of IFs can be pretty high. The Presidential Commission mentions, for example, a study that deals with CT scans conducted on patients at a trauma center, where 43 % of the patients ended up with at least one incidental finding (Munk et al. 2010) But this finding is exceptional; frequencies in the one-digit range are typically reported for this context (The Royal College of Radiologists 2011). Within the research context, IFs can additionally occur merely as a result of the examination methods themselves often being under control, which naturally influences the reliability of the results. Incidence numbers that are quoted in this context range from 3 to 12 % for IFs within neuroimaging and up to 30 % in imaging of the rest of the body (The Royal College of Radiologists 2011). The decision to clarify a suspicious finding using subsequent examinations depends on a range of factors and circumstances, including the potential benefits and costs in the clinical context as well as the study conditions in the research context. With considerations of this sort, we now finally arrive in the area of ethical considerations, which will be discussed below.

1.2 Typical Fields of Ethical Challenges

Irrespective of the context, the ethical challenges can be reduced to a few difficult-to-answer questions that typically arise in the field of IFs. To begin with, there is the question of who is interpreting the images, because this has remarkable influence on the number as well as on the reliability of the IFs. Secondly, and this is the question with the most implications, what happens with detected IFs? Will they be disclosed in the research context? Will findings revealed in the clinical context be communicated to the providers who requested the original examination? Should subsequent examination be recommended? This leads inevitably to the question, "Which kind of IFs should be communicated and which quality criteria should they meet?" Finally the question remains, how the patient or research participant should be informed about the findings and which conditions should be fulfilled according to best practice in breaking serious news?

IFs don't pose per se a critical ethical issue; they can be beneficial and lifesaving under certain circumstances. Under different circumstances though, such as when an IF turns out to be a false-positive, they can cause unnecessary and severe distress. It is mainly the handling of IFs, then, that determines whether an IF might be helpful or harmful, and therefore ethically critical or not.

Before recommendations on how to manage IFs are introduced, an attempt will be made to simply describe which concrete challenges might occur. This description will be based on critical questions and examples from practice. An assessment which of these should be avoided for ethical reasons and which sort of adverse consequences should at least be reduced requires in turn a short introduction of some relevant ethical principles, which likewise should precede the recommendations. Recommendations always have normative character; therefore a justifiable and mutually agreeable foundation is needed to legitimately demand their implementation.

1.3 Potential Outcome Resulting from the Question "Who Should Interpret the Images?"

Two different critical issues may follow the decision about *who* is responsible for interpreting the results of specific examinations; both of them are the outcome of a situation where the images in question are examined by persons that don't have the necessary expertise. For example, a survey regarding practice in the UK revealed that 43 % of research imaging is undertaken by research scientists without medical training (Booth et al. 2012). It might also happen that even when radiologists are responsible for the interpretation, an ambiguous result would make it necessary to consult an expert of a particular discipline to ultimately determine whether the finding is significant or not. Regardless of the situation, it might happen that on the one hand information relevant for the health of the concerned person is overlooked and on the other hand, just the opposite, the concerned person is either inundated with irrelevant or unreliable information, which, in the worst case, can cause not only anxiety and discomfort but also costly, invasive, and unnecessary interventions. The overlooking of severe findings or the misinterpretation of data that leads to the disclosure of false-negative results both pose problems and for two reasons: (1) curative actions that could contribute to the recovery or at least to a delay of the disease are not taken and (2) besides that, especially in the research context, a false sense of security might arise, since the concerned person might ignore existing symptoms because he or she fails to recognize the scientific purpose of the examination and therefore spuriously assumes not only that the examination would have identified anything severe but also that any such findings would have been communicated.

1.4 Disclosure and Non-disclosure of IFs in the Research Context and Communication of Suspicious Findings in the Clinical Context

More and more studies prove that most participants who take part in research studies believe that concerned researchers are obliged to disclose any suspect findings (Bjugn 2015; Cole et al. 2015; Erdmann 2015a, b). Participants even want to receive results of no clinical significance, as this is apparently connected to the notion of autonomous control over personal health information. The passively receiving patient is more and more replaced by "the information-seeking patient/participant," who actively gathers health information (Brothers 2015). And in many cases, the desire to get health information appears to be the main reason for participating in research studies (Erdmann 2015a). Aside from having a number of adverse consequences for both the participant and the researchers conducting the study, this tendency is also an implicit indicator of the diagnostic misconception (Appelbaum et al. 2004). Negative effects for the concerned person resulting from a disclosure of IFs could include, as noted above, psychological distress across a spectrum of types and magnitudes as well as disadvantages regarding financial, insurance, and job matters. The costs of subsequent examinations can also become a problematic factor. In Germany, costs that originate from clarification are usually covered by publicly funded health insurance. In some countries, however, every individual is not a member of the statutory health insurance and even then this does not ensure that all kind of costs will be covered (Cole et al. 2015). Furthermore, merely the suspicion that one might suffer from a certain disease can impede the conclusion of a contract relating to credits, job offers, or life insurance policies. This can cause a variety of difficulties and negative side effects (Presidential Commission for the Study of Bioethical Issues 2013; The Royal College of Radiologists 2011). These potential negative outcomes do not prevent, of course, the widespread preference for receiving IFs. Disadvantages are obviously either not foreseen, their likelihood of occurring is estimated to be low, or, in weighing the risks and benefits, individuals tend to conclude that the potential advantages outweigh the potential disadvantages.

So what are possible positive outcomes from a disclosure? Mainly health-related benefits should be considered on the side of the advantages, if it is the case that the follow-up confirms the suspicion and treatment is available, affordable, and effective. Another reason for a disclosure could be respect for the person, as withholding information in opposition to the preference of the individual could be considered as paternalistic. The subjects' autonomy is also the gravest argument that is adduced for disclosing results regarding diseases that are untreatable. In this case it makes no difference whether a treatment does not exist at all or the concerned person wouldn't benefit from it. Being aware that one suffers from a life-threatening and untreatable disease might enable this person to put their personal affairs in order, and in best cases, he or she may succeed to establish a eudemonistic attitude of living their remaining life span (Charmaz 1993; Erdmann and Langanke 2016). Recently, a study conducted by Cole et al., which deals with expectations, preferences, and specific needs of persons involved in the return of IFs from neuroimaging, added another argument in favor of disclosing IFs: increased trust in research (Cole et al. 2015).

Taken as a whole, the arguments related to participants' deliberation on IFs have been widely discussed in the literature (Erdmann 2015a; Christenhusz et al. 2013; Schmücker 2012). However, the perspectives of other stakeholders in this discussion have been examined less exhaustively. This gap is also closed by the examination of Cole et al., who considers the perspectives of investigators, IRB members, and physicians, among others. These stakeholders also feel a moral obligation to report IFs to participants, but as a whole, they estimate the benefits of disclosure more carefully and keep the disadvantages in perspective. Specifically, they focus on the waste of time and other resources; the worthlessness of certain information, accompanied by unnecessary psychological burdens; and also the detrimental effects that an unrestricted disclosure of IFs would pose, both to the healthcare system in general and to specific research enterprises in particular (Cole et al. 2015). Another argument, which alludes to the ethics of best practice in research, is sometimes quoted with regard to long-term epidemiological research: the bias that is generated when cohort members seek treatment they would not otherwise have pursued had they had not received the corresponding IF (Hoffmann 2014).

Many of the aforementioned considerations from the research context also apply to the direct-to-consumer context. In both cases, the conditions are set by the particular conductor or provider, and the participant can be seen as agreeing to these terms by signing the informed consent or the contract of purchase. In the context of medical care, the question of disclosure arises in a different way. In both the clinical and research contexts, there are no binding regulations related to IFs. No statutes or guidelines, for example, explicitly list the duties of clinicians regarding the management of IFs (for the US context, see Presidential Commission for the Study of Bioethical Issues (2013); for the UK context, see The Royal College of Radiologists (2011)). On the other hand, the relation between physician and patient relies on a contract governing medical treatment. This contract entails certain conditions that are not negotiated anew in each case. Analyses based on this provider-patient relationship, at least in the US and German contexts, indicate that physicians do not necessarily have a responsibility to report all kinds of IFs, although it is expected that relevant IFs with clinical utility will be communicated and that subsequent examinations, where required, will be recommended (Rudnik-Schöneborn et al. 2014). A violation of this responsibility is likely to be considered medical malpractice (Presidential Commission for the Study of Bioethical Issues 2013). This again complicates the critical challenge of differentiating between IFs with clinical utility and those that are clinically irrelevant, as well as the importance of defining the criteria that guide such decisions (Presidential Commission for the Study of Bioethical Issues 2013).

Before moving on to the topic of the proper criteria for identifying IFs with clinical utility, we should briefly mention the difficulties raised by uncertainty. This difficulty is explicitly noted in the report from the Presidential Commission for the Study of Bioethical Issues. "Better safe than sorry" is the more or less implicit attitude behind the tendency to pursue too many IFs rather than too few. Also, concerns about legal liability for overlooking information relevant to health can be a driving force for this behavior (Presidential Commission for the Study of Bioethical Issues 2013). The report correctly notes that conducting further diagnostic tests or procedures might lead to new – sometimes even life-threatening – risks or adverse psychological effects, including the risk of further incidental findings without any corresponding benefits. Just as a suspicious finding might help improve a patient's health or even save his or her live, it might instead be unnecessary and harmful, as well as costly (Presidential Commission for the Study of Bioethical Issues 2013). Up to now, however, there are no reliable numbers regarding the cost-effectiveness of IFs (Erdmann et al. 2015). It would lead us too far afield to examine this matter, but we can at least say that in times of limited resources considerations about the cost-effectiveness of interventions and the meaningful allocation of medical resources are clearly relevant to ethical analyses.

1.5 Positive and Negative Effects That May Arise from Decision About Which IFs Will Be Disclosed

We have examined a range of risks associated with returning or withholding IFs, including the risks that relevant health information might be withheld; that patients or research subjects might be burdened by unnecessary, awkward, costly, or even risky procedures to clarify the relevance of a finding; and that they may even experience psychological distress and/or financial disadvantages by either a too restrictive or too lenient disclosure strategy. In light of this, we can see that, if at all possible, IFs should only be disclosed if they would be beneficial to the concerned subject. Although this sounds trivial, the poor state of knowledge regarding IFs regularly results in an implementation that fails to achieve the outcomes desired. The Presidential Commission points out that there is a major need to increase knowledge about IFs that would enable the development of evidence-based practice guidelines. This demand is therefore the content of one of their overarching recommendations, including a recommendation that professionals within different contexts should not only participate in the development of such guidelines but also share them among communities of practitioners (Presidential Commission for the Study of Bioethical Issues 2013). Given the current state of knowledge, however, it remains the case that certain examinations are likely to produce IFs and that some anticipated (secondary) findings are even actively sought, while the reliability of these IFs often remains unclear. This forces researchers and practitioners to make non-evidence-based decisions regarding the reporting of IFs which might be beneficial, unnecessary, or even harmful. The Presidential Commission describes this tightrope walk in their report portraying both classes of cases, those where IFs had lifesaving character and also those where the result was harmful and even life-threatening.

It is immensely important, then, to enable patients and potential participants to thoroughly weigh the pros and cons of receiving IFs when an examination is being performed. A patient's consent must be the result of individual deliberations that take into account promised benefits as well as the likelihood of associated risks. In the research context, therapeutic/diagnostic misconception is a well-known phenomenon for eroding the informed consent since participants tend to overweigh the benefits and underestimate the risks (Appelbaum et al. 2004).

1.6 The Approach to Disclosing IFs and Possible Consequences

Astonishingly, the question of how disclosure procedures should be designed is still not a major focus in debates about the ethical aspects of IFs, although there is evidence that inappropriate disclosure methods represent one of the most abundant stress factors regarding IFs (Erdmann 2015a; Levine 2010). Clinical algorithms for breaking-serious-news, such as those used in oncology, can be implemented to mitigate the stressful and occasionally even traumatic reactions that the disclosure of severe even life-threatening news might cause (Baile et al. 2000). An argument that is often raised against approaches to disclosure that are more deliberate, elaborate, and costlier is that IFs can be disclosed as merely suspicious and have not yet been validated. That might be true, but for the concerned person, this difference is not evident, especially when there is no opportunity to ask questions about the consequences the assumed abnormality might have. Even the attempt to avoid certain keywords (tumor, aneurysm, etc.) that could trigger anxiety and other psychological distress is insufficient here, since individuals who get their results in a written form, and therefore lack a suitable provider able to immediately give desperately needed answers, are mostly forced to consult the Internet to receive relevant information concerning the content of the letter. Although concerning words might have been avoided in the report of the IF, they will certainly be encountered here. The most dependable way to mitigate the fear and anxiety is to communicate results in a face-to-face conversation, which provide the opportunity to explain the possibility of a false-positive finding and the tentativeness of the result. Finally the high frequency of IFs and the huge effort that would be necessary to communicate IFs personally is indeed an important consideration, but not one that would outweigh the ethical obligation to minimize foreseeable stress.

2 Ethical Prerequisites and Principles

This chapter is probably not the right site for fundamental examinations of the obligations that arise from ethical rationales. The reason why we nonetheless mention ethical principles here is that recommendations are normative in nature and thus need a foundation that makes it reasonably clear why one should apply them.

The debate about the handling of IFs including work to develop recommendations has been underway for a number of years. One reason, why a final agreement could never be struck, was that the discussion was missing a unifying ethical rationale. In the consequence, there were diverse proposals that tended to be either vague or contradictory. This again led to a situation in which researchers conducting studies bearing the risk to reveal IFs were forced to define local "stand alone" algorithms to deal with IFs. One example for such a study is the already mentioned SHIP study; the WB-MRI that was conducted in this context revealed about 30 % IFs. Based on the preliminary results of an empirical study with those persons who underwent this WB-MRI [(Langanke and Erdmann 2011), later versions in (Rudnik Schöneborn et al. 2014; Langanke et al. 2015)] Erdmann and Langanke devised a framework of ethical principles advocating for a moderate contractualism that ensures that the terms of a research study agreed to by participants through the informed consent process are binding for the investigators and must therefore be followed. Furthermore they proposed two imperatives based on the principle of fairness: the principle of transparency and the principle of minimizing foreseeable risks and harms.

The report of the Presidential Commission that was published in 2013 finally also comprehended ethical principles to underpin the recommendations. Those principles were supposed to accomplish a degree of universality that would be able to cover the challenges of medical care and research as well as DTC contexts, whereby the Commission admitted that scope, strength, and stringency of the principles might vary in order to bridge the gaps between all three contexts (Presidential Commission for the Study of Bioethical Issues 2013).

The following ethical considerations will introduce the "ethical basis" the Commission proposes, based on well-known and agreed-upon principles, so that we can subsequently explain why some clarification of those principles is needed. Any recommendation deduced from these principles would naturally need to be compatible with the relevant legal framework. This will be important later on when recommendations regarding the handling of IFs, especially the question of disclosure, are discussed.

Four principles were considered by the Commission as pertinent in the application to IFs:

Respect for persons, beneficence, justice and fairness, and intellectual freedom and responsibility (Presidential Commission for the Study of Bioethical Issues 2013). The principles are derived from two classic resources: Beauchamps' and Childress' Principles of Biomedical Ethics (Beauchamp and Childress 2009) and the Belmont Report (The National Commission for the Protection of Human Subjects of Biomedical and Behavioral Research 1978).

The principle of respect for persons is divided into two sub-issues in the Belmont report, the honoring of subjects' autonomy and the duty to protect vulnerable individuals whose autonomy is limited for whatever reason. In this context, "autonomy" incorporates the right and the capability for self-determined choices and decisions that enable individuals to direct the course of their life. The protection of persons with limited capacity to enact their own autonomy, while not mentioned explicitly in Presidential Commission's report, should be, based on the Belmont Report, adapted based on the risk of harm and the likelihood of benefit involved in research participation (The National Commission for the Protection of Human Subjects of Biomedical and Behavioral Research 1978). What is essential regarding this principle is that anything that would influence one's choices in either direction should be eliminated. In the present context, this pertains mainly to the information regarding the concerning examination and the consequences that might arise from the choice of participation or nonattendance. Without wanting to jump ahead, it shall be mentioned here that the recommendations of the Presidential Commission are deduced from this principle that prudence and deliberateness should govern the informed consent process of the potential patient or participant.

The second principle that is claimed by the Presidential Commission report is the principle of beneficence. This is meant as an appeal to professionals to take measures that assure the well-being of others. Non-maleficence is introduced here as a corollary from the principle of beneficence and is interpreted as not imposing harms on others. The latter will probably reach broad consent with the addressed professionals without any difficulty and across all three contexts (research, medical care, and DTC). On the other hand, however, the proposed obligation to maximize benefits is more controversial, except in the context of clinical care. The plain claim to not harm others may be seemingly agreeable at first glance, but – especially in the research context – can be hard to implement. The very minimizing of anticipated stress, a principle already adjusted by Erdmann and Langanke that refers to the principle of non-maleficence, would, so the objection, produce costs and efforts. For example, the disclosure of IFs in a way that mitigates the adverse psychological reactions should be done in a face-to-face communication and not in a written form. The costs of such a disclosure are often estimated inappropriately high. Obviously the answer to the question "what is appropriate" on the one hand and "reasonable" on the other must be the result of deliberation and is therefore heavily influenced by the interests of the person undertaking this deliberation.

Another heavily discussed aspect is the question of public beneficence. Here, the Presidential Commission refers to their first report *New Directions: The Ethics of Synthetic Biology and Emerging Technologies* where beneficence also includes interests of society and therefore quotes the duty to improve healthcare as a whole on the one hand and a more broadly weighing of costs and benefits for society on the other (Presidential Commission for the Study of Bioethical Issues 2013). In this way, a third component other than the interests of the participating person and the interests of those who conduct research becomes relevant: societal interests. Of course, it is important and legitimate to demand the best possible research practice that serves societal interest while balancing disproportionate costs and burdens for the healthcare system in total. Nevertheless, it should be noted that the individual beneficence should not be disregarded. And when personal risks cannot be avoided for reasons of costs and/or the effort required, the participating persons should at least be informed about this in order to ensure a valid consent.

The third principle of the Presidential Commission is the principle of justice and fairness, which demands fair and equitable treatment of all (Presidential Commission for the Study of Bioethical Issues 2013). The intention of justice and fairness in the interpretation of the Commission's report is, similar to the principle of beneficence, making sure that benefits as well as burdens are spread evenhandedly among affected parties. Additionally the principle suggests the equitable allocation of resources or the clarification of what one might reasonably and legitimately expect from others. Finally, this principle entails treating ethically similar cases alike (Presidential Commission for the Study of Bioethical Issues 2013), whereby the implications also meet concerns of rather societal character as the equitable supply of as many persons as possible with basic healthcare needs. This doubtlessly has to do with the fact that the report in question is edited in the USA, where access to affordable healthcare services is not guaranteed for all. For the application to IFs, the principle implies that especially an over-testing should be avoided, not only because of the costs but also because of the mental and physical health risks (Presidential Commission for the Study of Bioethical Issues 2013).

The fourth and final principle the Presidential Commission recommends is that of intellectual freedom and responsibility. This principle, which has no equivalent in either the principles of Beauchamp and Childress or the Belmont report, represents the interests of researchers and scientific progress and entails the responsible use of the associated rights and obligations. The Commission especially emphasizes the point that this principle can be seen as "a rejection of the technological imperative" (Presidential Commission for the Study of Bioethical Issues

2013). In terms of IFs, the principle alludes to the fact that not everything that can technically be done is useful, because limited resources might be wasted for results that are neither on behalf of individual well-being nor in the interest of the public.

Ethical recommendations are not assertive by definition; their status is different and depends on the strength of the principles on which they are based. At least in free and democratic societies, those principles are not simply enforced by those who might have the power to do so. Ethical principles mainly need the agreement of those who are affected by them in any way; higher liability is not achievable on this level. Choosing predominantly principles that originate in the already well-established principles of Beauchamp and Childress and the Belmont Report has the advantage that they are already seen as generally accepted. The fourth principle of intellectual freedom and responsibility proposed from the Presidential Commission however was probably specifically generated as a result of the examination of those challenges professionals encounter when dealing with IFs.

Erdmann and Langanke had a similar approach when designing their principles. Erdmann's empirical ethics study revealed that certain aspects regarding the IFs that were expected to be problematic from an ethical perspective turned out to be marginal or at least lesser in extent than expected. However, other unanticipated aspects were more challenging for the participants than originally assumed. The ethical framework that was the outcome of this study attempted to consider both theoretical aspects as well as evidence from the practice in the development of ethical principles. Thus the premise of contractualism and the two fairness imperatives of transparency and minimizing anticipated stress evolved from these deliberations. In light of the Presidential Commission's report, those principles seem to be mainly covered: the overall premise of contractualism as well as the fairness imperative from Erdmann/Langanke could be subsumed under the principle of justice. The demand for transparency can be found in the first principle of respect for persons. Finally, minimizing anticipated stress could be seen as an interpretation of the principle of beneficence. It might, however, be reasonable to adjust the principles of the Presidential Commission so that these issues are mentioned more explicitly. The recommendations below that virtually evolve from the principles might therefore eventually reveal, if scope, strength, and stringency of the principles are narrow enough to be not only beneficial but also sufficient in the application.

3 Recommendations

There are certainly a variety of ways to structure recommendations regarding IFs. The Presidential Commission's report differentiates between overarching recommendations and those of the different contexts in which IFs might occur (Presidential Commission for the Study of Bioethical Issues 2013). Here we attempt to structure recommendations not so much depending on the context of the IFs; instead the structure follows concrete procedure measures and their accompanying ethical challenges. Therefore, it will begin with recommendations that treat disclosure algorithms and aspects of clarification of IFs and end with recommendations that handle which sort of IFs to disclose at all. The background of this approach is the conviction that the more effort is invested in advance, the better is the chance that a handling of IFs will be achieved that complies with the abovementioned principles. The content of the recommendations presented here is mainly derived from two works: the report of the Presidential Commission, which we already have discussed in detail, and the report "Management of Incidental Findings Detected During Research Imaging" from the UK (Presidential Commission for the Study of Bioethical Issues 2013; The Royal College of Radiologists 2011).

The recommendations below represent a careful attempt to move the discussion about the handling of IFs forward by matching a variety of theoretical considerations with empirical data comprising the experiences and expectations of the persons involved.

3.1 Disclosure Algorithms

Depending on the severity of the finding, the approach to disclosure should be adjusted (to minimize distress, which can be anticipated). In the medical care context, this is probably unnecessary to recommend, but in the contexts of research and DTC testing, findings with a life-threatening outcome are still sometimes disclosed exclusively in writing. The justification for this is the provisional character of the finding that might turn out to be a false-positive result. For the person involved, however, the difference between a diagnosis and a suspicion might be not perceivable in that moment (Erdmann 2015a). A face-to-face communication offers at least the chance to point out this difference and to mitigate fear and anxiety caused by the disclosure. Furthermore, an appropriately trained person should be able to offer options and subsequent steps that should be undertaken and thus avoid the eventual traumatizing feelings of helplessness and hopelessness (Levine 2010). The report by representatives of research imaging centers goes one step further, recommending that unverified findings should not be disclosed without an action plan and that specialists able to provide informal advice should be identified in a timely manner as well as referral pathways provided (Recommendation no. 20 and no. 21). Otherwise participants have to bother with the clarification themselves, which can last weeks without official support, sometimes even months. This time of ambiguity is often experienced as even more stressful than the diagnosis of a severe disease itself, since coping processes are somewhat suspended (Erdmann 2015a).

3.2 Disclosure or Non-disclosure of IFs in the Research Context or the Communication of Suspicious Findings in the Clinical Context

To devise recommendations regarding this issue is problematic. The US and the UK recommendations that are used as a source for the present considerations and for orientation are rather vague on this issue. The UK report points out, for example, that at the moment, there is no possibility to formulate one single optimal strategy. Therefore, research imaging centers should continue to review their practices and proceed within a range of strategies with an acceptable minimum standard as long as circumstances and available resources change in a way that facilitates higher standards (The Royal College of Radiologists 2011). The report of the Presidential Commission, however, gives the very general advice in the overarching recommendation no. 1 that patients and participants should be informed "about the plan for disclosing and managing incidental and secondary findings, including what findings will and will not be returned" (Presidential Commission for the Study of Bioethical Issues 2013). However, there are neither instructions on how this plan could be compiled nor concrete decision aids or criteria that could be helpful deciding if IFs should be disclosed at all, and if so, which kinds should be disclosed in the recommendations concerning medical care and the research context, where advice of this sort is given again in a more context-specific way. Instead, recommendation no. 2 just mentions the need for further investigations and lacks any concrete advice: "Professional representative groups should develop guidelines that categorize the findings likely to arise from each diagnostic modality; develop best practices for managing incidental and secondary findings; and share these guidelines among practitioners in the clinical, research, and direct-to-consumer contexts" (Presidential Commission for the Study of Bioethical Issues 2013). Surely this is crucial and overdue, but for researchers and practitioners that have to deal with IFs now, and not sufficiently helpful. Therefore, a short introduction to the discussion of different disclosure algorithms is given:

Different types of "disclosure plans" have emerged in the research context where a complete non-disclosure strategy cannot be pursued for a variety of reasons, although this would certainly carry benefits, including being the most effective way to avoid the diagnostic misconception. The most apparent reasons are due to legal constrictions: In Germany, for example, there is an obligation located in the criminal care to

Table 1 Recommended classification of IFs by Wolf et al. originally the table contained both imaging and genetic IFs; the author deleted content that refers to genetic IFs (Wolf et al. 2008)

Category	Relevant incidental finding	Recommended action
Strong net benefit	Information revealing a *condition likely to be life-threatening* Information revealing a *condition likely to be grave that can be avoided or ameliorated [...]*	*Disclose* to research participant as an incidental finding, unless she or he elected not to know
Possible net benefit	Information revealing a nonfatal *condition that is likely to be grave or serious but that cannot be avoided or ameliorated, when a research participant is likely to deem that information important [...]*	*May disclose* to research participants as an incidental finding, unless she or he elected not to know
Unlikely net benefit	Information revealing a *condition that is not likely to be of serious health or reproductive importance* Information whose *likely health or reproductive importance cannot be ascertained*	*Do not disclose* to research participants as an incidental finding

render necessary and reasonable assistance in case of emergencies §323c StGB (Strafgesetzbuch 1998). This subsequently demands in the context of IFs that in the case that something is revealed which obviously demands immediate treatment, one is obliged to initiate appropriate steps regardless of whether the researcher involved is part of the medical staff. The only way to ensure the possibility of a complete non-disclosure strategy is to quarantine the imaging results long enough (Puls et al. 2010). As far as we know, however, this is only a theoretical solution that has never actually been implemented in research protocols.

Another way to handle the disclosure issue, which tries to combine the advantages of a high degree of transparency for the participants (to avoid false expectations such as the perception that a participant has been given a "clean bill of health") with a careful use of the work force and budget of the study, is the so-called positive list. Such lists contain a number of foreseeable and significant health-related findings, and participants are informed during the consent process that only the listed findings will be disclosed. There are at least two problems with this kind of "positive list": first, the decision about which criteria are applied to identify findings that is worth being disclosed and therefore listed and, second, what happens when findings that are not listed but seem to be of high significance and relevance for the concerned person are revealed?

And finally there is the very general strategy to communicate anything of relevance, whereby we again end up with the definition of relevance, which comes up in medical care and DTC contexts as well.

Due to the ambiguous character of information per se – as already pointed out, information with uncertain significance can lead to risky and costly and most notably unnecessary follow-up examinations as well as adverse psychological reactions – the key issues regarding the disclosure or the withholding of IFs, respectively, are on the one hand the informed consent process that should enable patients/participants to do a reasonable weighing of risks and benefits (q.v. recommendation no. 5, 6, 11 of the US report, but therefrom later) and on the other hand, on the professionals' side, the reliable appraisal of relevance and significance of the concerning information. To get more clarity concerning the latter, the UK report presents the following classification matrix that was developed by Wolf and her colleagues in the USA and delivers a system on how to define different classes of IFs (from imaging as well as from the genetic context) and proposals regarding the courses of action (Table 1) (Wolf et al. 2008).

Principally, the content of this table is already very suitable advice as a basis for recommendations regarding the question, which IFs should be communicated. There are two critical points that catch the eye just on second sight, which should nevertheless be mentioned at least shortly: To begin with, there is a discussion in progress about the question, what happens if a participant/patient chooses the right not to know and the inspection of the imaging scans reveals life-threatening information? Particularly, the question, if there is a "duty to communicate" in order to guarantee the protection of third party interests, is heavily discussed (Schmücker 2012). One way to avoid conflicts of this kind is the exclusion of persons choosing the right not to know from the possibility of participation. An in-depth discussion of this issue is not possible at this point. But at least the adumbration may be permitted that choosing this procedure would mean that particularly those persons actually participating for altruistic reasons are excluded and "punished" in a way for this attitude. Furthermore the decision only to disclose conditions which can be avoided or at least ameliorated might be estimated as violation of the principle of respect for persons. Withholding information lacks a comprehensible justification at least for validated information regarding severe conditions.

Besides that, the classification and the corresponding recommendations of Wolf and her colleagues seem to be very applicable not even for the research context but also for the medical care and DTC context. The issue why they are not included in the recommendation compilations, neither the US nor the UK report, therefore, remains unsettled. We presume that this has to do with the impact of Wolf's proposal not to disclose information "whose likely health importance *cannot be ascertained*." Currently, imaging examinations, even in the clinical context, produced a high number of IFs with indeterminate value. The ascertainment of importance for health is not always verifiable without vast effort particularly of radiologists' expertise, and even then, there would remain information whose significance could only be validated by the conduction of subsequent examinations. As the UK report mentions in its recommendations, there is a "lack of evidence on some key areas" which can only be eliminated by further research, which explains the vagueness of current regulations on the one hand and the demand for further activity which is mirrored in recommendation no. 3 of the Presidential Commission's report on the other hand: "Federal agencies and other interested parties should continue to fund research regarding incidental and secondary findings. This research should consider the types and frequency of findings that can arise from various modalities; the potential costs, benefits, and harms of identifying, disclosing, and managing these findings; and recipient and practitioner preferences about the discovery, disclosure, and management of incidental and secondary findings" (Presidential Commission for the Study of Bioethical Issues 2013).

3.3 Who Should Interpret the Images and Decide About the Disclosure of IFs?

Altogether the previous considerations should have made apparent that once the decision is made and that at least certain IFs will be disclosed, the decision which ones in particular has to be the result of a thorough assessment to ensure a minimal amount of false-positive as well as false-negative results and can't be committed by persons without appropriate qualification, training, and knowledge. Naturally, in medical care contexts as well as in DTC contexts, the reporting will be conducted by clinicians/radiologists. In the research context, different ways are established to implement radiologist expertise in the reporting process, e.g., in SHIP (Study of Health in Pomerania, see Chap. 5), a population-based study including a whole-body MRI, two radiologists examine the imaging scans independently of each other, whereas ambiguous cases are presented to a senior radiologist. Findings of unclear significance and without precedent are regularly discussed by an interdisciplinary advisory board, comprising radiologists, clinicians of different fields, epidemiologists, and ethicists before a decision regarding the question of disclosure is rendered (Langanke and Erdmann 2011; Schmidt et al. 2013). But also other sound solutions are conceivable. For example, the UK report mentions a research study group from the University of California conducting brain MRIs that established a web-based system in which board-certified neuroradiologists review scans of unclear value (The Royal College of Radiologists 2011). The idea to centralize the review process would not only have the advantage of greater unity of results. In this context, Berland, the chair of the American College of Radiology, points to the fact that currently there is a lack of standardized reporting which could lead to different interpretations as a result of the fact that the backgrounds and experiences of the concerned radiologists differ (Presidential Commission for the Study of Bioethical Issues 2013). Additionally this would insofar correspond with the issue of the overarching recommendations no. 3, no. 4, and no. 10 of the Presidential Commission's report as those include the claim that efforts should be undertaken to achieve more knowledge and transparency regarding the handling of IFs which again is provided as guidance to clinicians and researcher. This is surely associated with lots of effort, but investing less is probably incompatible with the demand to treat participants in accordance with the ethical principles of respect, the minimization of harm, etc.

3.4 Informing About the Handling of IFs/Consent Processes

The recommendations in regard to informing the patients, participants, and consumers are absolutely clear: Persons that consider taking part in any examination that bear the risk of IFs have to be informed about this. This means in detail that they have to be informed about:

- The risk that IFs will be detected and their prevalence
- The handling of IFs
- Risk of false-positive and false-negative results
- Negative consequences that might result from the disclosure (job chances, insurance issues, etc.)
- The fact that clarification again might be accompanied by own risks and psychological distress
- Possibilities to deny receiving certain findings

In case that the examinations take place in the research context, they additionally have to be informed in a way that prohibits the occurrence of therapeutic/diagnostic misconception.

The ethical principles of respect and beneficence as well as justice and fairness demand that consent procedures are designed in a way that guarantees transparency about examination conditions and enables the concerned persons to conduct a weighing considering benefits but also risks plus the corresponding chances of either. The Presidential Commission's report emphasizes especially the responsibility of the informing persons to provide guidance and support in making informed choices in all three contexts (e.g., recommendation no. 5, no. 7, and no. 15). Therefore informing should include the use of decision aids, graphical representations, etc., and can in certain cases require to point out or to respect that the waiving of certain examinations or denying to receive certain results, respectively, might be the more beneficial decision for the individual. By the way, possibilities and restrictions to ensure a valid informed consent are currently an own matter of controversial discussions.

3.5 Designing a Study Protocol in Research

The designing of a study protocol in research should, so the Presidential Commission, comprise the anticipation of IFs that are "predictably associated with a particular modality or type of research" and a corresponding and detailed plan on how to handle them. For cases in which clarification and therefore subsequent examinations are necessary, the plan should provide sufficient guidance concerning health insurance and therefore the safeguarding of treatment. Furthermore the Commission claims that this plan for ethical management of IFs should be submitted to an IRB, which reviews the plan and gives its approval (Presidential Commission for the Study of Bioethical Issues 2013).

Another issue that stands in connection with the design of the study protocol is the choice of the appropriate modality and adjustment fitting to the hypothesis or question, respectively, that shall be proved or examined. It makes a difference whether one conducts a whole-body MRI for epidemiological purposes or to satisfy in the DTC context people's wish for early detection of any pathological process that might go on or if the purpose of the examination is the clarification of some specific question and focuses on one selected area. Apparently the rate of false-positive and false-negative findings will depend on the chosen procedure and therefore controversial opinions exist regarding the question if, e.g., for MRIs, only limited sequences should be used or clinical standard scans should be added to reduce the risk of false-positive findings (The Royal College of Radiologists 2011).

4 Final Considerations

On the dealing with risks, burdens, and benefits of medical practice and research, the Declaration of Helsinki states:

> 16. In medical practice and in medical research, most interventions involve risks and burdens. Medical research involving human subjects may only be conducted if the importance of the objective outweighs the risks and burdens to the research subjects.
> 17. All medical research involving human subjects must be preceded by careful assessment of predictable risks and burdens to the individuals and groups involved in the research in comparison with foreseeable benefits to them and to other individuals or groups affected by the condition under investigation. Measures to minimise the risks must be implemented. The risks must be continuously monitored, assessed and documented by the researcher.
> 18. Physicians may not be involved in a research study involving human subjects unless they are confident that the risks have been adequately assessed and can be satisfactorily managed. When the risks are found to outweigh the potential benefits or when there is conclusive proof of definitive outcomes, physicians must assess whether to continue, modify or immediately stop the study (WMA Declaration of Helsinki 2013).

The abovementioned considerations about the handling of IFs should have made apparent that a careful and deliberate management of IFs, that is not only in accordance with general ethical principles, is expressed in the DOH, but also with those particularly concerning the challenges of IFs, based on a decision to be highly aware of the accompanied challenges and on the commitment to handle them in a way that at least minimizes the risks and burdens of those involved. If the planning process reveals that high efforts, particularly in regard to personal and financial resources, have to be invested to ensure ethically desirable conditions from the informing procedure up to the disclosure and clarification processes, the weighing should also include the benefit that can be achieved by the study itself. Meeting ethical standards of research includes the duty to fulfill standards of good scientific practice. Recently, the approach to reduce waste and increase value in biomedical research attracted a great deal of attention (Chalmers et al. 2014). Representatives of this approach argue that for different reasons the scientific value of many biomedical studies does not legitimize costs and efforts that originate from their conduction. Therefore, the deliberate weighing of costs, risks, and benefits should take place during all stages of study conduction, from the planning process to the reviewing of an ethics committee up to the handling of IFs. Different perspectives should be considered particularly concerning the question which risks and costs emerge, who has to carry them, and finally if the possible benefit for science and society resulting from the study legitimizes those.

The weighing between costs/risks and benefits naturally also takes place in the medical care context. Since the main interest of the attending physician should be the well-being of the patient, the challenge is to identify what serves patients' benefit best. The individual weighing which precedes the decision about attending a certain examination or the non-/disclosure of certain IFs, respectively, has to be supported, particularly by depicting the relevant information not only in a comprehensible way but also respecting the individual situation. The disclosure of all revealed IFs is not necessarily always in the interest of the concerned person, although almost all patients/participants wish to receive as much information as possible. The ambiguity of information, particularly the risks of subsequent examinations for clarification, therefore, has to be content of the consenting process.

The utilization of imaging examinations provided in the DTC context often takes place because healthcare insurances won't cover the costs, but the consumer hopes that this way eventually ongoing pathological processes are revealed in a stage in which they can be healed or at least adverse effects can be softened. In this context, obligations are rather due to legal than to moral considerations; therefore, it should at least be ensured that providers of those offers have the duty to inform their potential consumers appropriately, particularly about the risks of false-positive and false-negative results and the subsequent consequences. The Nuffield Council on Bioethics has compiled an evaluation of different DTC offerings which includes a chapter about "direct-to-consumer body imaging" (Bioethics 2010). In view of those offerings, they are very critical about the ability of individuals to pursue their interests especially with regard to full-body CT scans. They argue that the risks justify "the introduction of coercive state powers to prohibit the provision of such services" (Bioethics 2010). Additionally they estimate the risk/benefit ratio of other types of imaging as unclear and therefore propose different measures which include among others the attempt to regulate those services and plead for more transparency and information (Bioethics 2010).

Acknowledgments This publication originates from within the framework of the research network MENON – medical theoretical, ethical, and economical evaluation of System Medicine. The MENON Consortium is financed by the Bundesministerium für Bildung und Forschung (federal ministry of education and research) (01GP1408A and 01GP1408B).

References

Appelbaum PS, Lidz CW, Grisso T (2004) Therapeutic misconception in clinical research: frequency and risk factors. IRB Ethics Hum Res 26(2):1–8. doi:10.2307/3564231

Baile WF, Buckmann R, Lenzi R, Glober G, Beale EA, Kudelka AP (2000) SPIKES – a six-step protocol for delivering bad news: application to the patient with cancer. Oncologist 5:302–311

Beauchamp TL, Childress JF (2009) Principles of biomedical ethics. Oxford University Press, New York

Nuffield Council on Bioethics (2010) Medical profiling and online medicine: the ethics of 'personalised healthcare' in a consumer age, Chapter 10. Direct to consumer body Imaging. http://nuffieldbioethics.org/wp-content/uploads/2014/07/Personalised-healthcare-Chapter-10-Direct-to-consumer-body-imaging1.pdf. Accessed 07 Mar 2016

Bjugn R (2015) Research findings with clinical implications. Tidsskr Nor Legeforen 135(8):755–758. doi:10.4045/tidsskr.14.0861

Booth TC, Waldman AD, Wardlaw JM, Taylor SA, Jackson A (2012) Management of incidental findings during imaging research in "healthy" volunteers: current UK practice. Br J Radiol 85:11–21

Brothers KB (2015) Wie konnte das passieren? Die US-amerikanische Perspektive auf Zufallsbefunde in den ACMG-Empfehlungen. In: Langanke M, Erdmann P, Robienski J, Rudnik-Schöneborn S (eds) Zufallsbefunde bei molekulargenetischen Untersuchungen. Medizinische, juristische und ethische Perspektiven. Springer, Heidelberg, pp 178–190

Brothers KB, Langanke M, Erdmann P (2013) Implications of the incidentalome for clinical pharmacogenomics. Pharmacogenomics 14(11):1353–1362

Chalmers I, Bracken MB, Djulbegovic B, Garattini S, Grant J, Gülmezoglu AM, Howells DW, Ioannidis JP, Oliver S (2014) How to increase value and reduce waste when research priorities are set. Lancet 383(9912):156–165

Charmaz K (1993) Good days, bad days: the self and chronic illness in time. Rutgers University Press, New Brunswick

Christenhusz GB, Devriendt K, Dierickx K (2013) To tell or not to tell? A systematic review of ethical reflections on incidental findings arising in genetic contexts. Eur J Hum Genet 21:248–255

Cole C, Petree LE, Phillips JP, Shoemaker JM, Holdsworth M, Helitzer DL (2015) 'Ethical responsibility' or 'a whole can of worms': differences in opinion on incidental finding review and disclosure in neuroimaging research from focus group discussion with participants, parents, IRB members, investigators, physicians and community members. J Med Ethics 41(10):841–847. doi:10.1136/medethics-2014-102552

Erdmann P (2015a) Zufallsbefunde aus bildgebenden Verfahren in populationsbasierter Forschung. Mentis, Münster

Erdmann P (2015b) Handling incidental findings from imaging within IM related research. In: Fischer T, Langanke M, Marschall P, Michl S (eds) Individualized medicine. Ethical, economical and historical perspectives. Springer, Heidelberg, pp 231–250

Erdmann P, Langanke M (2016) The ambivalence of early diagnosis – Dealing with the false-positive risk in current Alzheimer research. In: Current Alzheimer Research (accepted)

Erdmann P, Fischer T, Raths S, Fleßa S, Langanke M (2015) Systemmedizin – Herausforderungen eines aktuellen Ansatzes. Deutsches Ärzteblatt 112:A1330–A1334

Hoffmann M (2014) Zufallsbefunde in der epidemiologischen Forschung. In: Lenk C, Duttge G, Fangerau H (eds) Handbuch Ethik und Recht der Forschung am Menschen. Springer, Heidelberg, pp 305–311. doi:10.1007/978-3-642-35099-3_52

Kohane IS, Masys DR, Altman RB (2006) The incidentalome: a threat to genomic medicine. JAMA 296(2):212–215

Langanke M, Erdmann P (2011) Die MRT als wissenschaftliche Studienuntersuchung und das Problem der Mitteilung von Zufallsbefunden. Probandenethische Herausforderungen. In: Theißen H, Langanke M (eds) Tragfähige Rede von Gott. Festgabe für Heinrich Assel zum 50. Geburtstag am 9. Februar 2011. Verlag Dr. Kovač, Hamburg, pp 197–240

Langanke M, Fasold J, Erdmann P, Lorbeer R, Liedtke W (2015) Informed consent in Gani_Med – a sectional design for clinical epidemiological studies within individualized medicine. In: Fischer T, Langanke M, Marschall P, Michl S (eds) Individualized medicine. Ethical, economical and historical perspectives. Springer, Heidelberg, pp 183–208

Levine PA (2010) In an unspoken voice. How the body releases trauma and restores goodness. North Atlantic Books/ERGOS Institute Press, Berkley

Munk MD, Peitzmann AD, Hostler DP, Wolfson AB (2010) Frequency and follow-up of incidental findings on trauma computed tomography scans: experience at a level one trauma center. J Emerg Med 38(3):346–350

Presidential Commission for the Study of Bioethical Issues (eds) (2013) Anticipate and communicate. Ethical management of incidental and secondary findings in the clinical, research, and direct-to-consumer-contexts. http://bioethics.gov/node/3183. Accessed 12 Jan 2016

Puls R, Hamm B, Hosten N (2010) MRT ohne Radiologen – ethische Aspekte bei bevölkerungsbasierten Studien mit MR-Untersuchung. Fortschr Röntgenstr 182:469–471

Rudnik-Schöneborn S, Langanke M, Erdmann P, Robienski J (2014) Ethische und rechtliche Aspekte im Umgang mit genetischen Zufallsbefunden – Herausforderungen und Lösungsansätze. Ethik in der Medizin 26:105–119. doi:10.1007/s00481-013-0244-x

Al-Shahi Salman R, Whiteley WN, Warlow C (2007) Screening using whole-body magnetic resonance imaging scanning: who wants an incidentaloma? J Med Screen 14(1):2–4

Schmidt CO, Hegenscheid K, Erdmann P, Kohlmann T, Langanke M, Völzke H, Puls R, Assel H, Biffar R, Grabe HJ (2013) Psychosocial consequences and severity of disclosed incidental findings from whole-body MRI in a general population study. Eur Radiol 23:1343–1351

Schmücker R (2012) Zufallsbefunde – was gebietet die Menschenwürde? http://www.uni-muenster.de/imperia/md/content/kfg-normenbegruendung/intern/publikationen/schmuecker/36_-_schm__cker_-_zufallsbefunde_und_menschenw__rde.pdf. Accessed 07 Mar 2016

Strafgesetzbuch in der Fassung der Bekanntmachung vom 13. November 1998 (BGBl. I S. 3322), das durch Artikel 15 des Gesetzes vom 4. Juli 2013 (BGBl. I S. 1981) geändert worden ist. http://www.gesetze-im-internet.de/stgb/BJNR001270871.html#BJNR001270871BJNG000102307. Accessed 07 Mar 2016

The National Commission for the Protection of Human Subjects of Biomedical and Behavioral Research (1978) The Belmont report: ethical principles and guidelines for the protection of human subjects of research. Department of Health, Education, and Welfare, Washington (DC). http://www.hhs.gov/ohrp/humansubjects/guidance/belmont.html. Accessed 07 Mar 2016

The Royal College of Radiologists (eds) (2011) Management of incidental findings detected during research imaging. A report by representatives of research imaging centres, professional societies, regulatory bodies, funding organisations, royal colleges involved in research imaging and patient organisations, in the UK. https://www.rcr.ac.uk/sites/default/files/publication/BFCR%2811%298_ethics.pdf. Accessed 13 Jan 2016

WMA Declaration of Helsinki – Ethical principles for medical research involving human subjects. 64th WMA General Assembly, Fortaleza, Brazil, October 2013. http://www.wma.net/en/30publications/10policies/b3/. Accessed 07 Mar 2016

Wolf SM, Lawrence FP, Nelson CA, Kahn JP, Cho MK, Wright Clayton E, Fletcher JG, Georgieff MK, Hammerschmidt D, Hudson K, Illes J, Kapur V, Keane MA, Koenig BA, LeRoy BS, McFarland EG, Paradise J, Parker LS, Terry SF, Van Ness B, Wilfond BS (2008) Managing incidental findings in human subjects research: analysis and recommendations. J Law Med Ethics 36(2):219–248

Medicolegal Aspects and Informed Consent

Leonard Berlin

The ability to search for the truth implies also a duty: not to conceal any part of what one has found to be true.

Albert Einstein

Where ignorance is bliss, 'tis folly to be wise.

Thomas Gray

Any human being of adult years and sound mind has a right to determine what shall be done with his own body. (Schloendorff v The Society of New York Hosp 1914)

Contents

1 **Frequency Engenders a Dilemma** 26

2 **Standard of Care** 27

3 **Defending an Ignored Incidentaloma in the American Courtroom** 29

4 **Medicolegal Duties of Researchers When Scanning Healthy Volunteers** 30

5 **Cascade of Unnecessary Imaging, Exposure to Radiation, and Informed Consent** 30

6 **Informed Consent** 31

7 **Conclusion: Incidentalomas and the Medicolegal Environment, 2016** 31

8 **Author's Advice** 32

References 32

Abstract

With the advent of high resolution CT, MRI, and ultrasound scanning, the frequency of radiologists' serendipitous discovery of incidental findings (colloquially referred to as "incidentalomas") on radiological examinations is increasing. Incidentalomas account for approximately 20% of all findings, due to two reasons: (a) the number of hi-tech imaging exams (primarily CT) performed today, and (b) the increasing sophistication of the technology. In the early 1980s when CT scanning was in its infancy, 3 to 5 million scans were performed annually in the US. In the past few years, the annual number of CT scans performed in the US has increased exponentially to well over 80 million. In addition, the specificity of the equipment has advanced geometrically such that abnormalities and/or pseudo-abnormalities 1 mm or a fraction of 1 mm in size that were virtually "invisible" before can now be seen quite easily.

Statistically only 1% or less of these incidentalomas represent an early malignancy or other severe pathology. Thus, radiologists are faced with a dilemma: if they report every incidentaloma, many patients will be subjected to a cascade of costly testing, sometimes leading to biopsies or other invasive procedures, all of which on occasion may lead to

L. Berlin, MD, FACR
Radiology Department, Skokie Hospital,
9600 Gross Point Road, Skokie, IL 60076, USA

Rush University, Chicago, IL, USA

University of Illinois, Chicago, IL, USA
e-mail: lberlin@live.com

Med Radiol Diagn Imaging (2016)
DOI 10.1007/174_2016_35, © Springer International Publishing Switzerland
Published Online: 29 Mar 2016

complications and cause harm to the patient who was completely healthy and was never ill to begin with. On the other hand, should the radiologist decide not to report the presence of an incidentaloma, and it is later discovered that it was indeed an early malignancy and thus a fatal delay in diagnosis and treatment ensued, the patient could be permanently harmed or even die, and a medical malpractice lawsuit would almost certainly follow.

What, if anything, should the radiologist report to the patient or the referring physician, when faced with an incidentaloma? Should, or must, informed consent be required? This Chapter will focus on both the moral-ethical, and the medico-legal, aspects of the incidentaloma dilemma faced everyday by radiologists as well as treating physicians.

Incidentalomas (colloquial term for incidental findings), defined as an incidentally discovered mass or lesion detected by CT or other imaging modality performed for an unrelated reason (Berland 2011), are becoming increasingly prevalent in everyday radiologic practice because there has been a massive increase in utilization and improved resolution of such high-tech imaging modalities as ultrasound, positron emission tomography (PET), magnetic resonance (MR), and computed tomography (CT). Incidentally discovered benign thyroid nodules are now commonplace on ultrasound studies of the neck (Hoang et al. 2015), false-positive findings suggesting Alzheimer and related neurodegenerative diseases that cause dementia are increasing in amyloid PET imaging (Dubroff and Nasrallah 2015), and uncertain findings questionably related to schizophrenia and related various neuropsychiatric and traumatic disorders are being found on MR scanning and its variants such as functional magnetic imaging and diffusion tensor imaging (Nucifora 2015). Recent radiology literature is replete with reports of clinically insignificant incidental CNS findings in patients undergoing brain screening MR scanning (Salman et al. 2007; Vernooij et al. 2007), MR cardiovascular screening (McKenna et al. 2008), whole-body MR screening (Hegenscheid et al. 2013), and MR research studies (Morin et al. 2009; Booth et al. 2010). Notwithstanding these references to ultrasound, PET, and MR imaging, however, the major cause of the unrelenting and problematic rise in incidentalomas is CT scanning.

CT has the advantages of being accessible, quick, and relatively inexpensive. Its only potential downside is that it exposes patients to ionizing radiation, a topic that will be discussed later in this chapter. In 1980, fewer than three million CT scans were performed in the USA, but since then, CT imaging has increased at a rate of 10 % per year; by 2009, the number of CTs performed in the USA annually reached 80 million (Brenner and Hricak 2010). The rise in utilization of CT in the emergency departments (EDs) is even greater. A recent study of EDs in the State of California disclosed that between 2005 and 2013, the probability of a patient with minor trauma undergoing at least one CT scan before discharge doubled, from 3 % to more than 7 % (Tong et al. 2016). Concurrent with increasing utilization, a plethora of major advances in spacial and contrast resolution of CT and MR scanners has occurred, thus allowing radiologists to "see" tiny possibly abnormal findings that were not discernible on equipment manufactured in previous decades.

1 Frequency Engenders a Dilemma

The increasing frequency with which incidentalomas occur has become a worldwide problem. Here are just a few percentages from various nations that quantify the frequency of incidentalomas among specific patient groups: Greece, 34 % of patients with stable blunt trauma (Sgourakis et al. 2011); the Netherlands, 35 % of patients with thoracoabdominal blunt trauma (van Vugt et al. 2012); Ireland, 67 % of patients undergoing emergency abdominal CT scans (Redmond et al. 2015); and the USA, 49 % of patients undergoing aortoiliac CT angiography (Apfaltrer et al. 2012), 82 % of patients being imaged by CT for staging of prostate cancer (Elmi et al. 2012), 40 % of patients undergoing research imaging exams at the Mayo

Clinic (Orme et al. 2010), 34 % of patients undergoing MR imaging in a large neuroimaging research project (Shoemaker et al. 2011), and up to 67 % of patients undergoing ultrasound of the neck (Hoang et al. 2015). Welch has summarized the appearance of incidentalomas as follows: 50 % in the lungs on chest CTs, 23 % in the kidneys and 15 % in the liver on abdominal CTs, and 67 % in the thyroid gland on ultrasound of the neck (Welch et al. 2011). His comprehensive review of the radiologic literature disclosed that less than 4 % of lung nodules and overall less than 1 % of incidentalomas elsewhere evolve into a lethal carcinoma.

The growing incidence of incidentalomas presents an increasingly serious dilemma for radiologists throughout the world: if there is reasonable belief that the incidentaloma is of no clinical significance, then mentioning it will likely lead to a cascade of expensive tests, some of which occasionally result in iatrogenic complications. However, if radiologists decide not to report an incidentaloma and in the unlikely event the incidentaloma later turns out to have been an early carcinoma or other serious disease that jeopardizes the patient's health, medical malpractice litigation could well ensue. Let us look more closely at this dilemma from medicolegal and ethical perspectives. The judicial statement that "Any human being of adult years and sound mind has a right to determine what shall be done with his own body" (Schloendorff v The Society of New York Hosp 1914), quoted at the beginning of this chapter, was rendered 102 years ago. In subsequent years, American appeals courts strengthened patient's rights of self-determination by imposing upon their physicians a duty to disclose to the patient all pertinent medical information:

> A physician undertaking a physical exam has a duty to disclose what he has found and to warn the examinee of any finding that would indicate the patient is in any danger. (Betesh v United States of America 1974)

> Those who place themselves in the hands of a person who is skilled in the medical profession have a reasonable expectation that the radiologist will warn of any dangers of which he is cognizant. By failing to inform the patient of the abnormality, the radiologist prevents the patient from halting the progress of his disease. (Daly v United States of America 1991)

> A doctor who undertakes to read x-rays, on which he observes abnormalities, must act reasonably in reading the x-rays and reporting the results. What constitutes reasonable reporting must be determined by a jury. (Stanley v McCarver 2004)

Emphasizing that ethical duties often surpass legal duties, the *Code of Ethics of the American Medical Association* states: "The physician's obligation is to present the medical facts accurately …and disclose all relevant medical information to patients" (American Medical Association Council on Ethical and Judicial Affairs 2015).

To what degree are these court decisions and the *AMA Code of Ethics* applicable to incidentalomas? Does an incidentaloma "indicate the patient is in any danger?" Is an incidentaloma a "danger of which the physician is cognizant?" Does a physician have knowledge that an incidentaloma might harm the patient if no warning is given? Can an incidentaloma be considered "relevant medical information?" The absence of a definite answer to these questions contributes to the dilemma faced by radiologists.

2 Standard of Care

Physicians in all nations are legally and morally obligated to adhere to a standard of care (SOC). There is no single written definition of SOC, but courts throughout the USA and elsewhere have generally agreed on what conduct does, and does not, constitute the standard of care (Berlin 1998). The following American court commentaries give the readers a reasonable understanding of the term standard of care:

> When a person assumes the profession of physician and surgeon, he must…be held to employ a reasonable amount of skill and care. For anything short of that degree of skill in his practice, the law will hold him responsible for any injury that may result from its absence. While he is not required to possess the highest order of qualification, to which some men attain, still he must possess and exercise that degree of skill, which is ordinarily possessed by members of the profession. (Richie v West 1860)

> Every person who enters the medical profession must exercise a reasonable degree of care and skill. He does not undertake to use the highest possible degree of skill, for there may be persons who, for having enjoyed a better education and greater advantage, are possessed of greater skill in their profession; but he undertakes that he will bring a fair, reasonable and competent degree of skill. (Smith v Overby 1860)

> Proof of a bad result or a mishap is not evidence of lack of skill or negligence. If a doctor has given a patient his best judgment, assuming that judgment is equal to that ordinarily used by reasonably well-qualified doctors in similar cases, he is not liable for negligence. (Spike v Sellett 1981)

> Perfection is a standard to which no profession can possibly adhere. Doctors are required to exercise reasonable care; they are not required to be perfect. (Blake v Gunderson Clinic, Ltd 1989)

> The term "standard of care" is generally understood to mean conduct against which a defending doctor's actions is to be measured…The established standard of care is stated as "use of the same degree of knowledge, skill, and ability as an ordinarily careful physician would exercise under similar circumstances." (Advincula v United Blood Services 1996)

Although the source of the above descriptions of the SOC is American courts, similar wording appears in courts worldwide. The SOC as described here is international.

Inasmuch as SOC is considered usual and customary conduct practiced by physicians in the local community under the same or similar circumstances, the question arises as to what constitutes "usual and customary conduct" regarding how radiologists handle incidentalomas. The SOC would be very clear if virtually all "reasonable and ordinary" radiologists managed incidentalomas in the same manner. However, data reveal that there is no consistency; some radiologists report them, and some radiologists ignore them. A recently published survey of 27 radiologists at three well-known and prestigious medical centers in the USA – Johns Hopkins University, New York University, and Stanford University – disclosed the degree of agreement on whether, and if so how, to report incidental findings ranged as low as 30 % (Johnson et al. 2012). There was wide disagreement not only across the three academic institutions but among radiologists in the same institution as well. Furthermore, in an attempt to bring about general agreement on the reporting of incidentalomas, the American College of Radiology (ACR) published a "White Paper" containing guidelines that, based on specific characteristics of an incidentaloma, would lead radiologists to be consistent in deciding whether to report the finding if it was suspicious for a malignancy or to ignore it if it was clearly benign (Berland Berland et al. 2010). Not surprisingly but nonetheless still disappointedly, one survey disclosed that as few as 29 % of radiologists adhered to guidelines published by the Fleischner Society, an internationally known society of thoracic radiologists (Esmaili et al. 2011). In a survey of 14,200 radiologists, inquiring about their knowledge of and adherence to guidelines of the ACR White Paper (WP) regarding recommendations on the reporting of abdominal incidental findings, 2865 (20 %) responded. Of these respondents, 1088 (38 %) indicated that they had read the WP, and of these, close to 90 % indicated that they at least sometimes adhere to the WP recommendations. However, when compared to the total number who responded to the survey, the percentage of respondents who adhered to the guidelines drops to 34 %. If we use as the denominator the entire 14,200 who were contacted, the percentage could drop to as low as 7 %. When asked with the question of whether their concern for being sued for malpractice leads them to increase recommendations for additional imaging of incidentalomas, 76 % answered affirmatively (Berland et al. 2014).

Notwithstanding that 99 % of all incidentalomas are benign and are not in the least bit a threat to the health of the patient, most radiologists are reluctant to ignore them because of the fear of being sued, given the unpleasant malpractice environment that exists in the USA and which, unfortunately, seems to be spreading to other nations as well. This fear is exemplified by a published lamentation of a well-known expert in obstetrical ultrasound, Dr. Roy Filly. He pointed out that in 10 % of normal pregnancies, sonograms contain apparent abnormalities that can be interpreted as markers of Down syndrome; however, in reality, almost all turn out to be clinically unimportant.

Filly opines that if he informed all parents of this so-called abnormality, "enjoyment of the anticipation of the birth" of their baby would be replaced by "anxiety and concern" (Filly 2000). Statistically, the likelihood that the fetus would be born with Down syndrome is extremely rare, and thus informing the parents of the marker would put 10 % of all pregnant women with perfectly normal fetuses through a great deal of worry. Filly asked himself, "Should I have the courage of my conviction and ignore these features?" He concluded that he wished he had the courage, but does not, because the American medicolegal climate is not conducive to his unilaterally ignoring such findings. If Filly, a well-known and prestigious expert in radiology, fears ignoring incidentalomas because of potential legal consequences, it is no surprise that most radiologists share the same fear. One American university disclosed that even when incidental findings that were not considered important enough to require medical follow-up were discovered, all patients were notified nevertheless because of "medical legal concerns" (Sperry et al. 2010).

3 Defending an Ignored Incidentaloma in the American Courtroom

There have not been any appeals court decisions rendered in the USA specifically focusing on malpractice issues regarding radiologists' reporting of incidentalomas. However, a small number of malpractice lawsuits related to incidentalomas have been filed, and some have proceeded to a courtroom trial. Contrary to most nations where civil litigation is tried by a judge only, in the USA, such litigation invariably is tried before a jury of laypeople. In one lawsuit, a radiologist was sued for failing to report on a chest CT exam a tiny benign appearing nodule that later turned out to be cancer. At the trial, the plaintiff's attorney addressed the defendant radiologist as follows:

> As a radiologist, you do not make a diagnosis of lung cancer. However, is not what you do similar to screeners in the security lines at the airports? A suitcase comes through the x-ray machine, something shows up, it might be a gun, it might not be a gun, they do not know, so they pull the bag off the line for someone else to examine. Isn't that what radiologists do—they question a finding on an x-ray, report it, and then someone else—the patient's physician—will then investigate the abnormality, just as security people in the airport investigate the suitcase? So is not the radiologist's duty simply to alert the ordering physician that there may be a problem, and then the physician undertakes further tests to determine whether the finding is significant and must be treated?

The defendant radiologist had no choice but to answer "yes." Notwithstanding the attorney's unrealistic if not ridiculous comparison between a radiologist and a security employee at an airport, the jury found in favor of the patient.

In another case in which a radiologist was sued because she decided not to report an incidentaloma because it was almost certainly a benign finding, but which later turned out to be carcinoma, the plaintiff's attorney questioned the radiologist at a jury trial as follows:

Question: Doctor, why didn't you report the potentially abnormal finding?

Answer: Because I thought the finding was almost certainly of no significance and would have led to a number of unnecessary and possibly dangerous tests.

Question: Could it have represented an early cancer?

Answer: Yes, but probably no more than a 1 % chance.

Question: Well, Doctor, in this case, it was 100 %. Shouldn't you have let the patient and his private physician decide whether further testing was indicated? Did you not deprive the patient, who is now dying of cancer rather than living and cured, of his inalienable right to make his own decisions about his health?

Once again, the radiologist had to answer in the affirmative and the jury found in favor of the patient.

In yet another case with similar details, the plaintiff's attorney asked the defendant radiologist, "Would you agree that when issuing a report that there is the benign incidentaloma of no significance, it's probably going to cause the referring physician receiving the report to engage in no further testing, which means that if it is cancer, it will continue to go undetected?" The radiologist answered "Yes," and then the attorney continued, "If judgments are to be made about whether the doctor should or should not follow up with a questionable finding, is it not your responsibility to leave the judgment making in the hands of the patient and the patient's physician? Did you not prevent the patient from undergoing further testing and getting an early diagnosis and cure of cancer?" Once again, the defendant radiologist had no recourse, answering "yes," and the jury found in the patient's favor.

A hypothetical case described in a fictional novel entitled *Handle with Care* very much resembled reality. In the book, a pregnant woman underwent a routine obstetrical ultrasound exam (Picoult 2009). The physician (an obstetrician rather than a radiologist in this case) noted a *marker* that remotely suggested osteogenesis imperfecta, but because he believed that the finding was insignificant, he did not inform the patient. The woman later delivered a child with osteogenesis imperfecta, and the child later died at a very young age. A malpractice lawsuit was filed against the obstetrician. The patient's attorney addressed the jury as follows: "This case is about the fact that the obstetrician knew that there was a potential problem but did not inform the patient. No one is blaming the obstetrician for the child's condition, or that the obstetrician caused the illness. However, the obstetrician is to blame for not giving the family all of the information she had, and when a physician withholds information from a patient, that is malpractice" (Picoult 2009).

4 Medicolegal Duties of Researchers When Scanning Healthy Volunteers

Although a comprehensive discussion pertaining to the management of potentially abnormal incidental findings discovered during research studies in which MR or CT scanning is performed on healthy volunteers is beyond the scope of this chapter, nonetheless, a few words are in order. There is little consistency in the laws among nations, nor in specific nations, regarding this issue, but generally, it is required that volunteers be informed during the consent process about whether a process exists for identifying abnormal incidental findings that may appear on research images and how and by whom such findings will be disclosed to the subjects (Booth et al. 2010).

5 Cascade of Unnecessary Imaging, Exposure to Radiation, and Informed Consent

As mentioned earlier, one of the potential harms of a patient's undergoing a cascade of tests, especially CT scans in order to ascertain whether an incidentaloma can adversely affect the health of the patient, is exposure to ionizing radiation. A recent article estimated that 1 in 460 women who undergo a CT scan of the abdomen and pelvis will develop a radiation-induced cancer (Smith-Bindman et al. 2009). Other articles have asserted that 29,000 cancers every year, half being fatal, can result from past CT use (deGonzales et al. 2009). The editor of *Archives of Internal Medicine* editorialized, "Large doses of radiation from the 19,500 CT scans performed every day in the US will translate into additional cancers" (Redberg 2009). Newspaper headlines such as "2 or 3 CT Scans = Hiroshima Radiation" (Chicago Tribune 2011) and "Overuse Of Diagnostic CT Scans May Cause 3 Million Excess Cancers In US Over The Next 2–3 Decades" (USA Today 2007) and a magazine article claiming that "15,000 People Are Estimated to Die Each Year Because of Cancers Caused by Radiation in CT Scans Alone" (Consumer Reports Magazine 2015) have been widely circulated. Although being challenged by many radiation physicists, nevertheless, these claims create unwarranted great concern among the public. In actual fact, radiation dose from abdominal-pelvic CT scans ranges from 15 to 25 mSv (millisieverts). It has not been scientifically proven that there is any risk from radiation dose under 100 mSv (McCullough et al. 2009). Other radiation physicists agree, concluding that the fear of carcinogenesis from diagnostic x-ray examinations is unjust, pointing out that there is no evidence of carcinogenic effect on humans or experimental animals from exposure to radiation at doses less than 100 mSv (Tubiana et al. 2009). A recent review of current reports from the International Atomic Energy Agency and studies from researchers at UCLA in Los Angeles, California, and Albuquerque, New Mexico, concluded that "Fear of radiation, even when diluted to homeopathic portions, unjustifiably compels some people to forgo live-saving diagnostic tests….Trying to avoid the horrors we imagine, we risk creating ones that are real" (Johnson 2015).

6 Informed Consent

There are two types of consent: (a) implied consent, given by a patient's actions rather than spoken words, e.g., voluntarily climbing on an exam table for a CT scan or extending an arm for an IV injection, and (b) informed consent, explicitly stated, required for patients about to undergo procedures that are not considered simple (Reuter 1987). When obtaining informed consent for a radiologic procedure, radiologists must inform the patient what they will do, why they will do it, and what are the risks, benefits, alternative options, and risk of not doing the procedure. In order to obtain legally acceptable informed consent, radiologists must inform patients of facts regarding the risks and complications and likelihood of their occurrence. The word "fact" is defined as "something that has been objectively verified" (The American Heritage dictionary and Second College 1985). The claim that cancer will develop as a result of radiation exposure to diagnostic radiological examinations is not, nor based on, a fact. If a patient asks what the likelihood is of a complication from a specific radiological procedure such as developing a pneumothorax following a thoracentesis, hemorrhage following an arteriogram, anaphylactic reaction from contrast media, a perforation of the colon from colonography, etc., the radiologist can quickly consult the radiologic literature and find actual statistics, i.e., facts, that can be given to the patient. However, with regard to the relationship between diagnostic-level radiation and the development of cancer, there are *no facts*. Rather, there are only hypotheses, queries, conjectures, estimates, projections, extrapolations, statistical probabilities, and opinions. Without facts, there can be no true informed consent. This was supported by a lawsuit brought by a group of employees who claimed that they developed cancer resulting from exposure to radiation emitted from radium dials; a US federal court dismissed the lawsuit stating (Johnston v US 1984):

> The court must reject the testimony of plaintiff's experts ….The law requires that causation must be proven to a reasonable degree of medical certainty….The experts' analyses that these plaintiffs' cancers were caused by radiation are not a medical opinion but are statistical sophistry. In matters of determining cancer risk from low doses of radiation, scientists deal with what exists in fact and can be measured or experimentally proven. They do not deal with theory, hypothesis and assumption. Such an approach cannot be used to establish legal cause.

Thus, current law does not require informed consent regarding possible harm from radiation exposure to patients undergoing CT exams or other diagnostic radiological exams utilizing radiation (Berlin 2011).

7 Conclusion: Incidentalomas and the Medicolegal Environment, 2016

Radiologists are faced with two questions regarding incidentalomas: (1) Should all incidentalomas be reported or just those that appear suspicious for a malignancy? And (2) if a radiologist fails to report an incidentaloma and it does develop into a malignancy that injures the patient, what is the likelihood of his or her being sued for malpractice?

As for Question 1, one group of physician-ethicists believes that clinicians should withhold information that is likely to overwhelm and distress patients if their having the information would provide no obvious benefit and they don't ask for it. "Information overload—especially if the information is not clinically relevant—may render more important discussions impossible.… We propose simple rules: If the patient asks, the clinician should tell. If the clinician is anxious about what would happen if the patient discovers that information has been withheld, then the decision to withhold should be reconsidered" (Epstein et al. 2010).

Welch contends that radiologists should report only those incidentalomas which they reasonably believe to represent a potential malignancy or other serious illness: "Balance the benefits and harms for patients. Do not say we are powerless because of lawyers. Ask yourself what is the right thing to do for patients and help your profession set a standard of practice" (Welch 2015). Welch continues that the problem is not confined to radiology: "All physicians need to shift their thresholds for diagnosis and intervention, knowing that patients with little chance to benefit from a diagnosis and treatment are also the ones at the highest risk for net harm."

As for Question 2, no physician wants to be sued, but more importantly, no physician wants to harm a patient (Warshauer 2010). Let us assume that a radiologist fails to report an incidentaloma that later is diagnosed as a carcinoma, the likelihood of which is no more than 1 %. In the USA, only a small minority of people who incur medical injury file malpractice lawsuits, and the percentage is probably much lower outside the USA. Thus, realistically, the likelihood of being sued for underreporting an incidentaloma is less than one-half of 1 %.

As already discussed in this chapter, a few malpractice lawsuits have been filed alleging negligence on behalf of radiologists for failing to report and inform the referring physicians of the presence of an incidentaloma, which later was diagnosed as a carcinoma. However, virtually all are either resolved at trial before a jury or a judge or settled out of court, and thus none has as yet been evaluated by an appeals court. Juries and judges determine the outcome of a specific malpractice trial, but only appellate and supreme courts determine precedence and law upon which the standard of care is based. None has yet ruled specifically on the incidentaloma issue, and therefore, we do not know how a court would rule if and when such lawsuits are filed. Therefore, radiologists must use their own best judgment in determining whether they should report an incidentaloma and, if so, recommend a CT or other examination to evaluate the finding.

8 Author's Advice

It is very hard to ignore something once it has been found – even if ignoring it is the right thing to do (Welch et al. 2011). Nevertheless, if the radiologist decides that a particular incidentaloma believed to almost certainly be of no clinical significance should be reported, I suggest the following phraseology: "An incidental density (or lesion) measuring xx mm is noted in the liver (or the kidney, lungs, etc.). The likelihood that this represents a malignancy is highly remote." In this manner, the radiologist has expressed his or her professional opinion and leaves it up to the referring physician and patient to decide whether follow-up studies, if any, should be undertaken.

References

15,000 people are estimated to die each year because of cancers caused by radiation in CT scans alone. Consumer Reports Magazine, Mar 2015

2 or 3 CT scans = Hiroshima Radiation. Chicago Tribune. 7 Jan 2011

Advincula v United Blood Services, 678 NE2d 1009 (Ill 1996)

American Medical Association Council on Ethical and Judicial Affairs (2015) Code of medical ethics of the American Medical Association Council on Ethical and Judicial Affairs, 2014–2015 edn. American Medical Association, Chicago, pp 8.08, 8.082

Apfaltrer P, Schymik G, Reimer P et al (2012) Aortoiliac CT angiography for planning transcutaneous aortic valve implantation: aortic root anatomy and frequency of clinically significant incidental findings. AJR Am J Roentgenol 198:939–945

Berland LL (2011) The American College of Radiology strategy for managing incidental findings on abdominal computed tomography. Radiol Clin North Am 49:238–243

Berland LL, Silverman SG, Gore RM et al (2010) Managing incidental findings on abdominal CT: white paper of the ACR Incidental Findings Committee. J Am Coll Radiol 7:754–773

Berland LL, Silverman SG, Megibow MD et al (2014) ACR members' response to ACR white paper on the management of incidental abdominal findings. J Am Coll Radiol 11:300–335
Berlin L (1998) Standard of care. AJR Am J Roentgenol 170:273–278
Berlin L (2011) Communicating the harmful effects of radiation exposure from medical imaging: malpractice considerations. Health Phys 101:583–588
Betesh v United States of America, 400 F Supp 238 (US Dist dc 1974)
Blake v Gunderson Clinic, Ltd., 152 Wisc. 2d 210 (1989)
Booth TC, Jackson A, Wardlaw JM (2010) Incidental findings found in "healthy" volunteers during imaging performed for research: current legal and ethical implications. Br J Radiol 83:456–465
Brenner DJ, Hricak H (2010) Radiology exposure from medical imaging: time to regulate? JAMA 304: 208–209
Daly v United States of America, 946 F2d 1467 (9th cir 1991)
deGonzales AB, Mahadevappa M, Kim KP et al (2009) Projected cancer risks from computed tomographic scans performed in the United States in 2007. Arch Intern Med 169:2071–2077
Dubroff JG, Nasrallah IM (2015) Will PET amyloid imaging lead to overdiagnosis of Alzheimer dementia? Acad Radiol 22:988–994
Elmi A, Tabatabaei S, Talab S et al (2012) Incidental findings at initial imaging workup of patients with prostate cancer: clinical significance and outcomes. AJR Am J Roentgenol 199:1305–1311
Epstein RM, Korones DN, Quill TE (2010) Withholding information from patients – when less is more. N Engl J Med 362:380–381
Esmaili A, Munden RF, Mohammed TL (2011) Small pulmonary nodule management: a survey of members of the Society of Thoracic Radiology with comparison to the Fleischner Society guidelines. J Thorac Imaging 26:27–31
Filly RA (2000) Obstetrical sonography: the best way to terrify a pregnant woman. (Editorial). J Ultrasound Med 19:1–5
Hegenscheid K, Seipel R, Schmidt CO et al (2013) Potentially relevant incidental findings on research whole-body MRI in the general adult population: frequencies and management. Eur Radiol 23:816–826
Hoang JK, Nguyen XV, Davies L (2015) Overdiagnosis of thyroid cancer: answers to five key questions. Acad Radiol 22:1024–1029
Johnson G. When radiation isn't the risk. New York Times, 22 Sept 2015:D3
Johnson PT, Horton KM, Megibow AJ et al (2012) Common incidental findings on MDCC: survey of radiologist recommendations for patient management. J Am Coll Radiol 8:762–767
Johnston v US, 597 FSupp 374 (D. Kansas 1984)
McCullough CH, Guimaraes L, Fletcher JG (2009) In defense of body CT. AJR Am J Roentgenol 193:28–39
McKenna DA, Laxpati M, Colletti PM (2008) The prevalence of incidental findings at cardiac MRI. Open Cardiovasc Med J 2:20–25
Morin SHX, Cobbold JFL, Lim AKB et al (2009) Incidental findings in healthy research subjects using whole-body MRI. Eur J Radiol 72:529–533
Nucifora PG (2015) Overdiagnosis in the era of neuropsychiatric imaging. Acad Radiol 22:995–999
Orme MM, Fletcher JGH, Siddiki HA et al (2010) Incidental findings in imaging research, evaluating incidence, benefit, and burden. Arch Intern Med 170:1525–1532
Overuse of diagnostic CT scans may cause 3 million excess cancers in the US over the next 2–3 decades. USA Today, 29 Nov 2007
Picoult J (2009) Handle with care. Simon & Schuster, New York, p 337
Redberg RF (2009) Cancer risks and radiation exposure from computed tomographic scans: how can we be sure the benefits outweigh the risks? Arch Intern Med 169:2049–2050
Redmond CE, Kelly ME, Winter DC et al (2015) Detection of incidental findings on emergency abdominal CT scans: a 1-year review. D I Eur:31:14–15
Reuter SR (1987) An overview of informed consent for radiologists. AJR Am J Roentgenol 148:219–227
Richie v West, 23 Ill 329 (1860)
Salman RAS, Whiteley WN, Warlow C (2007) Screening using whole-body magnetic resonance imaging scanning: who wants an incidentaloma? J Med Screen 14:2–4
Schloendorff v The Society of New York Hosp., 105 NE 92 (NY 1914)
Sgourakis G, Lanitis S, Korontzi M et al (2011) Incidental findings in focused assessment with sonography for trauma in hemodynamically stable blunt trauma patients: speaking about cost to benefit. J Trauma 71:E123–E127
Shoemaker JM, Holdsworth MT, Aine C et al (2011) A practical approach to incidental findings in neuroimaging research. Neurology 77:2123–2127
Smith-Bindman R, Lipson J, Markus R et al (2009) Radiation dose associated with common computed tomography examinations and associated lifetime attributable risk of cancer. Arch Intern Med 169:2078–2086
Smith v Overby, 30 Ga 241 (1860)
Sperry JL, Massaro MS, Collage RD et al (2010) Incidental radiographic findings after injury: dedicated attention results in improved capture, documentation, and management. Surgery 148:618–621
Spike v Sellett, 430 E2d 597 (Ill App 1981)
Stanley v McCarver, 92 P 3d 849 (ariz 2004)
William Morris The American Heritage dictionary, Second College Edition (1985) Houghton Mifflin Company, Boston, pp 484–485
Tong GE, Staudenmayer MD, Hsia RY (2016) Use of emergency department imaging in patients with minor trauma. J Surg Res. doi: http:lldx.doi.org/10.1016/J.Jss.2015.11.046. Accessed February 27, 2016

Tubiana M, Feinnendegen LE, Yang C, Kaminski JM (2009) The linear no-threshold relationship is inconsistent with the radiation biologic and experimental data. Radiology 251:13–22

van Vugt MD, Dekker HM, Deunk J et al (2012) Incidental findings on routine thoracoabdominal blunt trauma patients. J Trauma 72:416–421

Vernooij MW, Ikram MA, Tanghe HL et al (2007) Incidental findings on brain MRI in the general population. N Engl J Med 357:1821–1828

Warshauer DM (2010) The age of (over)discovery. J Am Coll Radiol 7:246–247

Welch HG (2015) Responding to the challenge of overdiagnosis. Acad Radiol 22:945–946

Welch HG, Schwartz LM, Woloshin S (2011) Overdiagnosed: making people sick in the pursuit of health. Beacon Press, Boston, p 95

Part II

IFs in Population Based Imaging/ Research Setting

Technical Prerequisites of Population-Based Imaging

Sergios Gatidis and Fabian Bamberg

Contents

1	**General Requirements**	37
2	**Imaging Modalities**	38
2.1	Magnetic Resonance Imaging	38
2.2	Computed Tomography	39
2.3	Ultrasound	39
3	**Data Storage and Data Distribution**	40
4	**Data Post-processing and Data Analysis**	40
Literature		41

S. Gatidis • F. Bamberg, MPH (✉)
Associate Chair, Department of Diagnostic and Interventional Radiology, University of Tuebingen, Hoppe-Seyler-Straße 3, 72076 Tübingen, Germany

The main goal of population-based imaging is to gain insight into physiological and pathophysiological processes of individuals by assessing corresponding morphological and functional changes in the general population using imaging techniques. This approach is fundamentally different from the usual clinical approach, where the individual examination is in the center of attention and usually not directly related or compared to population-based imaging data. Therefore, specific technical and organizational prerequisites have to be met in order to successfully conduct population-based imaging studies. In this chapter, these prerequisites will be discussed concerning the underlying imaging modalities as well as aspects of data storage and data processing.

1 General Requirements

In the context of population-based imaging, the focus of attention is not directed onto individual participants but rather on the whole population. The most important technical goal is thus to obtain comparable data from each included individual in order to allow for a valid epidemiological analyses.

Concerning the data acquisition step, the following requirements have to be met.

First of all, the image acquisition procedure has to be performed in a standardized manner in order to ensure reproducible results. Standardization has different implications for the

Med Radiol Diagn Imaging (2016)
DOI 10.1007/174_2016_74, © Springer International Publishing Switzerland
Published Online: 10 May 2016

different available imaging modalities that will be discussed in detail below. In general however, it is of importance that imaging protocols as well as underlying hardware and software are kept constant over the entire course of the study. It is thus crucial to establish and optimize these aspects in detail (e.g., in a smaller pre-study) before initiating the actual data acquisition.

Another technical prerequisite of data acquisition is the assurance of stable data quality over time and over different imaging sites in multicenter studies. Depending on the underlying imaging modality, different factors can cause qualitative and quantitative changes in imaging data over time including technical degradation of the scanner or replacement of imaging technicians. Most population-based studies are conducted over relatively long time periods. It is thus mandatory to repeatedly perform quality assurance tests and to intervene when deviations exceed acceptable levels.

Concerning the data processing step, the basic requirements are similar to the data acquisition step, and in many cases, these two steps are interwoven and cannot be entirely separated. Thus, data processing has to be performed in a standardized way, and quality assurance has to be performed constantly. More than in the data acquisition part, however, data analysis is often performed by a large number of individual researchers and research groups with heterogeneous backgrounds. As a result, data analysis procedures can vary largely. In order to ensure good data quality in this context, a precise documentation of the data analysis procedures has to be provided (e.g., in the form of defined standard operating procedures). As an alternative, data processing can be performed automatically using suitable algorithms.

2 Imaging Modalities

Numerous imaging modalities are used in daily clinical practice to establish clinical diagnoses for single patients including conventional x-ray examinations, CT, ultrasound, MRI, and PET. When considering abovementioned general requirements, the suitability of these modalities for population-based imaging studies is not the same. The ideal imaging modality for population studies would have the following properties:

- High informational content
- Reliable standardization and quantification
- Noninvasiveness (no radiation, no contrast agents, no adverse effects)
- Short examination times, low cost, wide availability

Especially noninvasiveness is an important aspect that has to be considered when examining healthy volunteers.

In reality, this perfect modality does not exist. The suitability and applications of available modalities are discussed in the following.

2.1 Magnetic Resonance Imaging

The majority of recent population-based imaging studies rely on MR imaging due to various reasons.

First of all, MRI is not associated with diagnostic radiation exposure which makes it easier to justify its use in healthy volunteers. When considering typical MR contraindications (metal implants, claustrophobia, etc.), the possible risks for participants are minimal. More attention to possible adverse events has to be paid when intravenous contrast agents are used in MRI, which increased the risk of adverse events (especially hypersensitivity reactions), and requires for prior exclusion of certain populations (especially patients with impaired renal function).

A crucially important advantage of MRI compared to alternative modalities is its versatility. Virtually all anatomical structures can be assessed in detail. In addition, MRI allows for the measurement of functional tissue properties such as perfusion, diffusion, or oxygenation which allows for a detailed characterization of physiological and pathophysiological processes. To a certain degree, these functional data can be acquired in absolute quantities and thus be compared within and among individual participants.

A drawback of MRI is the relatively long examination times. A comprehensive whole-body

MR study could easily last several hours. Typical whole-body protocols in ongoing population studies using MRI are restricted to about one hour of examination time which requires strict selection of single examination to be included. Novel MR imaging techniques promise accelerated examination, which may help to alleviate this challenge in the future.

A further limitation of MRI, especially compared to CT, is its susceptibility to artifacts resulting, e.g., from motion, magnetic field inhomogeneities, or sequence properties. Therefore, sequences included in an MR population study should be well tested and robust, and a good strategy for dealing with artifacts should be implemented.

In general, MR scanners are widely available and examination costs are high but manageable. It is however recommended that MR scanners within multicenter studies are of the exact same scanner type with the same field strength and hardware and software equipment. This is important as numerous studies have shown variations in image quality and quantitative imaging results between scanners of different vendors or even by the same vendor and different type. The scanner hardware and software setting should be kept constant during the entire course of the study in order to assure constant data properties even if this means that new technical developments from possible upgrades are missed.

Several possibilities exist in order to perform quality assurance on MR scanners, although this concept is not part of routine MR installations. The most widely accepted procedure is the repeated measurement of MR phantoms that allows for the analysis of scanner imaging properties. These phantom measurements can also be used for the purpose of cross-calibration between different scanner sites. Furthermore, basic image properties of study measurements (e.g., signal-to-noise ratio, signal intensities, etc.) can be quantified and compared.

2.2 Computed Tomography

CT is a possible alternative to MRI when it comes to whole-body applications. The main advantages of CT are its excellent quantifiability as well as speed and robustness of acquisition. This allows for precise assessment of moving organs (e.g., the heart). Furthermore, CT is very well suited for imaging of calcified structured (e.g., atherosclerosis) and lung tissue. Thus, CT has been used in several population studies in the past addressing specific questions.

The main drawback of CT is the associated radiation exposure that makes a wide use in healthy populations ethically difficult. Furthermore, application of intravenous contrast agents is necessary for many applications and is associated with a relevant risk for the occurrence of adverse effects (e.g., hypersensitivity reactions, renal impairment, etc.).

Compared to MR, the possibility of acquiring functional tissue information is relatively limited in CT. Novel technical developments (e.g., spectral CT) may open new possibilities in this direction but are not expected to reach the versatility that is provided my MRI in this context.

Taken together, CT is a suitable modality for population-based studies when specific questions are addressed and when the possible associated risks are carefully considered. In most population studies, however, especially when a broad range of possible scientific questions are addressed, MR is nowadays preferred.

2.3 Ultrasound

The third modality that is repeatedly used in population imaging studies is ultrasound.

Ultrasound has many advantages that allow a relatively simple implementation in population studies. In particular, it is noninvasive without known risks, it is associated with low cost, and it is widely accessible. In addition, ultrasound provides the possibility of assessing functional parameters, such as tissue perfusion or tissue elasticity.

However, several drawbacks limit the use of ultrasound in population imaging studies. The most important limitation is the relatively subjective nature of the acquired data as ultrasound allows for a high variation of examination techniques. This makes standardization difficult in most cases and results in low reproducibility, although exceptions have been reported for certain applications. Furthermore, data quality is highly dependent on the anatomical constitution of the participant which has a strong impact on image quality. In addition, only limited parts of the body can be examined, so that whole-body data cannot be realistically acquired.

Ultrasound is thus rather an add-on examination for specific questions (e.g., concerning the thyroid gland or vessel walls) and may be used in addition to whole-body modalities such as MRI. Compared to MRI and CT, it is crucially important that examiners receive standardized training concerning the specific study examinations in order to achieve a minimum of data standardization.

3 Data Storage and Data Distribution

The amount and complexity of data that are acquired in epidemiological imaging studies pose a challenge that is crucial to the successful conductance of the study. Multiple thousands of participants have been and are being included in recent and ongoing epidemiological MR studies, and in each single examination, dozens of three-dimensional, in some cases also higher-dimensional, datasets are acquired.

Specific expertise and experience are required to set up a hardware and software platform that enables storage and distribution of study data. Certain aspects are of central importance in this context. First of all, study data have to be stored safely in the sense that the risk of data loss should be excluded. To this end, data should, for example, be mirrored to at least one additional storage location. Data should in a second sense also be safe from unauthorized access. Appropriate encryption and security measures have to be planned and tested before initiating the study.

A major aspect of data security is connected to data anonymization or pseudonymization. Data privacy of single participants requires that the possibility of deducing the participants' identities from acquired imaging data should be excluded. Apart from consistent data anonymization, this requirement poses specific challenges in medical imaging as high-resolution imaging techniques may enable the identification of unique personal features such as facial morphology. These aspects have to be considered, and, if necessary, appropriate measures should be implemented (e.g., removing part of the imaging data if not necessary for the specific analysis).

While data security is a major aspect, efficient data distribution is of similar importance. Large epidemiological imaging studies are usually analyzed by many different research sites that all require access to study data. Two concepts of data distribution and analysis are possible in principle – a central and a peripheral concept. In the central concept, all imaging and demographic data are stored centrally, and the analyzing researchers are granted access to an online analysis platform where software tools are provided for remote data analysis. In the peripheral concept, actual study data (e.g., DICOM files) can be obtained by single research sites for the purpose of local data analysis. Both concepts have obvious advantages and disadvantages concerning data security, storage efficiency, and flexibility of data analysis. A combination of the two approaches is also conceivable. The process of data distribution should be defined prior to initiating analysis and may be adjusted to specific needs in the course of the study (Fig. 1).

4 Data Post-processing and Data Analysis

In order to deduce scientifically valid information from the complex data of epidemiological imaging studies, valid and efficient methods of data analysis are necessary.

Before actual data analysis is performed, certain post-processing steps may be required, especially in medical imaging. These steps include data normalization, computation of quantitative parameter maps from raw data, or segmentation of anatomical structures. It is advisable to perform this basic post-processing in a central and

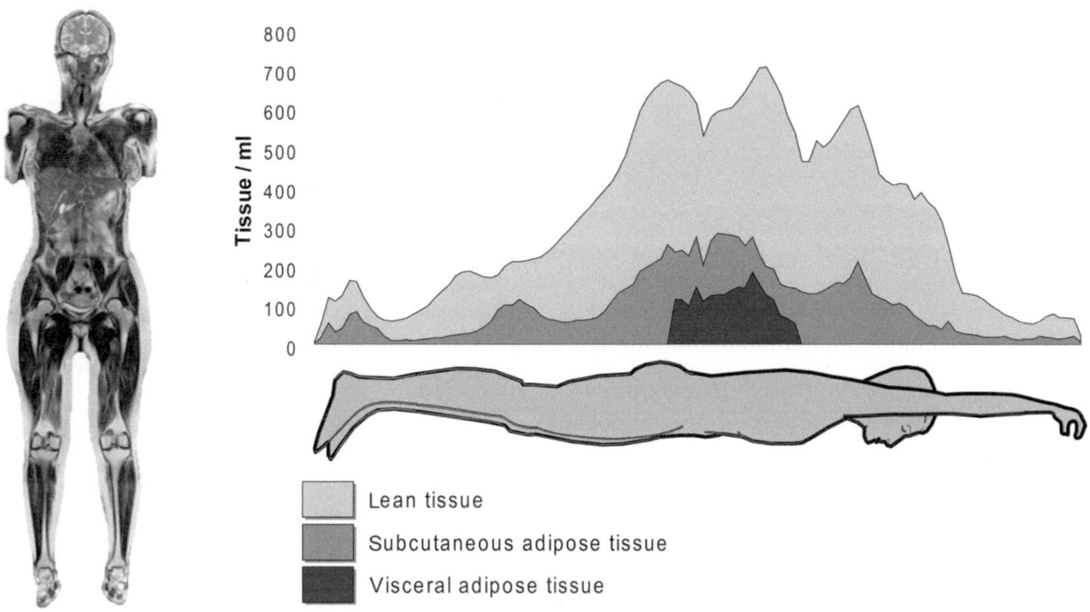

Fig. 1 Whole-body MRI and data processing. The *left part* of the figure shows a coronary view of a whole-body T1-weighted MR sequence used for depiction of anatomical structures. Automated analysis can be used for efficient and standardized quantification of MR sequences. The *right part* of the figure shows the results of automated quantification of adipose and lean tissue in a T1-weighted whole-body MR dataset (Courtesy of Dr. J. Machann, Tübingen)

standardized setting in order to provide researchers with the same database for further analyses. Depending on the context of the specific study, post-processing steps have to be specifically adjusted or even newly developed which should be taken into account.

The analysis of the acquired data poses a great challenge. Analysis should be valid and reproducible and at the same time efficient. Without efficient analysis methods, a comprehensive analysis of the vast amount of available data is not realistically achievable. A possible solution to this problem is automated and semiautomated computational approaches. The feasibility of automated analysis of medical imaging data using dedicated algorithms and machine-learning techniques has repeatedly been demonstrated in the past for a large variety of applications. Still, especially for MR data, reliable algorithms do not exist for many applications, and further research in this field is necessary. In this context, large epidemiological imaging studies may be a driver for innovative concepts of automated image analysis.

An important part of data analysis in population-based imaging studies is the statistical and epidemiological evaluation of connections and interrelations between acquired imaging and nonimaging parameters. These analyses can be highly complex and require specific expertise. This expertise should be provided in the form of a central statistical board in order to perform analyses and to support participating researchers.

Literature

Bamberg F, Kauczor HU, Weckbach S, Schlett CL, Forsting M, Ladd SC et al (2015) Whole-body MR imaging in the German National Cohort: rationale, design, and technical background. German National Cohort MRI Study Investigators. Radiology. 2015;277(1):206–220

Friedman L, Stern H, Brown GG, Mathalon DH, Turner J, Glover GH et al (2008) Test-retest and between-site reliability in a multicenter fMRI study. Hum Brain Mapp 29(8):958–972

Gatidis S, Schlett CL, Notohamiprodjo M, Bamberg F (2016) Imaging-based characterization of cardiometabolic phenotypes focusing on whole-body MRI-an approach to disease prevention and personalized treatment. Br J Radiol 89(1059):20150829

Hegenscheid K, Kuhn JP, Volzke H, Biffar R, Hosten N, Puls R (2009) Whole-body magnetic resonance imaging of healthy volunteers: pilot study results from the population-based SHIP study. Rofo 181(8):748–759

Medland SE, Jahanshad N, Neale BM, Thompson PM (2014) Whole-genome analyses of whole-brain data: working within an expanded search space. Nat Neurosci 17(6):791–800

Meyer J, Ostrzinski S, Fredrich D, Havemann C, Krafczyk J, Hoffmann W (2012) Efficient data management in a large-scale epidemiology research project. Comput Methods Programs Biomed 107(3):425–435

Petersen SE, Matthews PM, Bamberg F, Bluemke DA, Francis JM, Friedrich MG et al (2013) Imaging in population science: cardiovascular magnetic resonance in 100,000 participants of UK Biobank – rationale, challenges and approaches. J Cardiovasc Magn Reson Off J Soc Cardiovasc Magn Reson 15:46

Schlett CL, Hendel T, Hirsch J, Weckbach S, Caspers S, Schulz-Menger J et al (2016) Quantitative, organ-specific interscanner and intrascanner variability for 3 T whole-body magnetic resonance imaging in a multi-center, multivendor study. Invest Radiol 51(4):255–265

Thompson PM, Stein JL, Medland SE, Hibar DP, Vasquez AA, Renteria ME et al (2014) The ENIGMA Consortium: large-scale collaborative analyses of neuroimaging and genetic data. Brain Imaging Behav 8(2):153–182

Wurslin C, Machann J, Rempp H, Claussen C, Yang B, Schick F (2010) Topography mapping of whole body adipose tissue using a fully automated and standardized procedure. J Magn Reson Imaging : JMRI 31(2): 430–439

Part III

Handling/Management of IFs in Different Countries/Population Based Studies

Management of Incidental Findings in the Study of Health in Pomerania

Carsten-Oliver Schmidt and Katrin Hegenscheid

Contents

1 The Study of Health in Pomerania (SHIP): Cohort Description ... 45
2 Description of the Whole-Body MRI Implementation in SHIP ... 46
3 Informed Consent in SHIP and Perception of the Study ... 46
4 Assessment and Handling of Incidental Findings in SHIP ... 49
5 Distribution of Incidental Findings in SHIP ... 51
6 Impact of Incidental Findings: Empirical Evidence from SHIP ... 52
Conclusion ... 53
References ... 55

C.-O. Schmidt (✉) • K. Hegenscheid
Institut für Community Medicine – SHIP-KEF, Universitätsmedizin Greifswald, Walther-Rathenau-Str. 48, 17475 Greifswald
e-mail: carsten.schmidt@uni-greifswald.de

1 The Study of Health in Pomerania (SHIP): Cohort Description

The Study of Health in Pomerania (SHIP) is a population-based cohort study in north-east Germany, consisting of two independent cohorts, SHIP and SHIP-TREND (Volzke et al. 2011). Adults, selected from local population registries, aged 20–79, with their primary place of residence in the counties of Nordvorpommern and Ostvorpommern and the two cities of Greifswald and Stralsund, were eligible for participation. Baseline examinations of the first cohort were performed between 1997 and 2001 (SHIP-0) and follow-up examinations between 2002 and 2006 (SHIP-1), 2008–2012 (SHIP-2), and 2014–2016 (SHIP-3). A second cohort (SHIP-Trend) was conducted from 2008 until 2012; the first follow-up (SHIP-Trend 1) has started in March 2016.

SHIP comprises comprehensive examination programs to investigate the population-based burden of subclinical disorders and diseases, risk factors, and consequences as well as their progression over time. In addition, information on mortality is collected from population registries. Medical examination programs comprise, among others, somatometric and blood pressure measurements, ECG, a range of ultrasound examinations, sleep laboratory, and a dental examination. In addition, a wide range of biomaterials is collected.

Med Radiol Diagn Imaging (2016)
DOI 10.1007/174_2016_86, © Springer International Publishing Switzerland
Published Online: 26 Nov 2016

Whole-body magnetic resonance imaging (MRI) was first implemented in SHIP-2 and SHIP-Trend. An MRI follow-up has meanwhile been completed in the SHIP-3 cohort, and another one started in SHIP-Trend 1 (Hegenscheid et al. 2013, 2009). The main aims of the whole-body MRI study are to provide prevalence estimates for MRI findings in the general population, to establish reference parameters for various organs, and to associate MR findings with phenotypes from other examinations, as well as omics-related data.

This chapter presents results of the whole-body MRI implementation in SHIP-2 and SHIP-Trend, the management of incidental findings as well as empirical results on participants' attitudes, types of incidental findings, and their consequences.

2 Description of the Whole-Body MRI Implementation in SHIP

A standardized MRI protocol was performed using a 1.5-T MR imager (Magnetom Avanto; Siemens Medical Systems, Erlangen, Germany) (Hegenscheid et al. 2009). Each subject underwent a standardized whole-body MRI, consisting of a plain whole-body scan and contrast-enhanced modules. The detailed imaging protocols have been described previously (Hegenscheid et al. 2009). Subjects were placed in the supine position, and five phased-array surface coils were placed to the head, neck, abdomen, pelvis, and lower extremities. The spinal coil was embedded in the patient table. The whole-body MRI protocol had a total duration of ~90 min.

A contrast-enhanced cardiac MRI and MR angiography module was conducted in men, whereas a cardiac MRI and MR mammography module was conducted in women after the whole-body scan. Participation in the contrast-enhanced modules prolonged the duration of the MRI examination by another hour. All participants who agreed to intravenous secretin administration (Secrelux; Sanochemia Diagnostics GmbH; Neuss, Germany) underwent secretin-enhanced MR cholangiopancreatography. In case of known drug allergies or allergies to any kind of contrast agent, participants were excluded from the contrast-enhanced modules and secretin administration and underwent plain whole-body MRI only.

In SHIP-2 and SHIP-Trend, participation in the MRI was offered to all 6753 study volunteers, and 5330 were willing to take part. Almost 1000 of these were excluded according to exclusion criteria such as the presence of metal artifacts in the body, tattoos, or claustrophobia. Another 564 participants were excluded because no appointment could be made or the appointment was not kept. Ultimately, a total of 3640 participated in the whole-body MRI, but the examination had to be prematurely terminated in almost 300 subjects due to reasons such as claustrophobia or the detection of unknown artifacts in the fast scan. The latter indicates that an elaborate early assessment of exclusion criteria is important to avoid expensive empty examination slots.

3 Informed Consent in SHIP and Perception of the Study

A key challenge in the preparation of SHIP-2/SHIP-Trend was the proper development and implementation of an informed consent procedure to reduce risks such as therapeutic misconception (Appelbaum et al. 2004; Wolf et al. 2008; Erdmann et al. 2011) as we expected participants to be inclined to mistakenly conceive the research setting as a clinical diagnostic setting. Therefore, prior to the MRI examination, all participants underwent an extensive information and consent process:

1. All SHIP participants received an information brochure about the entire examination program including the whole-body MRI, explaining the examinations, research goals, and issues like data handling and data safety. Our explanations emphasized that research scans are not optimized for an ideal provision of clinical information and that their diagnostic meaning may be still unclear. Furthermore, we discussed potential benefits and harms of

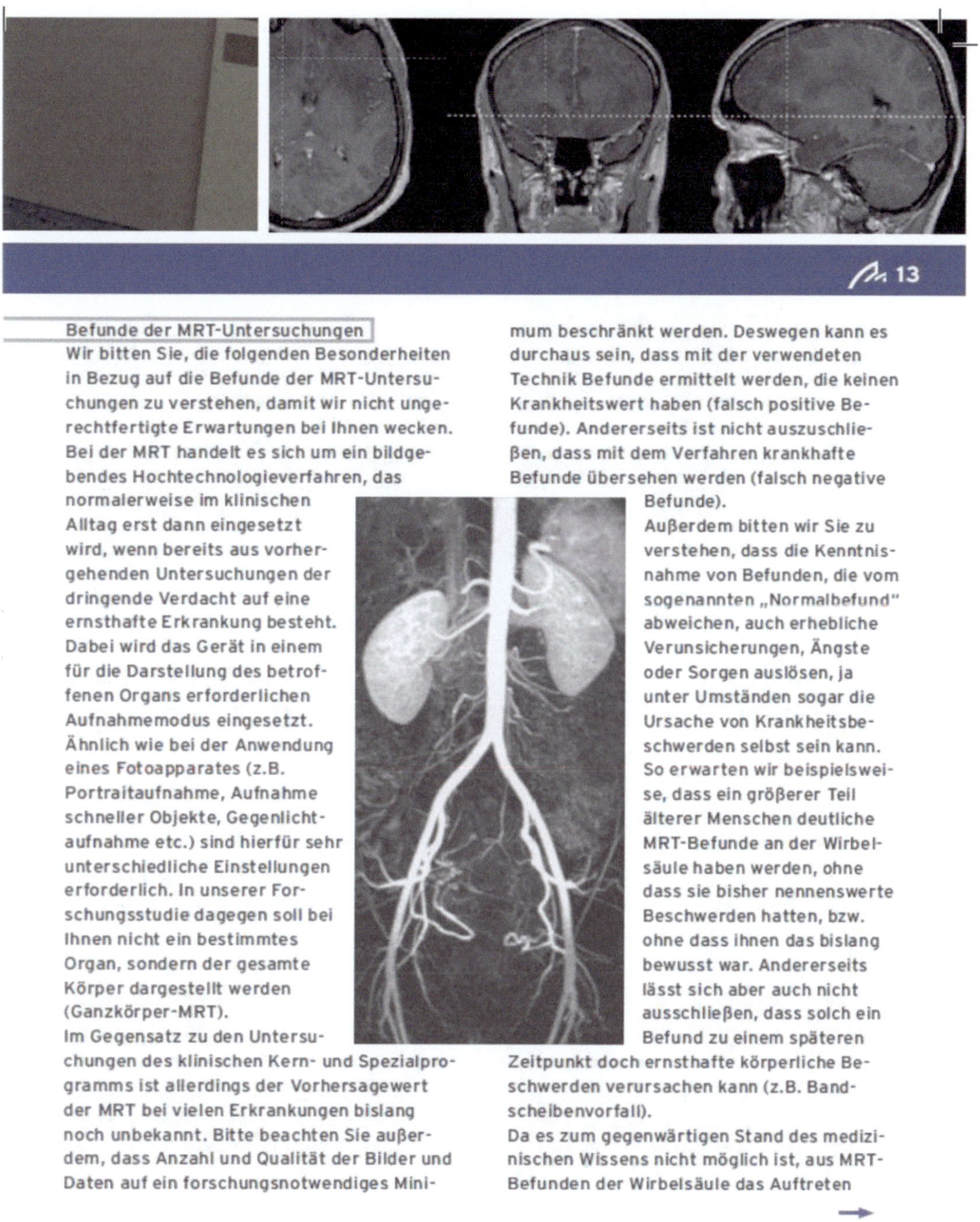

13

Befunde der MRT-Untersuchungen

Wir bitten Sie, die folgenden Besonderheiten in Bezug auf die Befunde der MRT-Untersuchungen zu verstehen, damit wir nicht ungerechtfertigte Erwartungen bei Ihnen wecken. Bei der MRT handelt es sich um ein bildgebendes Hochtechnologieverfahren, das normalerweise im klinischen Alltag erst dann eingesetzt wird, wenn bereits aus vorhergehenden Untersuchungen der dringende Verdacht auf eine ernsthafte Erkrankung besteht. Dabei wird das Gerät in einem für die Darstellung des betroffenen Organs erforderlichen Aufnahmemodus eingesetzt. Ähnlich wie bei der Anwendung eines Fotoapparates (z.B. Portraitaufnahme, Aufnahme schneller Objekte, Gegenlichtaufnahme etc.) sind hierfür sehr unterschiedliche Einstellungen erforderlich. In unserer Forschungsstudie dagegen soll bei Ihnen nicht ein bestimmtes Organ, sondern der gesamte Körper dargestellt werden (Ganzkörper-MRT).

Im Gegensatz zu den Untersuchungen des klinischen Kern- und Spezialprogramms ist allerdings der Vorhersagewert der MRT bei vielen Erkrankungen bislang noch unbekannt. Bitte beachten Sie außerdem, dass Anzahl und Qualität der Bilder und Daten auf ein forschungsnotwendiges Minimum beschränkt werden. Deswegen kann es durchaus sein, dass mit der verwendeten Technik Befunde ermittelt werden, die keinen Krankheitswert haben (falsch positive Befunde). Andererseits ist nicht auszuschließen, dass mit dem Verfahren krankhafte Befunde übersehen werden (falsch negative Befunde).

Außerdem bitten wir Sie zu verstehen, dass die Kenntnisnahme von Befunden, die vom sogenannten „Normalbefund" abweichen, auch erhebliche Verunsicherungen, Ängste oder Sorgen auslösen, ja unter Umständen sogar die Ursache von Krankheitsbeschwerden selbst sein kann. So erwarten wir beispielsweise, dass ein größerer Teil älterer Menschen deutliche MRT-Befunde an der Wirbelsäule haben werden, ohne dass sie bisher nennenswerte Beschwerden hatten, bzw. ohne dass ihnen das bislang bewusst war. Andererseits lässt sich aber auch nicht ausschließen, dass solch ein Befund zu einem späteren Zeitpunkt doch ernsthafte körperliche Beschwerden verursachen kann (z.B. Bandscheibenvorfall).

Da es zum gegenwärtigen Stand des medizinischen Wissens nicht möglich ist, aus MRT-Befunden der Wirbelsäule das Auftreten

Fig. 1 Sample page from the SHIP information brochure on the explanation of the meaning of MRI findings (page 16)

incidental findings as well as our disclosure policy. This is illustrated with a sample page of the brochure in Fig. 1. In addition to the brochure, all participants received a questionnaire on exclusion criteria to be filled out in case of the participants' consent for the MRI examination. Consent forms and the questionnaire were sent back by postal mail to the SHIP study center. Only a preliminary consent was requested at this time. The questionnaire

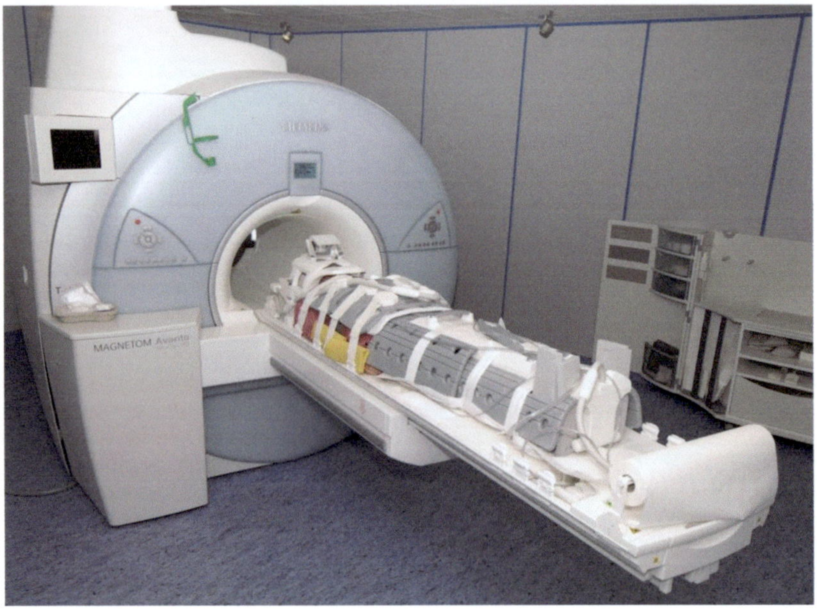

Fig. 2 Picture of a SHIP test volunteer being fully embedded by the coils before the start of the whole-body MRI examination

and consent form were reviewed upon receipt by the participant management. If the participant seemed eligible, an appointment was made for the MRI scan at the radiology department.

2. A video of the examination procedure was shown in the waiting area to all potential participants at the SHIP examination center, with the intent of familiarizing participants with the upcoming experience of a whole-body MRI, which requires the placement of coils along the entire body (Fig. 2). The video was recorded after repeated problems in the early phase of the study with participants feeling uncomfortable with and thus unable to handle the unexpected situation of being strapped up along their entire body.
3. Immediately before the MRI examination, a research radiologist personally described the whole-body MRI examination and the process of handling incidental findings to the study volunteer again and provided the opportunity to clarify any concerns regarding the examination. The participant provided his written final consent to take part in the MRI examination at this occasion.

It is important to note that almost 400 SHIP-2 and SHIP-Trend participants refused to take part in the MRI examination after expressing their initial willingness, indicating that in-depth information may change the attitude toward participation, potentially because of the high burden of the examination to the participant.

All participants could opt-out in written from receiving disclosure of incidental findings. This option was only chosen by two participants, while all others requested the commutation of findings. This reflects the genuine interest of most participants in knowing more about their health. There was one important limitation to the opt-out option. If a severe finding posed a serious potential threat of damage to a third party, its disclosure had to be accepted by the potential participant, and rejection would have resulted in the exclusion of a participant from the MRI examination. This did not happen.

Although we made extensive efforts to properly inform our study volunteers about the limitations of research MRI, therapeutic misconception could not be avoided (Erdmann et al. 2011; Schmidt et al. 2013). Nearly all participants (97 %) expected to find out whether they were healthy or not. This was surprising given the fact that we stated the opposite in written and oral form on several occasions before and after the examination. Furthermore, 22 % of males and

8 % of females believed that they no longer needed to participate in recommended routine screening examinations. Almost half stated that they sought to learn more about a pre-existing physical complaint. It seems that the demand for more information about one's own health is a key motivational factor for participation in a health study. This is implied by other studies as well (Kirschen et al. 2006).

4 Assessment and Handling of Incidental Findings in SHIP

The whole-body MRI implementation in SHIP was the first of its kind in a large general population cohort. The interpretation of findings was complicated for several reasons. First, the low pretest probability of serious pathologies (Volzke et al. 2012; Royal and Peterson 2008) in a general population sample likely reduces the positive predictive value of any finding. Second, the entire context of supporting clinical findings to aid in diagnosis is missing. Therefore an elaborated procedure was adopted to decide on the categorization and disclosure of MR findings. A primary goal was to protect participants from harms due to false-positive findings and from findings without forseeable therapeutic benefits. The assessment of incidental findings was conducted in two stages and has been described in detail elsewhere (Hegenscheid et al. 2013).

The procedure of assessing incidental findings began while the participant was present at the MRI unit. At that time, an ad hoc reading of the scans was performed by a trained radiologist to identify one of nine predefined life-threatening conditions requiring immediate referral, including acute brain infarctions, intracranial hemorrhage, or pneumonia. If present, these were disclosed to the participant immediately on site after the end of the MRI scan, and, if possible, the participant was referred to receive further diagnostics and treatment within the hospital.

Next, a comprehensive reading according to a standardized protocol that included a total of 670 items for whole-body MRI was conducted after the examination. At least two trained radiologists reviewed all scans independently. A three-point scale was used to rate the overall image quality (good, moderate, or poor) and artifacts (none, mild, or major). Additionally, readers evaluated images for the presence or absence of pathological findings and anatomical variants. All clinical judgements were exclusively made on the basis of MR images and performed using a digital picture archiving and communication system (IMPACS ES 5.2, Agfa HealthCare, Mortsel, Belgium). In case of a difference between the two first readings, a third reading was conducted by a senior radiologist to reach a consensus (Hegenscheid et al. 2013).

Incidental findings were classified and handled according to a standardized protocol approved by the institutional review board. Findings were classified into three categories for this purpose (Hegenscheid et al. 2013):

1. Category I findings were normal or common in asymptomatic subjects, e.g., anatomical variants, old brain infarcts, and sinusitis. This also included abnormalities without well-defined diagnostic and therapeutic consequences according to existing guidelines and best practice recommendations (e.g., disc herniation).
2. Category II findings were abnormalities needing further medical evaluation. Category II findings were disclosed to the participants by postal mail. Figure 3 lists selected precedents for Category II findings.
3. Category III findings required immediate referral. A list of nine potential category III findings was defined in advance of the study (Fig. 3).

Only findings requiring further medical attention were eligible for disclosure. Category I findings were consequently not disclosed to the participants. All detected Category II and III findings were passed on to an interdisciplinary advisory board. This board was established before the study began. Its permanent members comprised specialists from medical, surgical, neurological, epidemiological, and radiological departments. Depending on the detected abnormality, additional specialists were invited. Upon presentation of

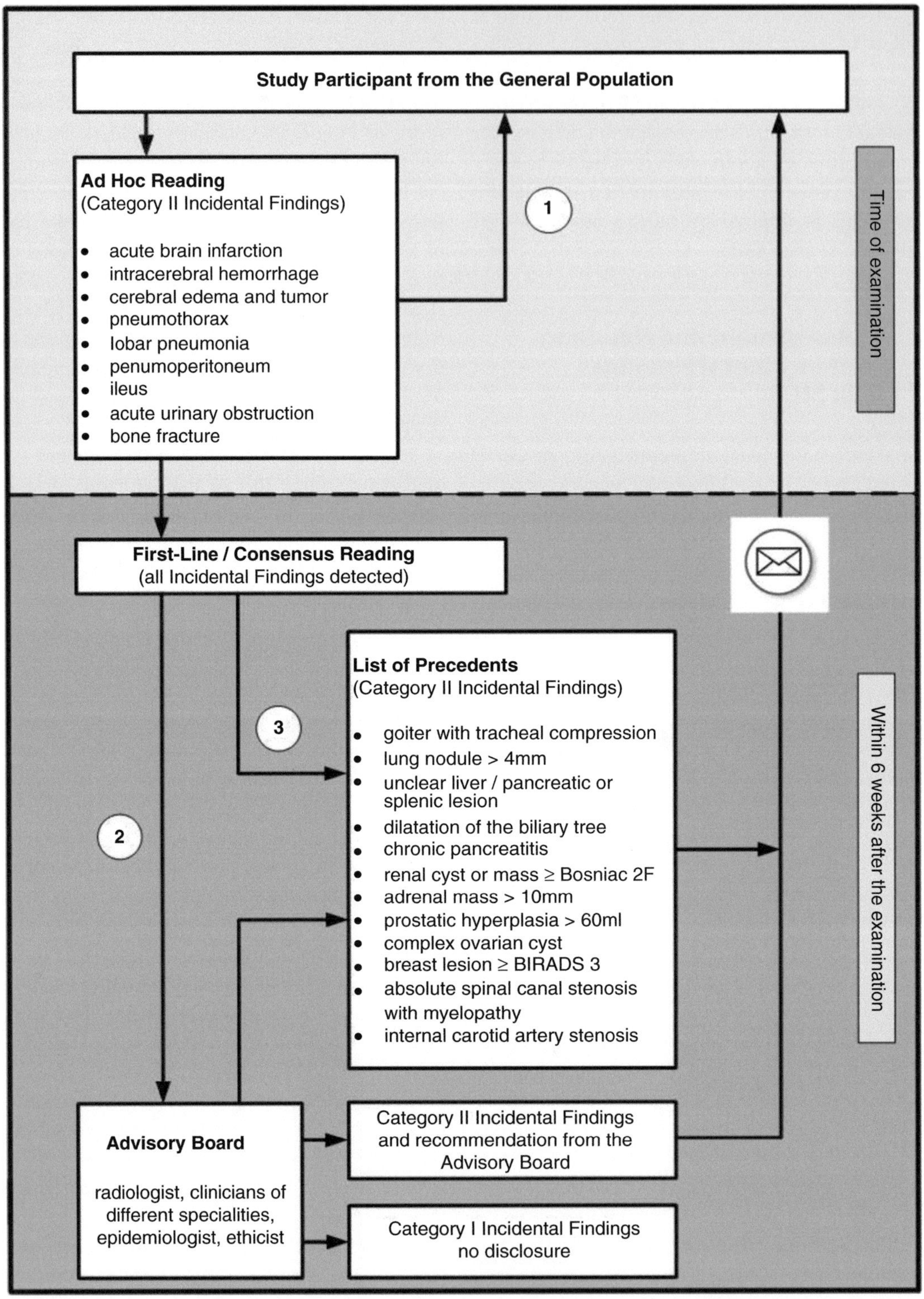

Fig. 3 Management protocol for the handling of incidental findings in SHIP. (*1*) Ad hoc reading with direct feedback to the participant in case of an acute finding requiring immediate referral (Category III). (*2*) Findings of potential clinical relevance were presented monthly to an interdisciplinary advisory board. The board subsequently recommend further clinical work-up (Category II) or not (Category I). (*3*) For frequent Category II incidental findings, the advisory board established precedents that were directly communicated to the participant

findings they reached a consensus about whether or not to recommend disclosure. If the board decided against disclosure the finding was reclassified to Category I. There was one exception to this procedure: for frequent findings of clinical relevance, a list of precedents was established to aid further decision-making. This list contained conditions such as lung nodules >4 mm, renal cysts (Bosniak$\geq$2), and others (Fig. 3). Any finding corresponding to a precedent could be handled without further involvement of the advisory board.

The entire reading and decision process, including the communication of findings by a postal letter to the study volunteer, was supposed to be completed within 6 weeks. The letter comprised a short description of the finding and specific recommendations for further diagnostic and clinical work-up. All notified participants received the option to contact research radiologists by phone for assistance in case of any questions or concerns. This option was used only by a very small minority.

The decision to use letters was mainly based on logistic considerations as disclosure in person was considered to require too many resources. Category II or III findings were not sent directly to treating doctors to respect the study volunteer's autonomy in the handling of their study findings. In addition, the feasibility of sending findings to doctors seemed low in the German medical system, where patients freely choose physicians of different specialities.

While a study might adopt a restrictive policy on the communication of findings, there are limitations. Study participants in Germany are entitled to receive all findings if they request them. In SHIP, MR images were not released to the participants routinely. However, study participants repeatedly requested them after the examination, and they were thus released to the participants.

5 Distribution of Incidental Findings in SHIP

Results from SHIP provide several important insights on the distribution and nature of findings in a general population cohort (Hegenscheid et al. 2013):

1. Incidental findings are very common.

   Among the first 2500 study volunteers, 13,455 findings and anatomical variants of any category were documented either on the plain whole-body MRI or the contrast-enhanced modules.
2. Most incidental findings are likely without medical importance.

   In total, 12,125 (90.1 %) of all findings belonged to Category I.
3. Severe findings requiring immediate medical attention are very rare. Only nine Category III findings among the first 2500 volunteers resulted in immediate medical action, some of which are shown in Fig. 4.
4. Findings of potential clinical relevance occur in a relevant minority of participants.

   In total, 1330 findings were presented to the advisory board, which subsequently decided to reclassify 278 of these findings to Category I. In total 1052 findings were disclosed to 787 participants. While only 10 % of all findings were considered to require further medical evaluation, almost every third (31.5 %) study volunteer was affected by them.
5. Most findings result from the plain whole-body MRI scan.

   In total, 893 (85 %) of the findings resulted from the plain whole-body MRI scan.
6. All body regions are affected.

In total, 46 findings occurred in the head (2 %), 69 (3 %) in the neck, 170 (7 %) in the abdominal organs and intestine, 170 (7 %) in the urinary tract, 212 (9 %) in the genital system, and 150 (6 %) in the spine or skeletal system. With regard to contrast-enhanced modules, most findings were breast lesions (BI-RADS $\geq$3), visible in the MR mammography (97 findings).A detailed overview is provided in (Hegenscheid et al. 2013).

7. Most findings are of an unclear nature.

   In total, 383 findings were considered benign, and 62 malignant while the remaining 607 (58 %) were of an unclear nature. This is probably the single most critical aspect, as the clinical importance of a finding

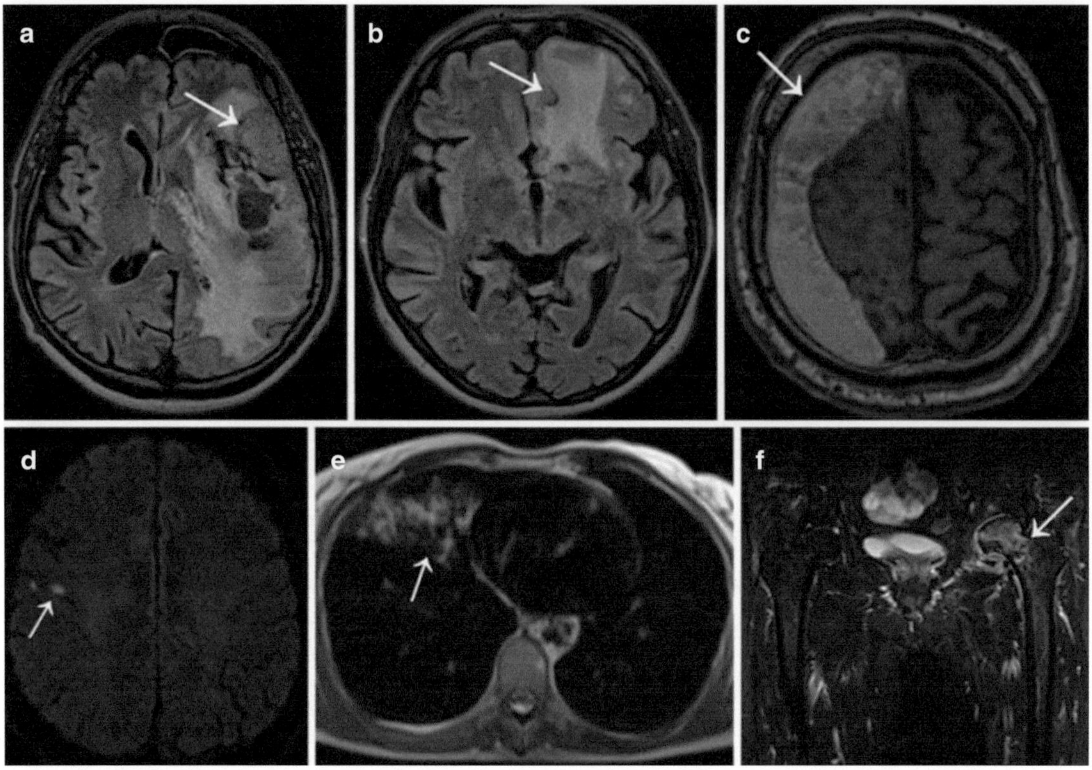

Fig. 4 Category III incidental findings on whole-body MRI. *Arrows* indicate the abnormalities. (**a**) Meningioma of the left sphenoidal wing (diameter 42 mm). (**b**) Metastasis (diameter 13 mm) of unknown primary in the left frontal lobe. Both show marked surrounding edema of the white matter on fluid-attenuated inversion recovery axial images. (**c**) A fluid-attenuated inversion recovery axial image shows a large subdural hematoma (diameter 30 mm) of the right hemisphere. (**d**) Diffusion-weighted echo-planar image shows a small area of acute cortical ischemia. (**e**) T2-weighted half-Fourier acquisition single-shot turbo spin-echo image displays lobar pneumonia of the right middle lobe. (**f**) Turbo inversion recovery magnitude coronal image shows extensive bone edema of the left femoral head and neck (Image and text taken from Hegenscheid et al. (2013))

can only be deducted from further diagnostic assessments but not from the MRI examination itself. Most study volunteers with a Category II finding are therefore confronted with the recommendation to seek additional diagnostics to exclude the possibility of a malignancy, which may place an enormous psychological burden on them. The proportion of unclear findings varied strongly across affected organ systems with most uncertain findings located in the breast (97 %), male genital system (91 %), and chest (91 %). In contrast, few uncertain findings occurred in the spine and skeletal system (8 %), and MR angiography (0 %). A detailed overview is provided in (Hegenscheid et al. 2013).

6 Impact of Incidental Findings: Empirical Evidence from SHIP

The management of incidental findings should be guided by a proper understanding about their consequences. SHIP follow-up studies after the MRI baseline examination provide important insights on potential consequences, harms, and benefits.

Based on a postal survey conducted on average 1 year after the examination, almost 10 % reported moderate to severe psychosocial distress while waiting for a finding (Schmidt et al. 2013). About 54 % stated that the disclosed finding was new to them. Almost one third (29 %) reported moderate to severe psychological distress after having received a finding. These findings corresponded to our expectations based on the unclear nature of most disclosed findings. Interestingly, the subjective experience of substantial distress endorsed by many participants had a minimal effect on the participants' overall positive evaluation of their MRI experience. Almost all (96%) stated being very content (Schmidt et al. 2013).

The consequences of the disclosed incidental findings weren't limited to psychosocial dimensions: they also influenced healthcare utilization to a substantial degree. About 75% of participants reported having made use of health services due to communicated findings and 50% stated that treatments were ongoing. From the perspective of an observational study, these "intervention" effects are highly concerning given the large proportion of SHIP participants with a disclosed finding (Schmidt ct al. 2013).

Our results provide further insight on the quality of our communications. We compared the perceived severity of findings from the participants' and radiologists' perspective. Findings were classified into one of three categories ranging from "life-threatening disease" via "non-life-threatening disease requiring medical attention" to "other." The agreement between participants and radiologists as measured by Cohen's Kappa was close to zero indicating almost a chance agreement. This indicates the necessity to better orient participants about the importance of findings (Schmidt et al. 2013).

Another important issue is whether our participants benefited from communicated incidental findings. This has been analyzed with regard to quality of life-related indicators, comparing MRI participants with nonparticipants. Based on a postal survey which was conducted on average 2.5 years after the baseline MRI examination (Schmidt et al. 2016), we estimated average treatment effects in 3745 SHIP-Trend participants for the SF-12 mental and physical health component summary score (Busija et al. 2011) as well as for the depression score, as measured with the PHQ-9 (Martin et al. 2006). Treatment effects were close to zero for all outcomes indicating a negligible effect on quality of life. MRI participants neither benefited nor were harmed on average.

Conclusion

Implementing whole-body MRI in a general population cohort is a complex endeavor not only because of the high costs and technical prerequisites. It also places a substantial burden on many study volunteers during and after study participation and may affect the natural course of health-related outcomes in undesirable ways due to the communication of findings in an observational study. Any whole-body MRI examination in a general population cohort must therefore be implemented with great caution to adequately balance participants' rights and researchers' interests. Below we target selected aspects of importance related to the handling of incidental MRI findings.

In implementing population-based MRI a large number of dropouts are likely. Little more than 60% of those initially willing to take part did complete at least the whole-body MRI scan due to a range of reasons including fulfilled exclusion criteria and refusal to participate after upon receiving more information about the examination. Dropout potentially threatens the generalizability of study results to the target population and must be taken into account.

It seems to be difficult for study participants to understand the diagnostic limitations of research imaging, and therefore therapeutic misconception is likely. Abstract explanations about false-negative or false-positive findings should therefore be complemented by lists of precise examples and, more importantly, by lists of findings that are not reported even if they are encountered. The latter may allow for a better understanding of what information might be missed.

Study volunteers commonly participate because they want to know more about their health. They expect to receive health information in return for their study participation. This must be respected from an ethical perspective (Schmidt et al. 2013; Viberg et al. 2014). On the other hand, researchers need to safeguard their study goals. As shown by our follow-up studies, any disclosure is an intervention and may bias longitudinal findings. With regard to healthcare utilization, there seem to be considerable effects, while less impact is observed on quality of life. Disclosure prioritizing the participants' point of view would result in maximizing the amount of disclosed information, the researchers' in minimizing it. This conflict can be resolved by a high degree of transparency regarding conditions under which volunteers participate (Langanke et al. 2011). These conditions are acceptable if adult participants understand and accept the potentially highly restrictive disclosure policy as well as potential harms related to disclosed findings.

It is the moral obligation of researchers to avoid harms to study volunteers (Langanke et al. 2011). The distress of waiting for results indicates that findings should be disclosed as quickly as possible. Communications should be made to all participants including those without a finding, and while most participants preferred a written communication, they should not only be conducted via postal mail (Erdmann et al. 2011; Schmidt et al. 2013). Rather, the mode of communication should correspond to the severity of a finding, and individual participant preferences may be taken into account (Erdmann et al. 2011; Shoemaker et al. 2011). This might also reduce discrepancies in the participants' evaluation of the results' importance versus that of the radiologists. Furthermore, if necessary, it would be desirable to support the scheduling of appointments for further diagnostic actions, to avoid stressful waiting times until a clarification is achieved (Erdmann et al. 2011).

We observed considerable distress in many of those receiving a finding, while benefits are much less clear. A restrictive communication policy may protect participants from dealing with many findings of questionable clinical utility. In fact, it seems likely that the vast majority of MRI findings are without beneficial value for participants and unusable to guide subsequent treatment decisions. A restrictive disclosure policy is therefore likely to reduce harms, but this assumption requires more empirical underpinnings. Nevertheless, a minority of findings have a high clinical utility and should be communicated to respect participants' autonomy in making their own health decisions (Schmidt et al. 2013; Viberg et al. 2014). Due to our experience in SHIP-2 and SHIP-Trend, we have adopted more restrictive communication policy for subsequent measurement waves. With our present knowledge, we consider the former SHIP-2/SHIP-Trend communication policy of findings as being too lenient.

It may be argued that not disclosing any MRI findings may be the best way to protect research interests. We perceive this assumption as erroneous. Nondisclosure likely increases nonresponse by a substantial margin as it contradicts the most important reason to participate (Schmidt et al. 2016). Resulting selection bias and the loss of statistical power may be a bigger problem than the restrictive disclosure of serious findings of high clinical utility. Such serious findings are rather rare in a general population cohort, and communicating them is unlikely to harm most research goals. The challenge rests in an adequate cutoff in deciding whether or not to disclose a finding. Furthermore, our health study is conducted at a medical school in cooperation with trained radiologists. Therefore, we perceive a moral obligation to not withhold knowledge about severe findings, particularly if they pose a potential threat of damage to a third party.

Finally, the terminology incidental findings itself requires some attention. Whether or not to call our findings incidental findings may be a matter of debate. The overwhelming majority of findings were identified and coded as part of a standardized protocol. In this sense, taking the researchers' perspective, they are clearly not incidental. However, findings were obtained outside a routine clinical context and without any clinical indication. Therefore, taking the participants' perspective, any novel finding may be regarded as incidental. Therefore we conceive the term incidental finding as applicable within the context of our study.

Acknowledgments SHIP is part of the Community Medicine Research net of the University of Greifswald, Germany, which is funded by the Federal Ministry of

Education and Research (grant No. 03ZIK012), the Ministry of Cultural Affairs, as well as the Social Ministry of the Federal State of Mecklenburg-West Pomerania. Whole-body MR imaging was supported by a joint grant from Siemens Healthcare, Erlangen, Germany, and the Federal State of Mecklenburg-Vorpommern. The University of Greifswald was a member of the "Center of Knowledge Interchange" program of the Siemens AG. Dynamic contrast-enhanced MR mammography research is part of the entire whole-body MRI study and was supported by Bayer Healthcare. The work was further supported by the DFG (grant No. SCHM 2744/1-1).

References

Appelbaum PS, Lidz CW, Grisso T (2004) Therapeutic misconception in clinical research: frequency and risk factors. IRB 26(2):1–8

Busija L, Pausenberger E, Haines TP, Haymes S, Buchbinder R, Osborne RH (2011) Adult measures of general health and health-related quality of life: Medical Outcomes Study Short Form 36-Item (SF-36) and Short Form 12-Item (SF-12) Health Surveys, Nottingham Health Profile (NHP), Sickness Impact Profile (SIP), Medical Outcomes Study Short Form 6D (SF-6D), Health Utilities Index Mark 3 (HUI3), Quality of Well-Being Scale (QWB), and Assessment of Quality of Life (AQoL). Arthritis Care Res 63(Suppl 11):S383–S412. doi:10.1002/acr20541

Erdmann P, Langanke M, Assel H (2011) Incidental findings – understanding of risks by research subjects and implications for research ethics. In: Collste G, Manzeschke A (ed) Proceedings from the Societas Ethica Annual Conference 2011, The Quest for perfection. The future of Medicine/Medicine of the future, Universita della Svizzera Italiana. Lugano/Linköping: Linköpiing University Electronic Press, p 26

Hegenscheid K, Kuhn JP, Volzke H, Biffar R, Hosten N, Puls R (2009) Whole-body magnetic resonance imaging of healthy volunteers: pilot study results from the population-based SHIP study. RoFo 181(8):748–759

Hegenscheid K, Seipel R, Schmidt CO, Volzke H, Kuhn JP, Biffar R et al (2013) Potentially relevant incidental findings on research whole-body MRI in the general adult population: frequencies and management. Eur Radiol 23(3):816–826. doi:10.1007/s00330-012-2636-6

Kirschen MP, Jaworska A, Illes J (2006) Subjects' expectations in neuroimaging research. J Magn Reson Imaging 23(2):205–209. doi:10.1002/jmri.20499

Langanke M, Brothers KB, Erdmann P, Weinert J, Krafczyk-Korth J, Dorr M et al (2011) Comparing different scientific approaches to personalized medicine: research ethics and privacy protection. Pers Med 8(4):437–444

Martin A, Rief W, Klaiberg A, Braehler E (2006) Validity of the brief patient health questionnaire mood scale (PHQ-9) in the general population. Gen Hosp Psychiatry 28(1):71–77

Royal JM, Peterson BS (2008) The risks and benefits of searching for incidental findings in MRI research scans. J Law Med Ethics 36(2):305–314, 212

Schmidt CO, Hegenscheid K, Erdmann P, Kohlmann T, Langanke M, Volzke H et al (2013) Psychosocial consequences and severity of disclosed incidental findings from whole-body MRI in a general population study. Eur Radiol 23(5):1343–1351. doi:10.1007/s00330-012-2723-8

Schmidt CO, Sierocinski E, Hegenscheid K, Baumeister SE, Grabe HJ, Volzke H (2016) Impact of whole-body MRI in a general population study. Eur J Epidemiol 31(1):31–39. doi:10.1007/s10654-015-0101-y

Shoemaker JM, Holdsworth MT, Aine C, Calhoun VD, de La Garza R, Feldstein Ewing SW et al (2011) A practical approach to incidental findings in neuroimaging research. Neurology 77(24):2123–2127. WNL.0b013e31823d7687 [pii]

Viberg J, Hansson MG, Langenskiold S, Segerdahl P (2014) Incidental findings: the time is not yet ripe for a policy for biobanks. Eur J Hum Genet 22(4):437–441. doi:10.1038/ejhg.2013.217

Volzke H, Alte D, Schmidt CO, Radke D, Lorbeer R, Friedrich N et al (2011) Cohort profile: the study of health in Pomerania. Int J Epidemiol 40(2):294–307. doi:10.1093/ije/dyp394

Volzke H, Schmidt CO, Hegenscheid K, Kuhn JP, Bamberg F, Lieb W et al (2012) Population imaging as valuable tool for personalized medicine. Clin Pharmacol Ther. doi:10.1038/clpt.2012.100

Wolf SM, Lawrenz FP, Nelson CA, Kahn JP, Cho MK, Clayton EW et al (2008) Managing incidental findings in human subjects research: analysis and recommendations. J Law Med Ethics 36(2):219–248. doi:10.1111/j.1748-720X.2008.00266.x, 1

Management of Incidental Findings in the German National Cohort

Robert C. Bertheau, Oyunbileg von Stackelberg, Sabine Weckbach, Hans-Ulrich Kauczor, and Christopher L. Schlett

Contents

1 **Introduction** 58

2 **Ethical Framework for IF-Reporting** 60

3 **Defining Problems in IF-Reporting** 60
3.1 Scientific Imaging Sequences 61
3.2 Limited Clinical Context 61
3.3 Disproportionate Increase of False Positives 61
3.4 Uncertainty Causing Out-of-Proportion Work-Up 62
3.5 Reliability, Reproducibility, and Consistency 62

4 **Translating the Ethical Framework into a Reporting Algorithm** 62
4.1 The List: An Approach to Define Clinically Relevant IFs 62
4.2 Technical Translation 65
4.3 Training and Certification of Radiologists 67
4.4 Quality Assurance 67

5 **Summary** 68

References 69

R.C. Bertheau • O. von Stackelberg
S. Weckbach • H.-U. Kauczor • C.L. Schlett (✉)
Department of Diagnostic and Interventional Radiology, University Hospital Heidelberg, Im Neuenheimer Feld 110, Heidelberg 69120, Germany
e-mail: christopher.schlett@post.harvard.edu

Abstract

The German National Cohort is a long term, multicenter, population-based cohort study currently undertaken in Germany with the goal of investigating the development of common chronic diseases. As part of this investigation, 30.000 out of the total of 200.000 participants are being subjected to a whole-body 3-Tesla MR imaging without contrast agents. To help with the implementation of national and international ethical guidelines a system was developed to classify and report incidental findings that might be detected on imaging and possibly pose a risk to the participant's health. This system focuses on guiding radiologists in the decision of reporting or not-reporting a finding in an attempt to balance the risk of over- and under-reporting, and thus, to minimize false positives and false negatives. The cornerstone of that process is a list specifying findings and separating them into report-worthy and not-report-worthy. For defining incidental findings, study specific limitations and confounders had to be taken into account. This book chapter details the necessary steps to develop such a system, illustrates the particular challenges and summarizes the ethical dilemmas with such a system. Further, technical and quality assurance tools are presented to guarantee high quality and consistency for incidental finding reporting in long-term, multicenter studies such as the German National Cohort.

Med Radiol Diagn Imaging (2016)
DOI 10.1007/174_2016_63, © Springer International Publishing Switzerland
Published Online: 18 May 2016

1 Introduction

The German National Cohort (GNC) is an interdisciplinary, multicenter, population-based cohort study currently undertaken by a network of over 25 institutions in Germany. Its main goal is to investigate the development of common chronic diseases including cancer, diabetes, cardiovascular, neurodegenerative/psychiatric, respiratory, and infectious diseases (German National Cohort (GNC) Consortium 2014; Wichmann et al. 2012). The GNC spans 18 study centers across Germany and will examine and follow about 200,000 subjects of the general population between the ages of 20 and 69 years with various examinations for a period of at least 25 years. Exams include interviews, questionnaires, a variety of physical exams, and the collection of biologic samples such as blood, urine, saliva, nasal swabs, and stool. While all 200,000 examinees undergo an initial exam which takes about 4 h, a subgroup of 40,000 examinees participate in an intensified 6-h exam (German National Cohort (GNC) Consortium 2014; Wichmann et al. 2012). A subgroup thereof—about 30,000 examinees—are being imaged by a 3 Tesla whole-body MR scanner conducted at five dedicated imaging centers across Germany (Bamberg et al. 2015). Imaging is comprised of scientific sequences which significantly differ from regularly deployed sequences in clinical settings, and no contrast agent is administered. Scan time is 60 min and the deployed sequences are listed in Table 1. Besides the five imaging centers, four imaging cores have been established to carry out central functions adjunct to large-scale, multicentric imaging. In detail, an

Table 1 MR sequences within the GNC (Modified based on Bamberg et al. (Bamberg et al. 2015)), which will be viewed by radiologists for IFs

MR sequence	Image resolution	Image contrast	Anatomic coverage
Neurodegenerative focus			
T1-3D-MPRAGE	1.0 mm isotropic; sagittal	T1w	Whole brain and upper spinal cord
2D-FLAIR	4.0 mm slice thickness; axial; 0.9 mm voxel size in-plane	T2w	Whole brain
Cardiovascular focus			
MRA 3D-SPACE-STIR	2.5 mm slice thickness; coronal; 1.2 mm voxel size in-plane	T2w	Lung apices to diaphragm
Cine SSFP LAX	6.0 mm slice thickness; 1.5 mm voxel size in-plane	SSFP	4-, 3-, 2-chamber view
Cine SSFP SAX	7.0 mm slice thickness; 1.7 mm voxel size in-plane	SSFP	12 short-axis stacks covering base to apex
Thoracoabdominal focus			
T2-HASTE	5.0 mm slice thickness; axial; 1.4 mm voxel size in-plane	T2w	Shoulder to epigastric region
T1-3D-VIBE-DIXON	3.0 mm slice thickness; axial; 1.4 mm voxel size in-plane	T1w	Neck to knee
Musculoskeletal focus			
PD-FS-3D-SPACE	1.0 mm isotropic; coronal	PD	Pelvis including iliosacral joint and both hips
T2-2D-TSE Spine	3.0 mm slice thickness; sagittal; 1.0 mm voxel size in-plane	T2w	Lumbar, thoracic, cervical spine

The entire MR sequence includes in addition a multiecho-3D-VIBE sequence of the liver, a MOLLI of the heart, a resting state EPI-BOLD of the brain. All three additional sequences have been excluded from IF-reading since they do not contain information relevant for IF identification and characterization

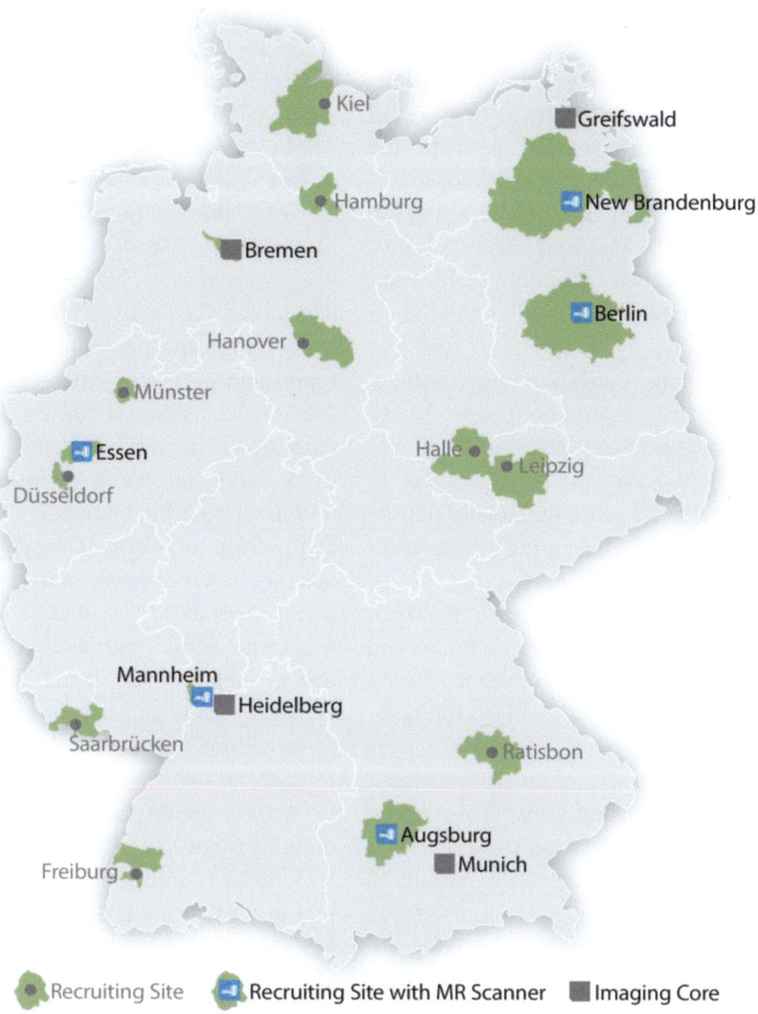

Fig. 1 Design of MRI study within the German National Cohort (GNC). While 200,000 subjects will be enrolled across 18 sites in Germany (*green areas*), about 30,000 subjects will undergo whole-body MR imaging. Thus, five dedicated MR scanners were installed (*blue squares*). In addition, four imaging cores have been established for central functions, in Munich for coordination and training, in Bremen for data management, in Greifswald for quality assurance, and in Heidelberg for incidental findings (*gray squares*). The imaging core for incidental findings has developed the basic concept for the management of MR-based incidental findings within the GNC. It provides daily support and advice to the five imaging sites and performs quality control regarding the reporting of incidental findings (Source: The German National Cohort Study)

imaging core for coordination and training has been established in Munich, an imaging core for data management in Bremen, an imaging core for quality assurance in Greifswald, and an imaging core for incidental findings (IFs) in Heidelberg (Fig. 1). The imaging core has prospectively developed the concept of reporting IFs as derived from the MRI exams within the GNC and has implemented the technical requisites. During the ongoing study, it provides quality assurance for IF-reporting, serves with advice in unclear cases and updates the standard operating procedures (SOPs) based on the latest clinical and scientific knowledge.

2 Ethical Framework for IF-Reporting

While most people of the general population could be considered fairly healthy, it is expected that imaging would occasionally lead to the discovery of illnesses of varying degree of medical importance (Lumbreras et al. 2010a, b). Based on the results of similar previous cohort studies, we estimated prospectively that "clinically relevant" IFs can be found in 10 % of the population undergoing MR imaging, considering the targeted age range and morbidity in Germany (Bamberg et al. 2015; Hegenscheid et al. 2013). Therefore, guidance was sought from the ethical commissions of the involved organizations to establish an ethical framework that would help in the management of any finding out of the ordinary, generally designated as IF.

General principles to be considered in the management of IFs were (Radiologists, T.R.C.o and Management of Incidental Findings detected during Research Imaging 2011; Weiner 2014) as follows:

- *Responsibility for the well-being of the participant:* A participant should be informed about health concerning IFs. This is in accordance with European and international ethical guidelines, for example, the Article 26 of the Additional Protocol to the Convention on Human Rights and Biomedicine, concerning Biomedical Research of the Council of Europe (Additional Protocol to the Convention on Human Rights and Biomedicine and concerning Biomedical Research 2007; Convention for the protection of Human Rights and Dignity of the Human Being with regard to the Application of Biology and Medicine: Convention on Human Rights and Biomedicine 1999).
- *Responsibility for the well-being of the society:* The general population might be affected from undisclosed illnesses a participant might suffer from. This includes, for example, illnesses that might carry an increased risk for the participant to cause a traffic accident. This is in accordance with the Article 26 of the Convention for the Protection of Human Rights and Dignity of the Human Being with regard to the Application of Biology and Medicine: Convention on Human Rights and Biomedicine of the Council of Europe (Convention for the protection of Human Rights and Dignity of the Human Being with regard to the Application of Biology and Medicine: Convention on Human Rights and Biomedicine 1999).

While these general ethical principles seem to be simple and straight forward, implementation presents certain challenges which will likely never be solved satisfactorily. The simple idea of classifying findings into reportable and non-reportable gets confounded by the definition of "IF" itself. While IF might ideally relate to a diagnosis, imaging by itself, even in clinical settings, rarely allows an abnormality to be specified down to a final diagnosis. IFs in MRI exams can present any form of untypical imaging characteristics, for example, a hyperintensity where it is not expected; a broad clinical description such as a cystic lesion; or a likely but not certain diagnosis such as an adrenal gland adenoma. Generally, only an accurate and established diagnosis allows for a reliable estimation of the impact for a participant's future health.

With ethical principles referring rather to diagnoses but imaging generally providing much less defined information, it becomes apparent that it is often unclear how to classify an IF into report-worthy or not. In clinical as well as in research settings, an innocuous finding wrongly reported as a false-positive illness may cause severe psychologic and bodily harm conflicting with the general bioethical principle of *primum non nocere* (do not harm). It may also unnecessarily increase health care spending, costs for society, and lead to occupational and insurance-related consequences.

3 Defining Problems in IF-Reporting

Following the ethical considerations set forth by international guidelines (Additional Protocol to the Convention on Human Rights and Biomedicine and concerning Biomedical Research 2007; Convention for the protection of Human Rights and Dignity of the Human Being with regard to the Application of Biology and Medicine: Convention on Human Rights and Biomedicine 1999; International Ethical Guidelines for Biomedical Research Involving Human Subjects 2002), a process dubbed "IF-reading" was established. IF-reading is a procedure described by SOPs developed by the researches of the GNC and approved by the ethical commissions of the involved organizations. Those SOPs are to ensure that every participant's imaging data is assessed by a board-certified radiologist within a certain time frame to detect IFs that might warrant a notification of the participant. Participants are only notified in case of "clinically relevant" IFs. This process poses some intricate difficulties different from IFs encountered during clinical exams. Considerations that need to be accounted for in the particular research setting of the GNC will be presented in the following paragraphs.

3.1 Scientific Imaging Sequences

Imaging sequences in the GNC, as in many other research projects, differ from clinically used sequences. They often do not have the particular purpose to obtain a certain clinical diagnosis. In the GNC, MR sequences were chosen with an emphasis on maximizing morphologic data acquisition in a restricted time frame, sacrificing some of the MRI-inherent benefits of analyzing a lesion based on a multitude of MR-characteristic tissue features. Therefore, IF-reading has to be based mostly on T1- and T2-weighted images without common, clinically applied sequences such as diffusion-weighted imaging (DWI), susceptibility-weighted imaging (SWI), etc. Due to their invasive nature, contrast agents, gut motility suppressing medications, bowel distending procedures, and endorectal/endovaginal coils have also been forgone. With the limited imaging set to characterize a finding, great uncertainty in specifying a finding and a large list of differential diagnoses including artifacts has to be expected.

While reacquisition of only one sequence is allowed, more reacquisitions, for example, because of motion or breathing artifacts, cannot be afforded due to time restrictions. Similarly, sequence protocols are fixed for comparability. No sequences can be swapped for, for example, less motion susceptible ones or more lesion appropriate ones, as it happens in clinical settings. This substantially reduces the sensitivity to pick up a lesion and hugely widens the gap between the ability to detect and characterize a finding.

3.2 Limited Clinical Context

To afford unbiased reporting, and because of strict German privacy and data protection laws, radiologists are blinded to personal and clinical information of the participant, except for gender and the year of birth. Moreover, no data from exams conducted in other areas of the GNC (e.g., blood tests) are shared with the radiologist in charge of the IF-reporting. This severely hampers guidance toward a probable diagnosis of an observed lesion.

3.3 Disproportionate Increase of False Positives

The probability of a lesion being a certain diagnosis is possibly distorted by the fact that examinees randomly selected from the general population are more likely to be healthy individuals, in contrast to patients with clinical indications for imaging. It is a mathematical phenomenon that the positive and negative predictive value of a particular imaging finding depends on the prevalence of the appendant disease in the examined population (Bender et al. 1998). Compared to a clinical setting where MRI is often applied to further characterize an already known or suspected lesion, a mostly healthy general population leads to a lower positive predictive value and accordingly to an increase in false-positive reports. Taking the generally poorer specificity of the applied scientific imaging sequences compared to clinical sequences into account, the report of a potentially harmful finding would come at the expense of an even larger number of false positives. Along with health care costs, physical and psychologic side effects of follow-up procedures would increase disproportionately, compared to true positive disease detection. The effect of false-positive reports is aggravated by the fact that possibly healthy individuals, that otherwise would not have been subjected to medical exams, might undergo harmful or side effect-stricken follow-up investigations.

3.4 Uncertainty Causing Out-of-Proportion Work-Up

The notification of a participant would likely trigger a clinical work-up outside the GNC. Participants would seek advice from their primary care physicians who would be forced, out of lack of more complete information, to follow up on IFs, likely starting with proper clinical imaging. While this is the intended purpose of the IF-reading to prevent harm from serious illnesses like cancer, for example, this would, under certain circumstances, lead to unnecessary and unnecessarily exaggerated work-up. While this is obvious for false-positive reports, this would also be the case for certain true positive reports, namely, when there is uncertainty about the clinical significance of findings. This includes minor ailments, anatomic variations within the normal range, illnesses that would usually be diagnosed and followed up on a less extensive and costly way, or illnesses that would not receive work-up at all at this point in time. Examples might be an *Arteria lusoria* occasionally leading to swallowing problems, a hiatal hernia that might or might not be clinically manifest, or the ubiquitous age-related degenerative joint or spine disease that might occasionally explain a participant's pain but otherwise would not need extensive or no work-up at all.

3.5 Reliability, Reproducibility, and Consistency

For the assessment of 30,000 MR scans acquired at five different sites, a relatively large number of radiologists are involved in reading the acquired data. Furthermore, with this imaging round expected to last at least 4 years, a significant fluctuation of involved radiologists is anticipated. Therefore, high-quality standards must be met to ensure consistency and reliability. It is well known from reproducibility studies that variability is induced by radiologists in image interpretation and diagnoses making (Robinson 1997). Considering the fundamental obligation to provide the same service and the same quality of service to each of the participants, variability should be limited as much as possible. This can be theoretically achieved by either reducing the number of involved radiologists, and/or by involving only highly and specifically trained radiologists, and/or by standardized reporting and/or by conducting quality assurance in IF-reporting.

4 Translating the Ethical Framework into a Reporting Algorithm

Considering the abovementioned restrictions, it became clear that reporting every possible disease would necessitate extensive clinical follow-up with significant over-reporting and disproportionate work-up. Individuals might thus come to harm from non-disclosure of disease states as well as from reporting every possible disease state. Therefore, the ethical framework was defined more precisely in an effort to find the possibly best balance between informing participants about relevant illnesses and avoiding reporting of irrelevant illnesses. To that end a robust system guiding radiologists in IF-reporting was established curtailing especially possibly minor illnesses with questionable relevance, normal variants, and highly uncertain diagnoses.

4.1 The List: An Approach to Define Clinically Relevant IFs

It was decided to develop a specified, categorized, and concise list of reportable findings, limiting uncertainty and false positives as well as establishing consistency. The ground work for this system was laid by expert radiologists familiar with the applied sequences and the ethical considerations.

The ratios of false-positive and false-negative findings are significantly determined by the applied MR sequences. As these ratios are specific to the set of sequences used, comparability with previous cohort studies using different imaging protocols might be severely hampered. Based on the extrapolation of extensive literature research data (excerpt (Abeloos and Lefranc 2011; Al-Shahi Salman 2007; Atalay et al. 2011; Ballantyne 2008; Beigelman-Aubry et al. 2007; Berland et al. 2010; Berlin 2011; Boland et al. 2008; Booth et al. 2012; Borra and Sorensen 2011; Bradley et al. 2011; Childs and Leyendecker 2008; Chow and Drummond 2010; Cordell 2011; Cramer et al. 2011; de Rave and Hussain 2002; Erdogan et al. 2007; Esmaili et al. 2011; Gore et al. 2011; Gross et al. 2010; Hartwigsen et al. 2010; Hoggard et al. 2009; Illes 2008; Irwin et al. 2013; Johnson et al. 2011; Kamath et al. 2009; Khosa et al. 2011; Ladd 2009; Lee et al. 2011; Legmann 2009; Lund-Johansen 2013; MacMahon et al. 2005; McKenna et al. 2008; Megibow et al. 2011; Milstein 2008; Morin et al. 2009; Morris et al. 2009; Nelson 2008; Orme et al. 2010; Pierce et al. 2009; Puls et al. 2010; Richardson 2008; Royal and Peterson 2008; Shoemaker et al. 2011; Subhas et al. 2009; van der Lugt 2009; Vanel et al. 2009; Vernooij et al. 2007; Zarzeczny and Caulfield 2012)), radiologic clinical experience and the knowledge and limitations of the applied sequences, a list of reportable IFs has been specifically tailored to the imaging data available (Table 2). Similarly, a list was created exemplarily specifying IFs that should not be reported.

The seemingly random combination of definitions based on clinical entities, morphologic and size criteria to assign findings to a specific IF-category was mainly determined by aforementioned limitations of imaging and the specific study settings. For example, using the available sequences (and likely a certain degree of motion artifacts), a lung nodule smaller than 1 cm could only be evaluated with great uncertainty—vessel flow artifacts or small dystelectases being so common. Therefore, a size cut off of 1 cm was chosen. Similarly, cervical lymphadenopathy was defined as at least three lymph nodes with a short-axis diameter of at least 1.5 cm, accounting for the fact that non-contrast-enhanced imaging of the neck would likely lead to an over-reporting of possibly enlarged lymph nodes. As reasoned above, some disease states have been excluded from reporting due to limited general significance, like diverticulosis. Others have been banned due to limited clinical significance specific to a non-targeted imaging setting, such as arthrosis or disk bulging, for which pre-symptomatic imaging is not an established proven method. Equally banned from reporting is, for example, cardiomyopathy, while being generally a significant disease, every participant undergoing MR imaging, has been subjected to echocardiography in another area of the GNC. Therefore, a possible cardiomyopathy would have been communicated already.

4.1.1 Separation into Acutely and Non-acutely Relevant IFs

Within this list, IFs were classified into acutely relevant and non-acutely relevant findings. Acutely relevant findings were defined as suspected disease for which the participant should receive immediate clinical care. Examples include possible stroke, pneumothorax, and aortic dissection. These findings not only have to be reported in a timely manner for the benefit of the participant but also to avoid danger to the public, for example, from causing a traffic accident. As of February 2016, the list contains 14 acutely relevant IFs.

4.1.2 Unlisted IFs

It is obvious that a list of a few dozen findings cannot encompass all report-worthy diseases. Therefore, a possibility to report unlisted findings was created. To limit over-reporting by radiologists, who out of professional habit are prone to rather over-report than under-report, a dedicated system has been established. It interposes an approval step before a report is sent out to a participant. Unlisted findings deemed report-worthy by the radiologist in charge are submitted for assessment to the imaging core facility in Heidelberg. All requests go through a standardized process (Fig. 2). Minor requests or technical errors, like an erroneously unlisted IF submission that already exists in the list, will be answered directly by the team of radiologists at the imaging core Heidelberg. More

Table 2 Excerpt of the IF-list for the MRI study of the GNC (by February 2015)

Organ system	Report category	IF	Literature
Nervous	Acutely relevant—report immediately	Suspected acute stroke	Hegenscheid et al. (2013), Lund-Johansen (2013), Vernooij et al. (2007)
Nervous	Acutely relevant—report immediately	Suspected intracranial/intraspinal hemorrhage (including subdural, epidural, subarachnoid, intracerebral, intraventricular hemorrhage)	Hegenscheid et al. (2013), Lund-Johansen (2013), Vernooij et al. (2007)
Nervous	Non-acutely relevant—report	Suspected cerebral lesion with edema and/or CSF obstruction and/or midline shift and/or lesion with a size or location prone for complications	Lumbreras et al. (2010a), Hegenscheid et al. (2013), Radiologists, T.R.C.o and Management of Incidental Findings detected during Research Imaging (2011), Morris et al. (2009), van der Lugt (2009)
Nervous	Do not report	Suspected unspecific white matter lesions	Radiologists, T.R.C.o and Management of Incidental Findings detected during Research Imaging (2011), Morris et al. (2009), van der Lugt (2009), Maia et al. (2012), Matsusue et al. (2006)
Vascular	Acutely relevant—report immediately	Suspected aortic dissection	(Lumbreras et al. (2010a), Hegenscheid et al. (2013)
Thoracic	Acutely relevant—report immediately	Suspected pneumothorax	Hegenscheid et al. (2013)
Thoracic	Non-acutely relevant—report	Suspected lung nodule/mass > 1 cm	Beigelman-Aubry et al. (2007), Esmaili et al. (2011), MacMahon et al. (2005)
Abdominal	Non-acutely relevant—report	Suspected adrenal mass > 2 cm	Lumbreras et al. (2010a), Hegenscheid et al. (2013), Berland et al. (2010), Gross et al. (2010), Legmann (2009)
Abdominal	Non-acutely relevant—report	Suspected solid or semisolid renal tumor > 2 cm	Lumbreras et al. (2010a), Hegenscheid et al. (2013), Berland et al. (2010), Gross et al. (2010), Legmann (2009)
Abdominal	Non-acutely relevant—report	Suspected complicated renal cyst (Bosniak ≥ 3)	Lumbreras et al. (2010a), Hegenscheid et al. (2013)
Abdominal	Do not report	Suspected liver cyst	(Lumbreras et al. (2010a), Hegenscheid et al. (2013), Radiologists, T.R.C.o and Management of Incidental Findings detected during Research Imaging (2011)
MSK	Do not report	Suspected non-acute fractures	(Lumbreras et al. (2010a), Hegenscheid et al. (2013), Radiologists, T.R.C.o and Management of Incidental Findings detected during Research Imaging (2011), Kamath et al. (2009), Lee et al. (2011)
MSK	Do not report	Suspected Scheuermann's disease	Hegenscheid et al. (2013), Lee et al. (2011)
MSK	Do not report	Suspected lipoma	Lumbreras et al. (2010a), Hegenscheid et al. (2013), Radiologists, T.R.C.o and Management of Incidental Findings detected during Research Imaging (2011)

The IFs are structured by organ system and stratified in "Acutely relevant," which must be reported immediately, in "Non-acutely relevant," which must be reported within 10 working days, and IFs which should not be reported. The entire list can be found at the bottom of the page at http://nako.de/studienteilnehmer/das-untersuchungsprogramm/mrt/. MSK denotes musculoskeletal

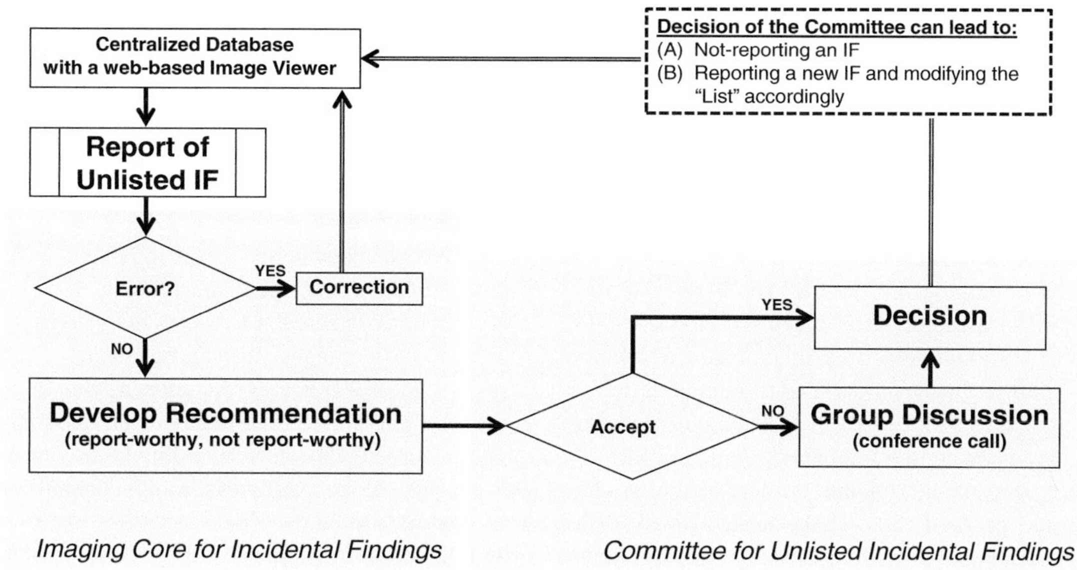

Fig. 2 Process of unlisted incidental findings (IFs). Findings deemed report-worthy by the radiologist and not been listed so far can be submitted to the imaging core facility in Heidelberg. Minor requests or technical errors will be answered directly by the imaging core. For all unlisted findings, which are more complex, the imaging core will sample the current scientific basic and clinical guidelines, estimate the diagnostic accuracy of the applied imaging technology for such a finding and develop based on this information a recommendation, which is discussed by the external committee. The external committee is composed of two radiologists, a general practitioner, an epidemiologist, and an ethicist; the committee makes the decision whether this finding is report-worthy on not report-worthy. Accordingly, the IF list will be updated

complex-to-judge submissions are referred to an external committee composed of two radiologists, a general practitioner, an epidemiologist, and an ethicist. Here, a final decision will be made, especially balancing the risk of over-reporting on a big scale for similar cases to come.

4.2 Technical Translation

4.2.1 Mode and Time Frame of IF-Reporting

Given the abovementioned restrictions for the interaction between the radiologists and the participants due to German privacy and data protection laws and study design of the GNC, communication is managed by a trust office, part of the study recruitment center. No identifying information (e.g., name, post address, etc.) is linked with any MR findings. Non-acute IFs will be reported via regular mail. Time frame for this scenario stipulates the completion of image reading within 5 working days and completion of mailing a letter to the participant within 10 working days after image acquisition.

Acutely relevant IFs require a more direct communication with the participant as soon as the radiologist in charge becomes aware of the situation. This situation may overrule some of the study design concerns. Thus, a detailed algorithm for getting hold of a participant has been developed, which includes immediate telephone contact. In that instance, personal data of the participant (name and phone number) will be provided to the radiologist by the study recruitment center. In case phone contact cannot be established within 24 hours, an expedited letter will be sent, informing the participant of the potentially dangerous condition with the advice to seek immediate medical attention. Participants without reportable IFs will not receive any letter.

In the event of unlisted IFs, the abovementioned time frame may be exceeded for non-acutely relevant unlisted IFs. Unlisted IFs, however, judged by the reading radiologist to be acutely relevant, will be reported in the aforementioned way, before consulting the imaging core Heidelberg. Thereafter, the imaging core Heidelberg will be informed about the unlisted IF and the communication with the participant. The imaging core will then decide if the unlisted IF will be added to the IF-list for similar cases to come.

The purpose of reporting IFs is not the assistance in ascertaining a diagnosis. How far GNC imaging could assist the primary care physicians in defining a diagnosis has been discussed during the initial stages of the GNC. It became obvious that time and manpower limitations would not allow for that. Key points were that primary care physicians would be hard to reach because of busy office hours, or that supplying primary care physicians with image data would require them to be technically and disease-specifically able to evaluate scientific image protocols, which is generally beyond the expertise and the time resources of primary care physicians. Furthermore, for practical and legal reasons, communication should be directed to the participant, especially since not all participants would have a regular primary care physician. Most importantly, the limited imaging information collected with scientific protocols would rarely, if ever negate the need for proper further imaging. Therefore, the purpose of IF-reporting is to call the participant's attention to a possibly concerning finding and provide anatomic location data to guide further work-up. Participants will be provided with a CD containing the imaging data when an IF is reported. While this may potentially facilitate further work-up, this is not meant to play a substancial role in establishing a diagnosis.

4.2.2 Data Processing

As imaging is taking place at five imaging centers across Germany and at MR scanners outside of a common hospital infrastructure, dedicated data management and image viewing tools were developed for the IF-reading. As already mentioned, the GNC requires a strict separation of identifying information and the exam results of the participant. Therefore, a dedicated software and hardware system was created that allows for blinded reading but automatically facilitates contacting the participant in the case of report-worthy IFs.

For image assessment, a web-based electronic case reporting form (eCRF) and an image viewer was developed. De-identified imaging data can be accessed on regular computers through a password-protected, encrypted gate, allowing the selection of listed IFs and submitting unlisted IFs. A standardized reporting tool as part of the image viewer has been developed by the imaging core in Bremen together with the management unit of the GNC's centralized database located in Greifswald. Within the MR images, IFs can be labeled by an arrow or a size indicator. As soon as the IF is marked, a pop-up window opens where the radiologists can select the corresponding finding from the list. The IF-report can be supplemented by anatomic location data where necessary, selected from the drop-down menus. The same pop-up window allows for submission of unlisted IFs which automatically triggers a notification to the imaging core in Heidelberg, including information on the unlisted IF that the reading radiologist has to fill in into preset fields.

Once the IF-reading has been finalized by the radiologist, all information regarding the reported IFs is being transferred via eCRF to the central database of the GNC. The eCRF allows for automatic generation of appropriate reports containing all selected IFs in a standardized, structured form without free text (Fig. 3). The report in PDF format, containing only the participant's study ID and no person-identifying information, will be automatically accompanied by a suitable cover letter. Specific cover letters exist to match different settings: (1) for notification of acutely relevant IFs, (2) for notification of non-acutely relevant IFs, and (3) for reporting non-acutely relevant IFs after the participant had already been contacted about acutely relevant IFs. The IF-report and the cover letter will be printed at the imaging site and sealed in an envelope labeled with the participant's study ID. Also enclosed will be a CD with the imaging data. This sealed envelope will be placed into another envelope containing the participant's address matched by the paticipant's study ID. This step is carried out at the recruitmet centers, as only those have access to person identifying data. From here letters will be sent out by regular or expedited mail according to the situation.

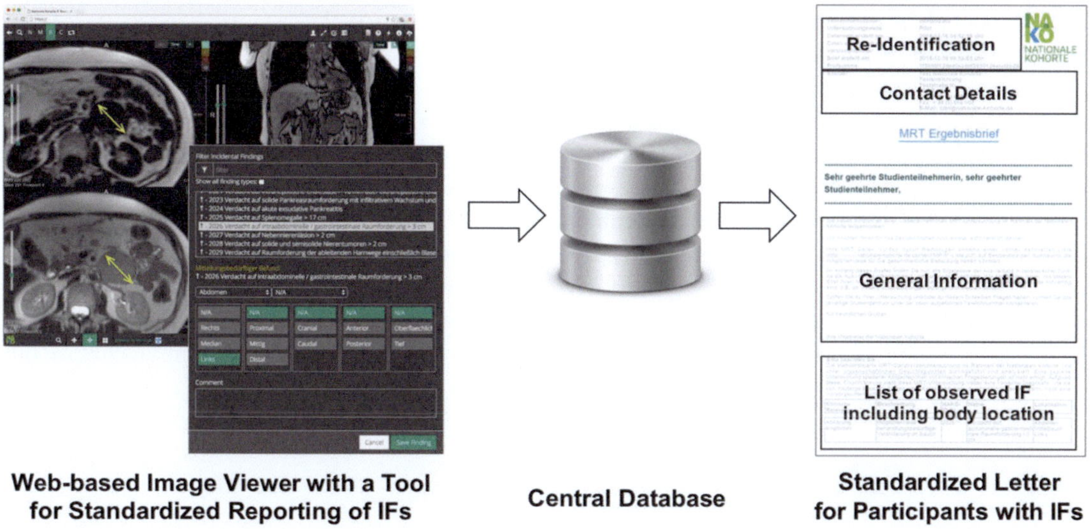

Fig. 3 Process of incidental findings (IFs) reporting in the German National Cohort (GNC). All images are reviewed by a board-certified radiologist using a web-based viewer. With a standardized reporting tool, the radiologist can highlight the findings (in this case an abdominal mass greater 3 cm). This information is saved in the central database, which automatically generates a standardized letter informing the participant regarding the detected IFs (here simplified on one sheet of paper). The letter contains the list of observed IFs, general information about IFs and the MR imaging as well contact details of the study site in case further consultation is necessary

4.3 Training and Certification of Radiologists

Training and certification of radiologists for the purpose of IF-reading is coordinated and implemented by the imaging core in Heidelberg. All IF-readings are performed only by board-certified radiologists. Initial reading can be done by radiologists in training with experience in MR imaging. However, their results have to be verified by board-certified radiologists similar to clinical settings in teaching hospitals in Germany. Only board-certified radiologists are able to finalize and sign-off on readings and trigger report letters. On top of that, all radiologists have to be trained and certified with respect to IF-reporting in the GNC. A multistep training system has been implemented requiring participation in a personal or videoconference-based teaching session and completion of a test. Instructions regarding image viewer operations and access to the database are given to the radiologist. All necessary SOPs are introduced as well. A dedicated training mode of the image viewer containing example cases with and without IFs is used for training purposes. Finally, a test including simulated cases must be passed in order to be certified as IF-reader for the GNC. Working as an IF-reader requires awareness of changing protocols and changes in the IF-list. Participation in yearly re-training and re-certification is mandatory. Training of the technicians operating the MR scanners is managed at the imaging core Munich.

4.4 Quality Assurance

To ensure consistency and inter-reader reliability, a protocol has been developed to monitor the performance of IF-reading across different imaging sites and different readers. A random subset of 10 % of all cases will be read again by radiologists of the imaging core in Heidelberg in a supervision reader mode. On top of that, the first 20 cases of each site and the first 5 cases of each reader will be subject to supervision reading. Discrepancies between primary reader and supervision reader will be recognized and recorded automatically. Analysis of those discrepancies may reveal problems in choosing the correct IF, in differently interpreting IFs, in following protocols or in correctly using the image viewer. Equally important, however, it may uncover poor phrasing of an IF, overlapping of IFs, or inadequacy of an IF. Depending on the type of discrepancy, several instruments can be used to solve problems. This includes personalized feedback to readers, discussion of cases at telephone conferences and meetings, especially to resolve structural or site-specific issues, and re-defining IFs or location options. As a last measure, readers can be subjected to re-training and re-certification, or be banned from participating in the GNC as IF-reader.

5 Summary

The concept of the German National Cohort for reporting IFs has been implemented since the start of the recruitment of MRI participants in spring 2014. At the current state, the recruitment is ongoing and will last for the next few years to achieve the targeted sample size. Based on the applied IF reporting concepts, several participants have been identified with IFs (Fig. 4) and informed accordingly. However, the clinical significance of our

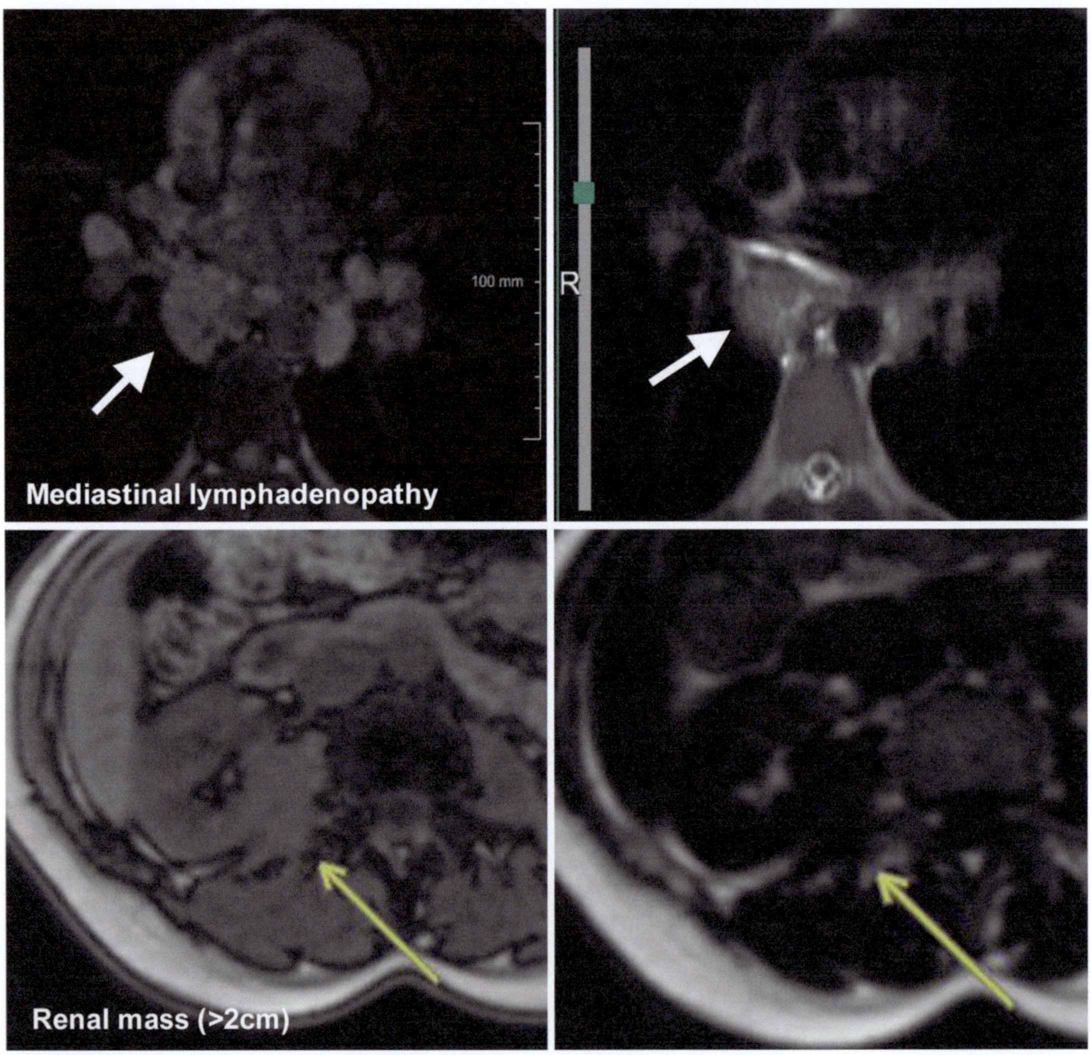

Fig. 4 Examples of common incidental findings (IFs) as observed in the German National Cohort (GNC). The two images on the *top* show a mediastinal lymphadenopathy (*white arrows*), the *left* one represents an image from the T1-3D-VIBE-DIXON sequence, and the *right* one an image from the T2-HASTE sequence. The two images on the *bottom* show a renal mass >2 cm without any fatty content (*yellow arrows*), on the *left* an opp-phase image and on the *right* a fat-image from the T1-3D-VIBE-DIXON sequence

reported IFs as well the performance of our implemented reporting system remains unknown at the current date and is subject to ongoing research. Our findings as well as results from other large-scale cohorts utilizing imaging continuously influence how we will report IFs in the future in research as well as in clinical settings.

References

Abeloos L, Lefranc F (2011) What should be done in the event of incidental meningioma? Neurochirurgie 57(2):78–81

Additional Protocol to the Convention on Human Rights and Biomedicine, concerning Biomedical Research (2007). Council of Europe Steering Committee on Bioethics, Strasbourg

Al-Shahi Salman R (2007) W.N. Whiteley, and C. Warlow, screening using whole-body magnetic resonance imaging scanning: who wants an incidentaloma? J Med Screen 14(1):2–4

Atalay MK et al (2011) The prevalence and clinical significance of noncardiac findings on cardiac MRI. AJR Am J Roentgenol 196(4):W387–W393

Ballantyne C (2008) To know or not to know. Nat Med 14(8):797

Bamberg F et al (2015) Whole-body MR imaging in the German national cohort: rationale, design, and technical background. Radiology 277(1):206–220

Beigelman-Aubry C, Hill C, Grenier PA (2007) Management of an incidentally discovered pulmonary nodule. Eur Radiol 17(2):449–466

Bender R et al (1998) Variation of sensitivity, specificity, likelihood ratios and predictive values with disease prevalence by H. Brenner and O. Gefeller, statistics in medicine, 16, 981-991 (1997). Stat Med 17(8): 946–948

Berland LL et al (2010) Managing incidental findings on abdominal CT: white paper of the ACR incidental findings committee. J Am Coll Radiol 7(10): 754–773

Berlin L (2011) The incidentaloma: a medicolegal dilemma. Radiol Clin North Am 49(2):245–255

Boland GW et al (2008) Incidental adrenal lesions: principles, techniques, and algorithms for imaging characterization. Radiology 249(3):756–775

Booth TC et al (2012) Management of incidental findings during imaging research in "healthy" volunteers: current UK practice. Br J Radiol 85(1009):11–21

Borra RJ, Sorensen AG (2011) Incidental findings in brain MRI research: what do we owe our subjects? J Am Coll Radiol 8(12):848–852

Bradley AJ, Lim YY, Singh FM (2011) Imaging features, follow-up, and management of incidentally detected renal lesions. Clin Radiol 66(12):1129–1139

Childs DD, Leyendecker JR (2008) MRI of the pelvis: a guide to incidental findings for musculoskeletal radiologists. Semin Musculoskelet Radiol 12(1):83–103

Chow A, Drummond KJ (2010) Ethical considerations for normal control subjects in MRI research. J Clin Neurosci 17(9):1111–1113

Convention for the protection of Human Rights and Dignity of the Human Being with regard to the Application of Biology and Medicine: Convention on Human Rights and Biomedicine. (1999). Council of Europe, Strasbourg Cedex

Cordell S (2011) The biobank as an ethical subject. Health Care Anal 19(3):282–294

Cramer SC et al (2011) A system for addressing incidental findings in neuroimaging research. Neuroimage 55(3):1020–1023

de Rave S, Hussain SM (2002) A liver tumour as an incidental finding: differential diagnosis and treatment. Scand J Gastroenterol Suppl 236:81–86

Erdogan D et al (2007) Management of liver hemangiomas according to size and symptoms. J Gastroenterol Hepatol 22(11):1953–1958

Esmaili A, Munden RF, Mohammed TL (2011) Small pulmonary nodule management: a survey of the members of the society of thoracic radiology with comparison to the fleischner society guidelines. J Thorac Imaging 26(1):27–31

German National Cohort (GNC) Consortium (2014) The German national cohort: aims, study design and organization. Eur J Epidemiol 29(5):371–382

Gore RM et al (2011) Hepatic incidentalomas. Radiol Clin North Am 49(2):291–322

Gross MD et al (2010) Incidentally-discovered adrenal masses. Discov Med 9(44):24–33

Hartwigsen G et al (2010) Incidental findings are frequent in young healthy individuals undergoing magnetic resonance imaging in brain research imaging studies: a prospective single-center study. J Comput Assist Tomogr 34(4):596–600

Hegenscheid K et al (2013) Potentially relevant incidental findings on research whole-body MRI in the general adult population: frequencies and management. Eur Radiol 23(3):816–826

Hoggard N et al (2009) The high incidence and bioethics of findings on magnetic resonance brain imaging of normal volunteers for neuroscience research. J Med Ethics 35(3):194–199

Illes J (2008) Brain screening and incidental findings: flocking to folly? Lancet Neurol 7(1):23–24

International Ethical Guidelines for Biomedical Research Involving Human Subjects. (2002). Council for International Organizations of Medical Sciences (CIOMS), Geneva

Irwin RB et al (2013) Incidental extra-cardiac findings on clinical CMR. Eur Heart J Cardiovasc Imaging 14(2):158–166

Johnson PT et al (2011) Common incidental findings on MDCT: survey of radiologist recommendations for patient management. J Am Coll Radiol 8(11):762–767

Kamath S et al (2009) Incidental findings on MRI of the spine. Clin Radiol 64(4):353–361

Khosa F et al (2011) Prevalence of noncardiac findings on clinical cardiovascular MRI. AJR Am J Roentgenol 196(4):W380–W386

Ladd SC (2009) Whole-body MRI as a screening tool? Eur J Radiol 70(3):452–462

Lee S, Joo KB, Ryu JA (2011) Subjective incidental findings of the lumbar spine at MRI. Am J Roentgenol 197(6):W1168–W1168

Legmann P (2009) Adrenal incidentaloma: management approaches: CT – MRI. J Radiol 90(3 Pt 2):426–443

Lumbreras B, Donat L, Hernandez-Aguado I (2010a) Incidental findings in imaging diagnostic tests: a systematic review. Br J Radiol 83(988):276–289

Lumbreras B et al (2010b) Unexpected findings at imaging: predicting frequency in various types of studies. Eur J Radiol 74(1):269–274

Lund-Johansen M (2013) Expect the unexpected: incidental findings on brain magnetic resonance imaging. World Neurosurg 80(5):e119–e120

MacMahon H et al (2005) Guidelines for management of small pulmonary nodules detected on CT scans: a statement from the fleischner society. Radiology 237(2):395–400

Maia AC Jr et al (2012) Incidental demyelinating inflammatory lesions in asymptomatic patients: a Brazilian cohort with radiologically isolated syndrome and a critical review of current literature. Arq Neuropsiquiatr 70(1):5–11

Matsusue E et al (2006) White matter changes in elderly people: MR-pathologic correlations. Magn Reson Med Sci 5(2):99–104

McKenna DA, Laxpati M, Colletti PM (2008) The prevalence of incidental findings at cardiac MRI. Open Cardiovasc Med J 2:20–25

Megibow AJ et al (2011) The incidental pancreatic cyst. Radiol Clin North Am 49(2):349–359

Milstein AC (2008) Research malpractice and the issue of incidental findings. J Law Med Ethics 36(2): 356–360, 214

Morin SHX et al (2009) Incidental findings in healthy control research subjects using whole-body MRI. Eur J Radiol 72(3):529–533

Morris Z et al (2009) Incidental findings on brain magnetic resonance imaging: systematic review and meta-analysis. BMJ 339:b3016

Nelson CA (2008) Incidental findings in magnetic resonance imaging (MRI) brain research. J Law Med Ethics 36(2):315–319, 213

Orme NM et al (2010) Incidental findings in imaging research: evaluating incidence, benefit, and burden. Arch Intern Med 170(17):1525–1532

Pierce SR et al (2009) Incidental findings during functional magnetic resonance imaging: ethical and procedural issues. Am J Phys Med Rehabil 88(4): 275–277

Puls R, Hamm B, Hosten N (2010) MRI without radiologists–ethical aspects of population based studies with MRI imaging. Rofo 182(6):469–471

Radiologists, T.R.C.o., Management of Incidental Findings detected during Research Imaging (2011). The Royal College of Radiologists, London

Richardson HS (2008) Incidental findings and ancillary-care obligations. J Law Med Ethics 36(2):256–270, 211

Robinson PJ (1997) Radiology's Achilles' heel: error and variation in the interpretation of the Rontgen image. Br J Radiol 70(839):1085–1098

Royal JM, Peterson BS (2008) The risks and benefits of searching for incidental findings in MRI research scans. J Law Med Ethics 36(2):305–314, 212

Shoemaker JM et al (2011) A practical approach to incidental findings in neuroimaging research. Neurology 77(24):2123–2127

Subhas N et al (2009) Incidental tumor and tumor-like lesions around the knee. Semin Musculoskelet Radiol 13(4):353–370

van der Lugt A (2009) Incidental findings on brain magnetic resonance imaging. BMJ 339:b310

Vanel D et al (2009) The incidental skeletal lesion: ignore or explore? Cancer Imaging 9(Spec No A):S38–S43

Vernooij MW et al (2007) Incidental findings on brain MRI in the general population. N Engl J Med 357(18):1821–1828

Weiner C (2014) Anticipate and communicate: ethical management of incidental and secondary findings in the clinical, research, and direct-to-consumer contexts (December 2013 report of the presidential commission for the study of bioethical issues). Am J Epidemiol 180(6):562–564

Wichmann HE et al (2012) The German national cohort. Bundesgesundheitsblatt Gesundheitsforschung Gesundheitsschutz 55(6-7):781–787

Zarzeczny A, Caulfield T (2012) Legal liability and research ethics boards: the case of neuroimaging and incidental findings. Int J Law Psychiatry 35(2):137–145

Management of Incidental Findings on Multimodal Imaging in UK Biobank

Lorna M. Gibson, Jonathan Sellors, and Cathie L.M. Sudlow

Contents

1	**Introduction**	72
1.1	UK Biobank	72
1.2	The UK Biobank Imaging Study	72
2	**UK Biobank IF Protocol**	74
2.1	Development of the UK Biobank IF Protocol	74
2.2	Consent Processes	74
2.3	Identification of IF	75
2.4	Feedback of IF	75
3	**Evaluation of the Impact of the UK Biobank IF Protocol**	75
3.1	Evaluating Participants' Understanding of Consent	75
3.2	Comparing the UK Biobank IF Protocol with Full Review of Images by Radiologists	76
3.3	Qualitative Work	76
3.4	Ongoing Evaluation	76
4	**Summary**	77
References		77

Abstract

UK Biobank is a major national health resource which aims to improve prevention, diagnosis and treatment of a wide range of serious and life-threatening illnesses. UK Biobank recruited 500,000 people aged between 40 and 69 years in 2006–2010, who underwent a range of measurements and provided detailed information about themselves, donated biological samples for future analyses and agreed to have their health followed long term. Among a range of ongoing enhancements, the UK Biobank Imaging Study aims to perform brain, cardiac and body magnetic resonance imaging, dual-energy X-ray absorptiometry and carotid Doppler ultrasound in 100,000 participants, generating the world's largest multimodal imaging dataset.

As incidental findings (IF) are an expected consequence of its imaging study, UK Biobank developed a pragmatic, scalable protocol for handling IF, in which participants and their

L.M. Gibson
University of Edinburgh, Centre for Clinical Brain Sciences, Chancellor's Building, 49 Little France Crescent, Edinburgh EH16 4SB, UK
e-mail: lorna.gibson@ed.ac.uk

J. Sellors
University of Oxford, Clinical Trial Service Unit and Epidemiological Studies Unit, Nuffield Department of Population Health, Richard Doll Building, Old Road Campus, Oxford OX3 7LF, UK

UK Biobank Coordinating Centre, 1-2 Spectrum Way, Adswood, Stockport SK3 0SA, UK
e-mail: jonathan.sellors@ukbiobank.ac.uk

C.L.M. Sudlow (✉)
University of Edinburgh, Centre for Clinical Brain Sciences, Chancellor's Building, 49 Little France Crescent, Edinburgh EH16 4SB, UK

UK Biobank Coordinating Centre, 1-2 Spectrum Way, Adswood, Stockport SK3 0SA, UK
e-mail: cathie.sudlow@ed.ac.uk

Med Radiol Diagn Imaging (2016)
DOI 10.1007/174_2016_91,
Published Online: 17 Dec 2016

general practitioners receive feedback in limited circumstances: when, during image acquisition, a radiographer notices a potentially serious IF ('indicating the possibility of a condition which, if confirmed, would carry a real prospect of seriously threatening life span or of having a substantial impact on major body functions or quality of life') and a radiologist subsequently confirms a potentially serious IF.

UK Biobank has compared its IF protocol against a commonly used protocol (systematic review of all images by radiologists) and collected comprehensive data on the impact of feedback of potentially serious IF on participants and health services. The results will be published separately and will provide robust, empirical evidence to inform debates surrounding handling IF and designs of future studies' IF policies.

1 Introduction

1.1 UK Biobank

UK Biobank is a large, prospective epidemiological research resource which recruited approximately 500,000 people aged 40–69 between 2006 and 2010 (Sudlow et al. 2015). UK Biobank aims to enable studies of the prevention, diagnosis and treatment of common and serious diseases and is open to use by researchers from anywhere in the world for health-related research which is in the public interest (Collins 2012). The UK Biobank resource contains detailed baseline questionnaire and physical measurement data, genotyping and biochemical assay data, and biological samples from all participants (Sudlow et al. 2015). UK Biobank participants have agreed to have their health followed, and data on health outcomes are derived via linkages to routinely collected national healthcare datasets. Enhanced data collection is ongoing in subsets of participants, and in April 2014, UK Biobank embarked on its most ambitious enhanced data collection project to date: the UK Biobank Imaging Study.

We aim to describe the UK Biobank Imaging Study, the development of the UK Biobank incidental findings (IF) protocol and UK Biobank's programmes of evaluation of this protocol: (i) of participants' understanding of consent in relation to receiving feedback about a potentially serious IF (defined as one indicating the possibility of a condition which, if confirmed, would carry a real prospect of seriously threatening life span or of having a substantial impact on major body functions or quality of life) and (ii) the impact of the UK Biobank IF protocol on participants and health services, the results of which will be published separately.

1.2 The UK Biobank Imaging Study

Over the next seven years, UK Biobank will perform brain, cardiac and body magnetic resonance imaging (MRI), carotid Doppler ultrasound and dual-energy X-ray absorptiometry (DXA) in 100,000 of its participants and generate the world's largest multimodal imaging dataset. The data will enable researchers to investigate associations between imaging-derived phenotypes (IDP) and the wealth of exposure and outcome data from baseline and other enhanced data collections and health record linkages within the resource.

Research imaging is currently underway at the purpose-built imaging centre in Stockport, with further centres planned. On arrival at the imaging centre, participants undergo registration, prescreening and consent, followed by imaging. In order to provide contemporaneous non-imaging data, at the end of the visit, participants repeat the entire baseline assessment and an additional 12-lead electrocardiogram. Each participant's imaging visit lasts approximately four hours.

The UK Biobank Imaging Working Group collaborated with over 100 scientists to design the UK Biobank Imaging Study protocol, which aims to balance the acquisition of high-quality imaging data against feasible methods which are acceptable to participants (Matthews and Sudlow 2015; UK Biobank 2015e). These data enable UK Biobank to generate a wide range of IDP

(Table 1) and facilitate the development and testing of new image analyses methods, the results of which are being integrated into, and thus further enhancing, the UK Biobank resource (Matthews and Sudlow 2015).

Participants undergo an approximately 30-min 3.0 T brain MRI (Skyra, Siemens, Erlangen, Germany), which includes structural (T1, T2 fluid-attenuated inversion recovery, susceptibility-weighted imaging and T2*), functional and diffusion imaging (UK Biobank 2016). From these images, UK Biobank generates IDP including measures of volumes of total grey matter, cortical grey matter, total white matter, cerebrospinal fluid and structures such as the thalamus, detailed data on activation and statistical effect sizes in different regions during fMRI tasks and diffusion parameters such as fractional anisotropy in different white matter tracts (UK Biobank 2016; Miller et al. 2016).

A 20-minute non-contrast cardiac MRI is acquired using a 1.5 T Magnetom Aera scanner (Siemens Healthcare, Erlangen, Germany). Sequences include long and short axis cine, aortic distensibility cine, tagging and aortic valve flow images, from which IDP such as cardiac output, ejection fraction and end-diastolic, end-systolic and stroke volumes are calculated and from which a wide range of additional measures are being derived using novel, automated methods (UK Biobank 2015b; Petersen et al. 2013).

Participants are then repositioned within the 1.5 T scanner and undergo a 10-min body MRI. In total, these images cover tissues from the neck to the knees and include a T1 abdomen, T1 pancreas and a liver and pancreas multi-echo sequence. From these images, semiautomated measures of liver fat, fibrosis and haemosiderosis percentages can be made, in addition to body composition measurements of subcutaneous and visceral fat and thigh muscle mass (UK Biobank 2015a; West et al. 2016). Ongoing methodological developments will lead to the derivation of an increasingly wide range of measures.

Table 1 Summary of imaging modalities and imaging-derived phenotypes included in the UK Biobank Imaging Study

Imaging modality and references for further information	Scanner	Scan duration (min)	Imaging acquired	n IDP currently available	Examples of available IDP
Brain MRI (UK Biobank 2016)	3.0 T Skyra[1]	30	T1, T2 FLAIR, SWI, T2*, fMRI, DWI	749	Tissue volumes, activation during fMRI, fractional anisotropy
Cardiac MRI (UK Biobank 2015b)	1.5 T Magnetom Aera[1]	20	Cine (long axis, short axis, aorta), tagged, aortic valve flow	30	Cardiac output, ejection fraction, stroke volumes
Abdominal MRI (UK Biobank 2015a)	1.5 T Magnetom Aera[1]	10	T1 abdomen, T1 pancreas, liver and pancreas multi-echo, Dixon	5	Percentages of liver fat, fibrosis and haemosiderosis, body composition
DXA (UK Biobank 2015c)	iDXA[2]	20	Whole body, thoracolumbar spine, hips, knees	120	Bone area, mineral content and density, lean mass, fat mass
Carotid Doppler US (UK Biobank 2015d)	5–13 MHz linear array transducer and CardioHealth Station[3]	10	Video loops in longitudinal and transverse plane, CIMT measures	16	Minimum, maximum and mean CIMT

IDP imaging-derived phenotypes, *MRI* magnetic resonance imaging, *FLAIR* fluid-attenuated inversion recovery, *SWI* susceptibility-weighted imaging, *fMRI* functional MRI, *DWI* diffusion-weighted imaging, *DXA* dual-energy X-ray absorptiometry, *US* ultrasound, *CIMT* carotid intima-media thickness

[a]Siemens, Erlangen, Germany

[b]GE-Lunar, Wisconsin, USA

[c]Panasonic, Leicester, UK

Carotid Doppler ultrasound images are acquired during a 10-min examination using a 5–13 MHz linear array transducer and a CardioHealth Station (Panasonic, Leicester, UK). Two-dimensional transverse and longitudinal plane images of each carotid artery are saved as cine loops, followed by two measures of intima-media thickness per carotid artery. From these images, mean, minimum and maximum calculations of carotid intima-media thickness are generated, and additional measures of plaque characteristics will follow (UK Biobank 2015d).

DXA images of the whole body, thoracolumbar spine, hips and knees are acquired using an iDXA scanner (GE-Lunar, Wisconsin, USA). The scanner automatically generates multiple IDP of the bone area, mineral content and density and body composition measures of lean and fat mass (UK Biobank 2015c).

Descriptions of all available IDP from each modality, and non-imaging variables, are available from the UK Biobank showcase (http://www.ukbiobank.ac.uk/data-showcase).

2 UK Biobank IF Protocol

2.1 Development of the UK Biobank IF Protocol

Incidental findings (IF) are findings deemed beyond the aims of a study (Wolf et al. 2008). IF are particularly pertinent to the UK Biobank Imaging Study given the nature of IF which may be identifiable on multimodal imaging of 100,000 largely asymptomatic participants. The handling of IF in research imaging is the subject of widespread debates (Gibson et al. 2016 In Press), and while there is no 'one-size-fits-all' approach to detecting and feeding back IF, researchers should anticipate IF and design appropriate IF handling policies (Medical Research Council and Wellcome Trust 2014).

The UK Biobank IF protocol was developed following an extensive process which involved reviewing existing policies for feedback of findings to UK Biobank participants, published evidence and guidance on IF, received external legal advice on the scope of the duty of care and consultations with the independent UK Biobank Ethics and Governance Council, UK Biobank's major funders (Wellcome Trust and Medical Research Council) and with the Royal College of Radiologists and the Society and College of Radiographers. In addition, UK Biobank sought to learn from the experiences and approaches taken to handling IF used by several other large-scale research imaging projects, including the German National Cohort, the Rotterdam Scan Study, the Multi-Ethnic Study of Atherosclerosis (MESA), and the Reykjavik Heart Study. UK Biobank also consulted with relevant experts to explore the legal and ethical factors which were applicable to the development of the IF protocol.

The UK Biobank IF protocol was developed from first principles as a pragmatic protocol that could be implemented on a large scale with the objective of striking the optimum balance of most net benefit and least net harm to 100,000 largely asymptomatic participants (UK Biobank 2015e). Under this protocol, participants only receive feedback in specific, limited circumstances: when a radiographer identifies a potentially serious IF during the acquisition or quality assessment of images during the imaging visit and a radiologist subsequently confirms the presence of a potentially serious IF. UK Biobank defines a potentially serious imaging IF as 'as a finding which indicates the possibility of a condition which, if confirmed, would carry a real prospect of seriously threatening life span, or of having a substantial impact on major body functions or quality of life.'

2.2 Consent Processes

Before attending the imaging centre, UK Biobank provides participants with an information leaflet which includes a description of the IF protocol and what they should and should not reasonably expect (UK Biobank 2014b).

The information leaflet explains that the scans are not intended to diagnose an illness or identify a particular abnormality and that they will not be looked at routinely by doctors. Participants are informed that if, during the scan, the radiographer notices something which they think may be serious, only then will the scan be reviewed by a doctor; if the doctor thinks there may be a potentially serious finding, the participant and their GP will be informed. The leaflet gives examples of IF which would be fed back to participants (a tumour) and those which would not (gallstones or a simple cyst).

UK Biobank's consent form explicitly asks for participants' consent on the basis that (a) they understand that these scans are for research purposes only and that they will not be routinely examined by medical staff and should not be regarded as part of a 'health check,' (b) that they give permission for UK Biobank to contact them and their GP in the event that a potentially serious IF is found on a scan and (c) that a lack of contact from UK Biobank does not imply that no potentially serious IF exists, but simply that no such abnormality was noticed by the staff taking the scans (UK Biobank 2014a).

2.3 Identification of IF

UK Biobank modified a list of IF developed by the German National Cohort to detail those IF which may be detected on brain, cardiac or body MR or DXA which UK Biobank would consider potentially serious and warrant feedback to participants and their GPs and those which it would consider not serious and would not be fed back. It was deemed that carotid Doppler ultrasound conducted by radiographers would not produce any IF which would be considered potentially serious.

The list is not exhaustive, and in the event that an IF is detected which is not included in the list, radiographers and radiologists are guided by the UK Biobank definition of a potentially serious IF (those which indicate the possibility of a condition which, if confirmed, would carry a real prospect of seriously threatening life span or of having a substantial impact on major body functions or quality of life) to judge whether an IF is deemed potentially serious or not (UK Biobank 2014b).

2.4 Feedback of IF

If the reviewing expert decides that the IF is not serious, then no further action is taken. If, on the other hand, the reviewing expert confirms that the IF is potentially serious, then they provide a short summary for the participant and a more comprehensive summary for the participant's GP (UK Biobank 2015e).

The GP is informed that the images have not been optimised for the purpose of identifying abnormalities and have not been reviewed in a clinical setting. Further investigations and/or referrals are left to the discretion of the GP. As required, the participant's doctors are able to review the scans collected by UK Biobank (UK Biobank 2015e).

3 Evaluation of the Impact of the UK Biobank IF Protocol

3.1 Evaluating Participants' Understanding of Consent

Given that systematic radiologist review of all acquired images is not undertaken, the UK Biobank IF Protocol will inevitably fail to identify some potentially serious IF which represent serious diseases. Public expectations relating to feedback of IF may well be unrealistic, the public associate imaging with clinical diagnoses (Kirschen et al. 2006), and expect that images will be reviewed by experts (The Royal College of Radiologists 2011). It is therefore crucial to manage participants' expectations of what will be fed back, and what will not, and specifically to ensure that they understand that the imaging does not constitute a 'health check' and that lack of feedback of a potentially serious IF does not represent an 'all clear.' The intention of the UK Biobank information materials and consent process is to provide participants with a fair, reasonable and realistic expectation of the outcome of their visit for imaging in the UK Biobank Imaging Study. UK Biobank developed a questionnaire to assess participants' understanding of this consent, which is sent to imaged participants two days after their imaging visit.

Participants are asked whether or not they thought they consented to the following: return of scans and results at the end of the imaging visit; to choose whether they and their GP would be informed; that they and their GP would automatically be contacted; that they would receive feedback of a potentially serious IF during the imaging visit; whether they would receive feedback of an IF after the imaging visit. These data are periodically reviewed so that the design of the UK Biobank Imaging Study consent materials can be improved and results will be published separately.

3.2 Comparing the UK Biobank IF Protocol with Full Review of Images by Radiologists

There is no 'best' policy for handling IF detected during research imaging of healthy populations, and existing studies vary in their approach (The Royal College of Radiologists 2011). However, there are likely to be 'better' and 'worse' policies for handling IF, which will depend on the context of the individual research study. Imaging studies should develop IF policies which are appropriate to their context (Medical Research Council and Wellcome Trust 2014), and evaluation studies which directly compare different approaches to IF will guide decisions as to which policy is more appropriate.

UK Biobank therefore designed such an evaluation study, the methods and results of which will be published in a forthcoming research article. In brief, UK Biobank assessed the prevalence of potentially serious IF and the proportions of these which were finally diagnosed as serious (i.e. true positives) and not serious (i.e. false positives) as a result of the UK Biobank IF Protocol compared with a common approach to handling IF in other imaging studies: systematic review of images by radiologists. UK Biobank also investigated the rate of serious final diagnoses which were detected by radiologists but missed by the UK Biobank IF Protocol (i.e. false negatives). The impact of feedback of potentially serious IF on participants and health services was informed by questionnaires to participants and their GPs. This evaluation was encouraged by the main funders of UK Biobank (the Medical Research Council and the Wellcome Trust) and the UK Biobank's independent Ethics and Governance Council.

Results on the rates of prevalence of potentially serious IF, false positives, false negatives and the impact of feedback of potentially serious IF were crucial in guiding judgement of the potential net benefit and net harm of each protocol.

3.3 Qualitative Work

In order to provide context for and greater exploration of the results of the quantitative evaluation study of the UK Biobank IF Protocol described above, UK Biobank commissioned the research company TNS-BMRB to conduct a parallel qualitative study of participants' experiences of the imaging visit, understanding of the consent they had given, the process and opinions of receiving feedback of a potentially serious IF and the impact of receiving feedback of a potentially serious IF (TNS-BMRB 2015). These qualitative data were collected with the aim of informing the protocol on feedback of IF for the main phase of the UK Biobank Imaging Study. The detailed methods and results of this study will be made available in a separate report.

3.4 Ongoing Evaluation

UK Biobank continues to send questionnaires to participants two days following their imaging visit in order to evaluate their understanding of consent and to send questionnaires six weeks and six months following imaging to collect data on final diagnoses, clinical follow-up and impact on participants. In addition, UK Biobank continues to send questionnaires after six months to GPs in order to collect data on final diagnoses, clinical follow-up and GPs' opinions on the net benefit and harm of providing feedback of a potentially serious IF on their patients.

This systematic follow-up of participants will provide much-needed robust, empirical data on the impact on participants and health services and data on final diagnoses and false-positive rates. Such data, along with linkages to national healthcare datasets, will enable UK Biobank to continually monitor the impact of its IF protocol and to address additional questions raised by the UK Biobank evaluation study described which warrant further research: whether or not early diagnosis of serious disease results in net benefit for asymptomatic participants and what are the health economic consequences of the UK Biobank Imaging IF Protocol. These data will contribute evidence to the debates surrounding the management of IF in research imaging and inform the practical design of appropriate and feasible IF policies for future imaging studies.

4 Summary

The UK Biobank Imaging Study aims to image 100,000 healthy participants and will generate the world's largest multimodal imaging dataset. UK Biobank has developed a pragmatic, scalable protocol for handling IF during the Imaging Study which results in feedback of IF to participants and their GPs in only limited circumstances: where a radiographer notices a potentially serious IF, images are reviewed by a radiologist, and feedback given if the radiologist confirms the presence of a potentially serious IF. This approach differs from many studies, including other large national imaging projects, in which systematic review of images by radiologists for IF is undertaken. The impact of the UK Biobank IF protocol is under continuous evaluation, and data collection is ongoing of participants' clinical follow-up and final diagnoses and the impact on participants' emotional well-being, insurance and finances and work and activities. In addition, UK Biobank has performed a head-to-head comparison of its IF protocol against systematic review by radiologists, and following initial data analyses and revision of consent materials, it continues to assess participants' understanding of consent. Such analyses will be of value not only to UK Biobank, but will provide much-needed robust, empirical data on the impact of feedback of IF which will address current gaps in knowledge and inform the design of IF policies in future imaging studies.

References

Collins R (2012) What makes UK Biobank special? Lancet 379(9822):1173–1174. http://dx.doi.org/10.1016/S0140-6736(12)60404-8

Gibson LM, Sudlow CLM, Wardlaw J (2016) Incidental findings: current ethical debates and future challenges in advanced neuroimaging. In: Illes J, Hossain S (eds) Neuroethics: anticipating the future, 2 edn. Oxford University Press, Oxford (In Press)

Kirschen MP, Jaworska A, Illes J (2006) Subjects' expectations in neuroimaging research. J Magn Reson Imaging 23(2):205–209. doi:10.1002/jmri.20499

Matthews PM, Sudlow C (2015) The UK Biobank. Brain 138(12):3463–3465. doi:10.1093/brain/awv335

Medical Research Council, Wellcome Trust (2014) Framework on the feedback of health-related findings in research. www.mrc.ac.uk/documents/pdf/mrc-wellcome-trust-framework-on-the-feedback-of-health-related-findings-in-researchpdf/

Miller KL, Alfaro-Almagro F, Bangerter NK, Thomas DL, Yacoub E, Xu J, Bartsch AJ, Jbabdi S, Sotiropoulos SN, Andersson JLR, Griffanti L, Douaud G, Okell TW, Weale P, Dragonu I, Garratt S, Hudson S, Collins R, Jenkinson M, Matthews PM, Smith SM (2016) Multimodal population brain imaging in the UK Biobank prospective epidemiological study. Nat Neurosci 19(11):1523–1536. doi:10.1038/nn.4393

Petersen SE, Matthews PM, Bamberg F, Bluemke DA, Francis JM, Friedrich MG, Leeson P, Nagel E, Plein S, Rademakers FE, Young AA, Garratt S, Peakman T, Sellors J, Collins R, Neubauer S (2013) Imaging in population science: cardiovascular magnetic resonance in 100,000 participants of UK Biobank - rationale, challenges and approaches. J Cardiovasc Magn Reson 15(1):46–46. doi:10.1186/1532-429X-15-46

Sudlow C, Gallacher J, Allen N, Beral V, Burton P, Danesh J, Downey P, Elliott P, Green J, Landray M, Liu B, Matthews P, Ong G, Pell J, Silman A, Young A, Sprosen T, Peakman T, Collins R (2015) UK Biobank: an open access resource for identifying the causes of a wide range of complex diseases of middle and old age. PLoS Med 12(3):e1001779. doi:10.1371/journal.pmed.1001779

The Royal College of Radiologists (2011) Management of incidental findings detected during research imaging. https://www.rcr.ac.uk/system/files/publication/field_publication_files/BFCR%2811%298_ethics.pdf

TNS-BMRB (2015) Attitudes to and impact of the feedback of potentially serious incidental findings from UK Biobank's imaging pilot study.

UK Biobank (2014a) Consent form for the imaging assessment: UK Biobank. http://www.ukbiobank.ac.uk/wp-content/uploads/2016/06/consent_form_imaging.pdf

UK Biobank (2014b) Information leaflet: imaging assessment visit. http://www.ukbiobank.ac.uk/wp-content/uploads/2016/06/information_leaflet_imaging.pdf

UK Biobank (2015a) UK Biobank body (abdominal) MRI scan. http://biobank.ctsu.ox.ac.uk/crystal/docs/body_mri_explan.pdf

UK Biobank (2015b) UK Biobank imaging modality cardiovascular magnetic resonance (CMR). http://biobank.ctsu.ox.ac.uk/crystal/refer.cgi?id=349

UK Biobank (2015c) UK Biobank imaging modality DXA. http://biobank.ctsu.ox.ac.uk/crystal/refer.cgi?id=502

UK Biobank (2015d) UK Biobank imaging modality: carotid ultrasound. http://biobank.ctsu.ox.ac.uk/crystal/refer.cgi?id=511

UK Biobank (2015e) UK Biobank: report on feasibility of imaging assessments in 100,000 participants.

UK Biobank (2016) UK Biobank brain imaging documentation. http://biobank.ctsu.ox.ac.uk/crystal/refer.cgi?id=1977

West J, Dahlqvist Leinhard O, Romu T, Collins R, Garratt S, Bell JD, Borga M, Thomas L (2016) Feasibility of MR-based body composition analysis in large scale population studies. PLoS One 11(9):e0163332. doi:10.1371/journal.pone.0163332

Wolf SM, Lawrenz FP, Nelson CA, Kahn JP, Cho MK, Clayton W, Fletcher JG, Georgieff MK, Hammerschmidt D, Illes J, Kapur V, Keane MA, Koenig BA, Leroy BS, McFarland EG, Paradise J, Parker LS, Terry SF, Ness BV, Wilfond BS (2008) Managing incidental findings in human subjects research: analysis and recommendations. J law Med Ethics J Am Soc Law Med Ethics 36(2):211–219. doi:10.1111/j.1748-720X.2008.00266.x.Managing

Management of Incidental Findings on Neuroimaging in the Rotterdam Study

Daniel Bos and Meike W. Vernooij

Contents

1	**Setup of the Rotterdam Study**	79
2	**Neuroimaging in the Rotterdam Study**	80
3	**Hardware and Imaging Protocol**	80
4	**Protocol for Detection and Management of Incidental Findings**	81
5	**Review of Scans for Incidental Findings**	82
6	**Frequencies of Incidental Findings on Brain MRI in the Rotterdam Study**	82
7	**Feedback of Incidental Findings to Participants**	85
8	**Follow-Up of Incidental Findings on Brain MRI**	85
9	**Participants' Expectations and Experience**	85
Conclusion		86
References		86

Abstract

This chapter gives an overview of the management of incidental findings on neuroimaging in the population-based Rotterdam Study, in which brain MRI was introduced as part of the core study protocol in 2005 (1.5 T). To this purpose, a protocol for the management of incidental findings was defined by a group of experts from different fields. During the study, all brain scans are reviewed for incidental findings by group of trained researchers, under the supervision of a neuroradiologist. Only findings deemed of potential clinical relevance (according to the study protocol) are reported to the participants. Overall, incidental findings that require additional clinical review by a medical specialist, of which meningiomas and aneurysms are most common, occur in just over 3%. The vast majority of these undergo a watch and wait policy, indicating that clinical consequences are in most cases limited.

1 Setup of the Rotterdam Study

In response to the rapid increase in the number of elderly persons in the population, in 1990, the Rotterdam Study was initiated to study determinants and causes of common age-related diseases (Hofman et al. 2015). Examples include

D. Bos, MD, PhD • M.W. Vernooij, MD, PhD (✉)
Departments of Radiology and Epidemiology, Erasmus MC, University Medical Centre Rotterdam, P.O. Box 2040, Rotterdam 3000 CA, The Netherlands
e-mail: m.vernooij@erasmusmc.nl

Med Radiol Diagn Imaging (2016)
DOI 10.1007/174_2016_53,
Published Online: 07 May 2016

cardiovascular disease, neurologic diseases, locomotor disease, and ophthalmologic diseases. Using a prospective population-based design, 7983 persons aged 55 years or older and living in a well-defined district in the city of Rotterdam in the Netherlands were initially included in the study. Later, in 2000, the cohort was extended with another 3011 participants who had turned 55 years of age or moved into the study district. A further extension of the cohort was started in 2006 and consisted of 3932 subjects that were age 45 years and older, resulting in a total study population of 14,926 subjects. All participants are invited for extensive reexaminations every 4–5 years. As a result, persons from the first cohort are already participating in their sixth visit, the persons of the second cohort will shortly start the fourth visit, and the people of the third cohort will be invited for their third visit.

2 Neuroimaging in the Rotterdam Study

Common neurologic brain diseases in the elderly, especially dementia and stroke, put a huge burden on current healthcare, both in terms of patient suffering and healthcare costs (Prince et al. 2013; Mozaffarian et al. 2016). Still effective therapeutic and preventive strategies targeted at reducing these diseases remain scarce. A key element for successful development of such strategies is gathering in-depth knowledge on their etiology and pathophysiology. In this light, an important aspect of these neurological brain diseases is that subtle cerebral changes already develop long before the diseases become clinically overt. Using noninvasive magnetic resonance imaging (MRI), these early changes can be readily visualized, providing unique insight into these early stages of disease.

As one of the first population-based studies, in 1995, the Rotterdam Study introduced brain MRI to study the underlying structural brain changes of age-related neurologic diseases, in a subset of all participants (Ikram et al. 2015). Yet, especially during the last decade, rapid technological improvements in MRI have led to better image quality, shorter scanning times, and improved sequences. Moreover, significant improvements in post-processing techniques of MRI data have considerably increased possibilities for faster image processing, better visualization, and quantification of imaging findings. Following these developments, in 2005, a dedicated research scanner was installed in the Rotterdam Study research center, and brain MRI was incorporated in the core protocol of the Rotterdam Study (Ikram et al. 2015). From this time onward, all participants taking part in their regular visit to the Rotterdam Study center were invited to undergo brain MRI examinations during a separate visit to the research center. Persons with MRI contraindications or claustrophobia were considered not invited. Importantly, the scanner capacity allows examining 56 brain MRI examinations per week, which is more than the throughput of the regular Rotterdam Study center visits. Therefore, we were able to invite various subsets of participants for re-scanning. As a result, as of July 2015, we have performed over 12,000 brain MRI examinations in over 5800 subjects (overall response rate of over 75 %).

3 Hardware and Imaging Protocol

All brain MRI examinations in the Rotterdam Study are performed on a 1.5 T MRI machine (GE Healthcare, Milwaukee, USA) (Ikram et al. 2015). The MRI is equipped with a dedicated 8-channel head coil and the possibility of parallel imaging using the array spatial sensitivity encoding technique (ASSET). For data consistency and comparability during the study, all acquisition parameters have been unchanged since the beginning of the study, and no software or hardware upgrades have been performed.

The current imaging protocol consists of seven separate sequences, which will be discussed below, with a total examination time of 50 min (see also (Ikram et al. 2015)). This imaging protocol was carefully chosen while taking into account the quality of the imaging data, potential inconvenience for the participants, and the costs. From the scientific point of view, the choice of sequences in the imaging protocol was based on the primary study interests, namely, measures of brain atrophy, measures of cerebral small vessel disease (infarcts, white matter lesions, and cerebral microbleeds), measures of white matter microstructure, cerebral blood flow, and functional brain connectivity. In order to facilitate easy applicability of the MRI protocol by technicians, only standard brain imaging sequences as provided by the manufacturer are used.

The imaging protocol (Box 1) begins with a three-plane localizer, after which structural imaging is performed using T1-weighted (T1w), proton density-weighted (PDw), and fluid-attenuated inversion recovery (FLAIR) sequences. The combination of these three sequences allows for an accurate assessment of brain structure, the presence of infarcts, and the presence and amount of white matter lesions. Moreover, these sequences are well suited for automated segmentation and quantification of brain tissue. Diffusion tensor imaging (DTI) is performed to assess the microstructural integrity of the white matter. Next, a dedicated 2D phase contrast sequence is done in order to assess the total cerebral blood flow. A 3D T2*-weighted gradient-recalled echo scan is used to image cerebral microbleeds. Since 2012, the imaging protocol also includes a resting-state functional MRI sequence, in order to assess functional brain connectivity. The protocol is described in detail in (Ikram et al. 2015).

4 Protocol for Detection and Management of Incidental Findings

A protocol describing the review of acquired images for the presence of unexpected findings and the management and feedback of these findings was installed prior to the start of the study. To this end, an expert panel was formed that consisted of a neurologist, a neurosurgeon, a neuroradiologist, an endocrinologist, a medical decision-making expert, and an oncology epidemiologist (Vernooij et al. 2007). The purpose of this panel was to define a priori a list of findings that should be referred (Box 2) and a list of findings that would not need referral (Box 3, see also (Vernooij et al. 2007)). The panel based its decisions on best available evidence, for example, on rupture risk of incidentally discovered small aneurysms (ISUIA 1998; Wiebers et al. 2003). Handling of incidental findings is done according to these lists (see further below). Furthermore, the expert panel functions as ad hoc consultants for cases that come up and do not meet the a priori defined criteria.

During the course of the study, since the installment of the protocol in 2005, the full expert panel reconvened twice: once to redefine criteria for referral of small cerebral aneurysms (deciding not to refer small anterior circulation aneurysms <7 mm in size (Wiebers et al. 2003; ISUIA 1998)) and a second time to modify the referral criteria for

Box 1. Summary of the Sequences Used in the Imaging Protocol in the Rotterdam Study

Scout (positioning)
Scout (localizer)
Proton density-weighted sequence
2D phase contrast sequence
Resting-state functional MRI sequence
T1-weighted sequence
Fluid-attenuated inversion recovery sequence
Diffusion tensor imaging sequence
T2*-weighted sequence

Box 2. Findings on Neuroimaging That Require Referral

Pituitary macroadenoma
Meningioma (except <2 cm on convexity)
Vestibular schwannoma
Malignant primary brain tumors
Metastases
Aneurysms in the anterior circulation >7 mm in size in persons <80 years
Aneurysms in the posterior circulation in persons <80 years
Intracranial carotid occlusion
Colloid cyst

Box 3. Findings on Neuroimaging That Do Not Require Referral
Silent brain infarcts
White matter lesions
Microbleeds
Iron deposition
Atrophy
Arachnoid cysts
Intracerebral cysts not suspect for neoplasm
Sinusitis and other benign mucosal swelling in sinonasal cavities
Enlarged perivascular spaces
Cavernous angioma
Aneurysms in the anterior circulation ≤7 mm in size
Aneurysms in persons >80 years
Unruptured arteriovenous malformations
Vertebral artery occlusion

small meningiomas (deciding not to refer small convexity meningiomas <2 cm but rather offer a research follow-up). Also, in a separate meeting with only the endocrinologist consultant, criteria for referral of small intrasellar cysts were refined.

5 Review of Scans for Incidental Findings

All acquired research scans are transferred using secure data connection from the MRI scanner in the research center to a digital picture archiving system (PACS). All scans are reviewed for the presence of unexpected findings by a team of trained raters.

Raters are all PhD students in the neuroimaging group of the Rotterdam Study. Most (>90 %) of them have a medical background (MD training), though some do not (e.g., neuropsychology). All raters receive an extensive training in neuroanatomy, scan reading (including basic MRI technique), and basic detection of normal versus abnormal on brain imaging. The training consists of an introductory afternoon led by a neuroradiologist, 2 weeks of observing scan reading by one of the more experienced raters, and a 2-month period in which the rater is gradually working through a training set of 120 scans that were selected as a mixture of positive and negative for incidental findings (approximately 30 % positive for any finding). The training set is read blinded for the presence of findings, after which the findings are disclosed by a neuroradiologist and the results of the rater are supervised and performance is evaluated.

After the training period, the performance of the raters on the last half of the set is used to assess their ability to start rating research scans prospectively. If deemed necessary, the training period can be extended. For the first 2 weeks after training, the raters double read all scans with one of the more experienced raters. Only if no major discrepancies arise is the rater deemed qualified for independent rating.

All scans are reviewed for the presence of unexpected findings within 1 week after acquisition. In case a finding that is deemed of potential urgent nature is discovered (e.g., subdural hematoma, large brain tumor), the raters communicate their findings directly with a neuroradiologist attached to the Rotterdam Study. All other findings are recorded in an in-house developed database, using a structured format and the ability to add free text (Fig. 1). All entries in the database are discussed in a 6-weekly feedback meeting led by a neuroradiologist and attended by all raters.

6 Frequencies of Incidental Findings on Brain MRI in the Rotterdam Study

The overall prevalence of incidental findings on brain MRI examinations in the Rotterdam Study currently is 9.5 % (549 findings in 5800 participants; mean age 64.9 years; Bos et al. 2016). Of these, the most common are meningiomas and cerebral aneurysms (Figs. 2, 3, and 4). Examples of less frequent findings are pituitary abnormalities (i.e., cysts or macroadenomas), arachnoid cysts, or cavernous angiomas. Also, some rare findings such as vestibular or trigeminal schwannomas were found (<1.0 %, included in "Other" in Fig. 2; see also Vernooij et al. 2007).

Interestingly, the prevalence of incidental findings in our population is somewhat higher than reported in other studies (Morris et al. 2009). An

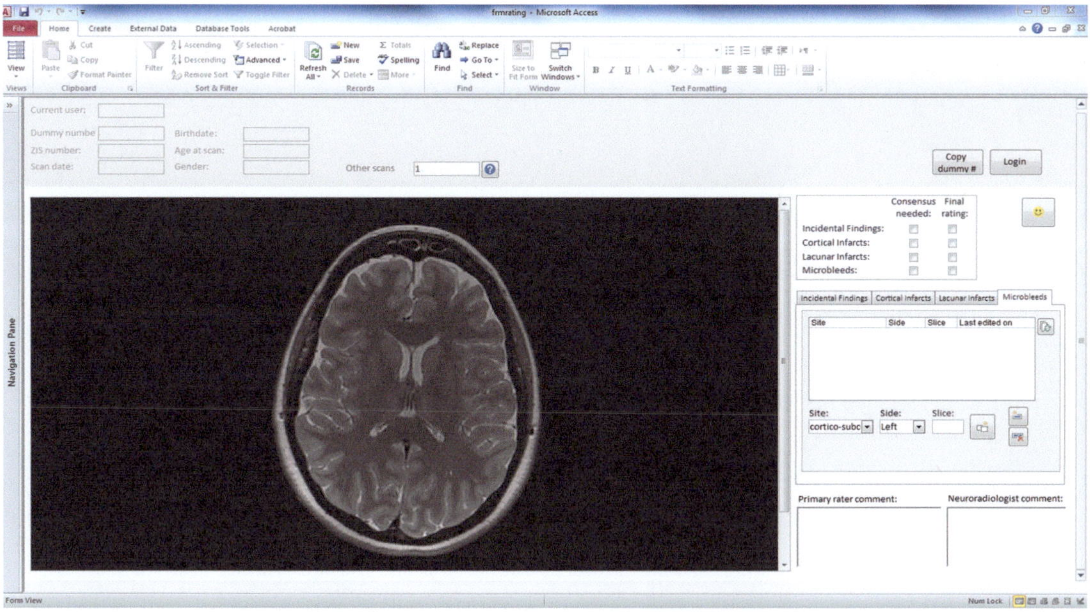

Fig. 1 Screenshot of in-house developed database to register incidental findings on brain MRI. In the *upper row*, the participant's basic characteristics will be filled out (e.g., scan date, date of birth). In the *left screen*, the scan will be displayed. The fields on the *right side* can be used to characterize potential incidental finding

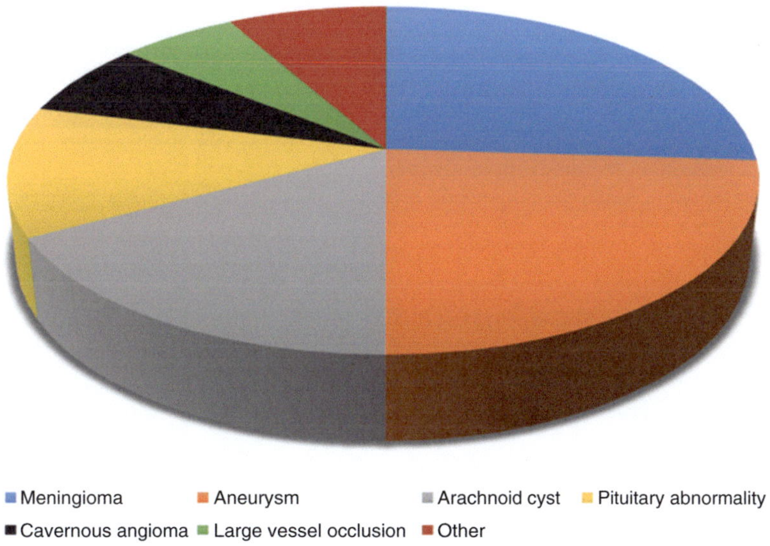

Fig. 2 Pie chart on the frequency of incidental findings on brain MRI in the Rotterdam Study. The section "Other" includes vestibular schwannoma, arteriovenous malformation, dural fistula, possible glioma, trigeminal schwannoma, orbital dermoid cyst, fibrous dysplasia, intracranial lipoma, atypical cerebellar lesion, ganglioglioma, subependymoma, metastasis, pineocytoma, pharyngeal mucosal asymmetry, colloid cyst of the third ventricle, and expansive lesion in the maxillary sinus

important topic to consider with respect to the detection – and thus the frequency – of incidental findings on brain MRI is that this is directly related to multiple nontechnical and technical issues. One of the most important nontechnical issues is the composition of the study population. Important differences in frequency estimates, especially with regard to meningiomas and aneurysms, may arise simply because of the age distribution of the population. In particular for aneurysms, it is well established that these are not present at birth, but develop during aging (Wiebers et al. 2003). Other reasons for differences in frequency estimates across different studies may be due to more technical aspects of the imaging procedure. Examples include the use of specific image sequences, the use of contrast

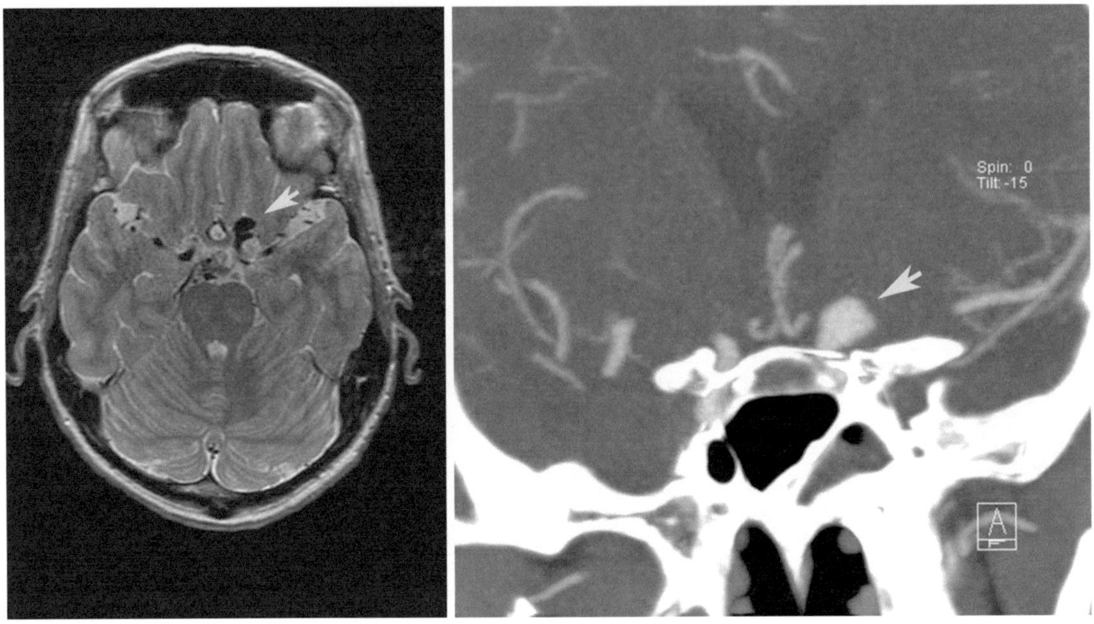

Fig. 3 Example of incidentally discovered aneurysm. T2w MR research scan (*left*) acquired in a 57-year-old female Rotterdam Study participant shows an aneurysm of the left intracranial internal carotid artery. After hospital referral for further workup, CT angiography (*right*) confirmed a 9 mm carotid tip aneurysm. The aneurysm was coiled successfully

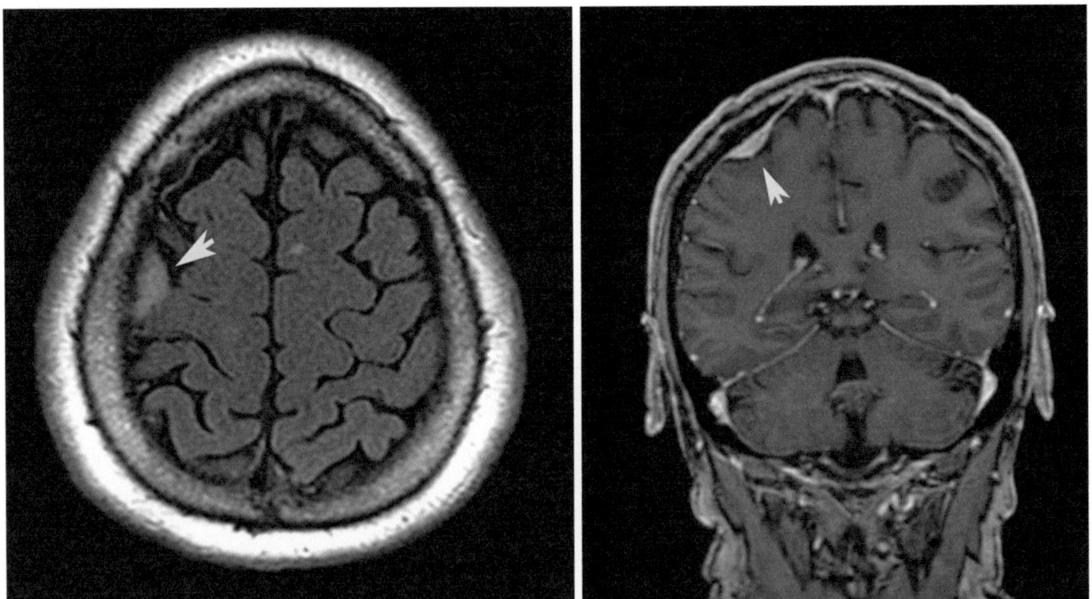

Fig. 4 Example of incidentally discovered meningioma. FLAIR scan (*left panel*) of this 68-year-old male Rotterdam Study participant shows a hyperintense broad-based dural mass, compatible with a meningioma. After hospital referral, the presence of a meningioma was confirmed on T1w-Gd scan (*right panel*). Clinical follow-up was conducted by yearly MRI for 5 years, during which the meningioma did not change and patient was discharged from further follow-up. In a later version of the Rotterdam Study incidental findings protocol, convexity meningiomas <2 cm in size were no longer referred

material, and the type of post-processing of the images (van der Lugt 2009). Importantly, in the Rotterdam Study, an optimized MRI protocol is used, and incidental findings are registered by experienced readers with additional review of all recorded incidental findings by a neuroradiologist. Also, the use of a high-resolution proton density-weighted sequence allows a good visualization of the circle of Willis compared to conventional T1-weighted and T2-weighted sequences (Vernooij et al. 2007) and improves the detection of aneurysms. Taken together, these factors may all contribute to differences in the prevalence of specific imaging findings.

7 Feedback of Incidental Findings to Participants

All study participants sign an informed consent upon study entry, which includes a paragraph on incidental findings: "(..) the study is not aimed at detecting diseases. (..) in addition, The Rotterdam Study does not examine everything in the entire body. This means that some diseases may remain undetected. Of course, many diseases and disorders are noticed during the research examinations. Diseases or disorders that are observed and are deemed of importance will be communicated to me and to my general practitioner, unless I have indicated that I object to this."

For all findings that meet the criteria for referral (Box 2), the informed consent of the participant is checked and how he/she filled out the option to receive information on incidental findings. In practice, >95 % of study participants indicate that they wish to receive feedback on important incidental findings.

Relevant findings are communicated back to the participant by telephone by one of the neuroradiologists involved in the Rotterdam Study. An appointment with a relevant medical specialist is scheduled within 1 week after this telephone conversation. Consent to feedback information to the participant's GP is explicitly confirmed during the telephone conversation, as well as approval to transmit the research scan to the hospital database. The participant also receives contact information of the neuroradiologist to reach him/her should any questions arise before or after the hospital visit. Explicit mention is made that the hospital visit is not research related, and thus insurance fees may apply.

8 Follow-Up of Incidental Findings on Brain MRI

As highlighted in the paragraph on the frequency of incidental findings on brain MRI, we found an overall frequency of 9.5 %. Of all persons with an incidental finding on brain MRI, 188 (34.2 %) were referred for clinical workup (Bos et al. 2016). Importantly, over 75 % of these underwent a watch-and-wait policy or were instantly discharged from further clinical workup after the first visit. This thus suggests that incidental findings on brain MRI are frequent among community-dwelling middle-aged and elderly persons, but in the vast majority without direct clinical consequences.

In light of the investigation of the natural course of meningiomas, those persons with meningiomas that did not meet the criteria for additional clinical workup are re-invited for a follow-up scan after 1–2 years. In combination with data from persons that were referred for clinical workup and were on a watch-and-wait policy (follow-up with imaging in the clinical setting), it was found that the vast majority remained stable in size over the years (Bos et al. 2016).

9 Participants' Expectations and Experience

As part of a research project in collaboration with the Department of Medical Ethics of Erasmus MC, in 2014–2015, several individual interviews and group focus sessions were held with participants of the Rotterdam Study to discuss the issue of incidental findings. For these interviews, a mixture of participants who had been fed back information on an incidental finding in the brain as well as persons without any findings were invited. Participants were questioned about their expectations prior to the research examination, their comprehension of the text in the informed consent, and their experience with management of incidental findings, if they had been fed back any. Results of these interviews are currently being processed and will be published separately. In general, the initial qualitative data indicate that a main motivation for participation in research is interest of the participant in his/her own health. With regard to the detection of incidental findings, the participants expect that "someone will be looking at the scans." Most of them prefer to know about any incidental findings. Those who have received feedback of an incidental finding in the Rotterdam Study say that they are content with knowing and feel fortunate for being monitored or taken care of. None reported serious or long-term psychological harm from knowing.

Conclusion

In conclusion, the Rotterdam Study uses a predefined protocol for detection and management of incidental findings on neuroimaging research scans. A two-step procedure, including the initial rating of all acquired scans by trained researchers and validation of these findings by a neuroradiologist, is applied. Feedback of findings to participants depends on a priori defined criteria. The reading of all scans for incidental findings provides interesting information on the prevalence and natural course of these asymptomatic lesions in community-dwelling subjects, which can be the basis for future guidelines for management.

References

Bos D, Poels MMF, Adams HHH, Akoudad S, et al (2016) Prevalence, clinical management and natural course of incidental findings on brain MRI: A population-based imaging study. Radiol. In press

Hofman A, Brusselle GG, Darwish Murad S et al (2015) The Rotterdam Study: 2016 objectives and design update. Eur J Epidemiol 30:661–708

Ikram MA, van der Lugt A, Niessen WJ et al (2015) The Rotterdam Scan Study: design update 2016 and main findings. Eur J Epidemiol 30:1299–1315

ISUIA (1998) Unruptured intracranial aneurysms – risk of rupture and risks of surgical intervention. International Study of Unruptured Intracranial Aneurysms Investigators. N Engl J Med 339:1725–1733

Morris Z, Whiteley WN, Longstreth WT Jr et al (2009) Incidental findings on brain magnetic resonance imaging: systematic review and meta-analysis. BMJ 339: b3016

Mozaffarian D, Benjamin EJ, Go AS et al (2016) Heart disease and stroke statistics-2016 update: a report from the American Heart Association. Circulation 133:e38–e360

Prince M, Bryce R, Albanese E et al (2013) The global prevalence of dementia: a systematic review and meta-analysis. Alzheimers Dement 9(63–75):e62

van der Lugt A (2009) Incidental findings on brain magnetic resonance imaging. BMJ 339:b3107

Vernooij MW, Ikram MA, Tanghe HL et al (2007) Incidental findings on brain MRI in the general population. N Engl J Med 357:1821–1828

Wiebers DO, Whisnant JP, Huston J 3rd et al (2003) Unruptured intracranial aneurysms: natural history, clinical outcome, and risks of surgical and endovascular treatment. Lancet 362:103–110

Incidental Findings in a Population Based Study Using Cardiac CT: Experience from the Multi-Ethnic Study of Atherosclerosis (MESA)

Sina Rahmani and Matthew J. Budoff

Contents

1 **Significant Alerts** 89

References 90

Abstract

The Multiethnic Study of Atherosclerosis (MESA) Study was initiated in July 2000 to investigate the prevalence, correlates, and progression of subclinical cardiovascular disease in a population-based sample of 6,814 men and women aged 45-84 years at 6 clinical centers. Coronary artery calcium has been measured in serial exams using Electron-beam and multi-detector row computed tomography scanners. Since 2000, there have been 5 exams and participants have undergone cardiac scans at the 6 clinical centers. The CT Reading Center for cardiac scans in the MESA Study is at Los Angeles Biomedical Research Center. In this chapter we discuss technical parameters of the CT studies, prevalence of different incidental findings and our approach in evaluating and reporting these findings.

The Multiethnic Study of Atherosclerosis (MESA) was initiated in July 2000 to investigate the prevalence, correlates, and progression of subclinical cardiovascular disease (CVD) in a population-based sample of 6,814 men and women aged 45–84 years at six clinical centers (Bild et al. 2002; Carr et al. 2005). Coronary artery calcium (CAC) (Agatston et al. 1990) has been measured in serial exams using electron-beam and multi-detector row computed tomography (CT) scanners (Detrano et al. 2005). Since

S. Rahmani, MD
Division of Cardiology, Los Angeles Biomedical Research Institute at Harbor-UCLA, Torrance, CA, USA
e-mail: srahmani@labiomed.org

M.J. Budoff, MD, FACC (✉)
Division of Cardiology, Los Angeles Biomedical Research Institute at Harbor-UCLA, Torrance, CA, USA
e-mail: mbudoff@labiomed.org

Med Radiol Diagn Imaging (2016)
DOI 10.1007/174_2016_49, © Springer International Publishing Switzerland
Published Online: 21 Apr 2016

2000, there have been five exams and participants have undergone cardiac scans at the six clinical centers. The CT reading center for cardiac scans in the MESA is at Los Angeles Biomedical Research Center.

CAC has been assessed on cardiac CT scans in relation to the risk of future cardiac events, and from repeated scans in selected individuals, the progression of coronary calcium is related to baseline risk factors and risk of future events. This study has shown that progression of CAC is associated with an increased risk for future hard and total coronary heart disease events (Budoff et al. 2013a, b).

Electron-beam CT and four-detector row CT were used in MESA exam 1 (Carr et al. 2005). The electron-beam CT system, Imatron C150, operated with an exposure time of 100 ms, a fixed peak voltage of 130 kVp, and a fixed tube current of 630 mA. The nominal section thickness was 3.0 mm. The volume zoom four-detector row CT system was operated in the axial scan mode with prospective ECG triggering, 140 kVp, and gantry rotation speed of 0.5 s. Standard tube current-time product was 50 mAs, and those who weighed more than 100 kg underwent CT with a tube current-time product of 63 mAs. With this scanner, four 2.5-mm sections were acquired per cardiac cycle and actual exposure time was 360 ms. LightSpeed Plus systems were operated in the axial scan mode (cine) with prospective ECG triggering with 120 kVp and gantry rotation speed of 0.5 s. Individuals who weighed 100 kg or less underwent CT with tube current of 320 mA, and those who weighed more than 100 kg underwent CT with a tube current of 400 mA, and four 2.5-mm sections were acquired simultaneously. Exposure time was 330 ms (Carr et al. 2005).

In exam 1, all noncardiac lung fields were reviewed within 2 weeks of receipt by a radiologist. If the radiologist felt that an alert is warranted, a report was written and was transmitted immediately to the field site principal investigator (PI) and coordinator, and a copy is sent to the coordinating center. Table 1 shows the prevalence of incidental findings in the 7,700 scans done in exam 1. Figures 1, 2, 3, and 4 show four different incidental findings in exam 1.

Table 1 Prevalence of incidental findings in MESA

Pathology	Number (of 7,700)	Percent
Aortic calcification	19	0.2
Mitral valve calcification	11	0.1
Pericardial effusion	72	0.9
Pericardial thickening	60	0.8
Aortic root dilation	6	0.1
Descending aorta dilation	2	0.0
Liver lesions	406	5.3
Pulmonary pathology		
Nodules	1,766	23
Calcified nodules	333	4.3
Nodules with irregular margins	110	1.4
Consolidations	70	0.9
Nonspecific interstitial changes	291	3.8
Adenopathy	27	0.4
Pleural effusion	573	7.4
Chest wall abnormality	64	0.8

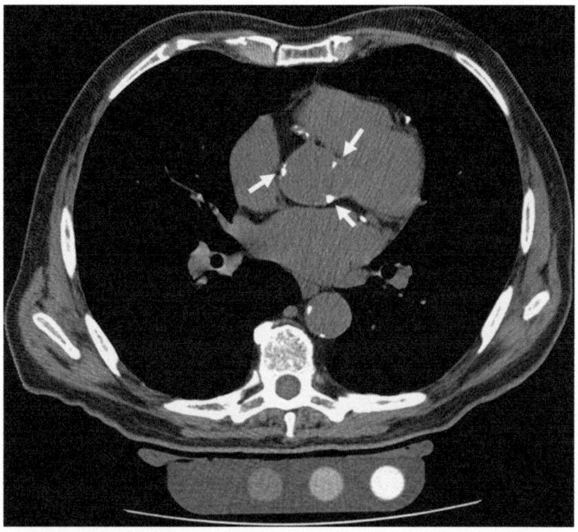

Fig. 1 Aortic valve calcification

In subsequent exams, the initial review of cardiac scans was performed at the Los Angeles Biomedical Research Center by a physician, with experience in CT imaging. If the review was negative for a significant noncardiac finding, the process ended, and a report documenting this was

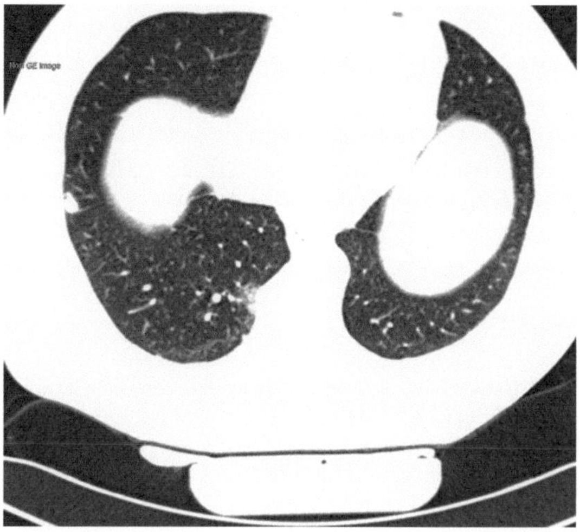

Fig. 2 Pulmonary nodule in the right lower lobe

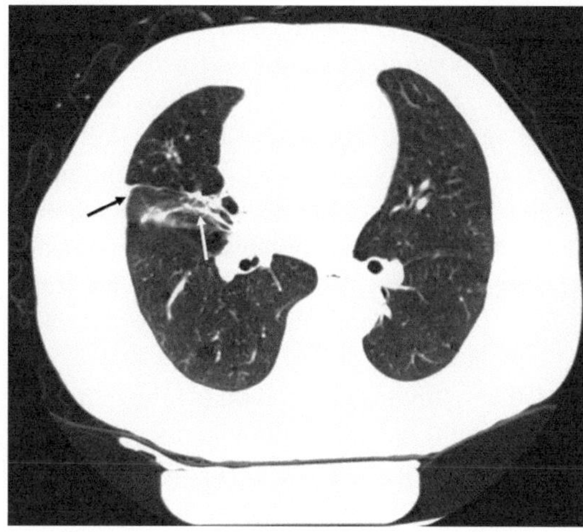

Fig. 4 Pleural thickening (*black arrow*), dense scar with calcification of the right middle lobe (*white arrow*)

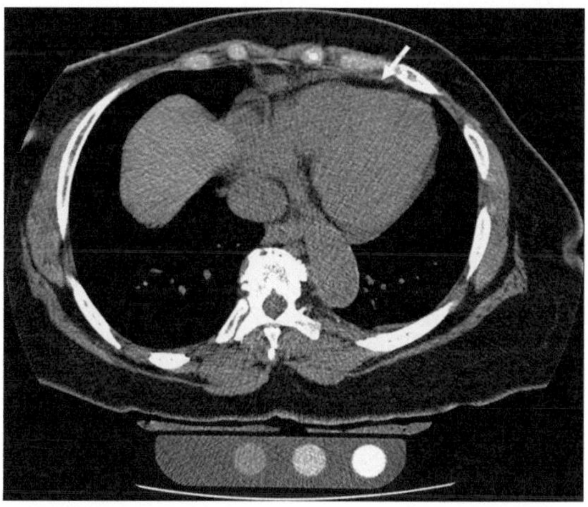

Fig. 3 Pericardial effusion

sent to the coordinating center. If on initial review, there was a significant or potentially significant finding, the report was then reviewed by a radiologist, experienced in the application of appropriate diagnostic criteria for an asymptomatic screening population. This second interpretation reviewed all initial clinical readings that were positive for any findings. This systematic approach allowed us to have timely reporting, while maintaining a consistent and evidence-based approach to the clinical reviews of the CT exams.

The reporting center provided the clinic and participant with a report on letterhead documenting the potential issue in clear language with a recommended next action. In addition to the reports, the CT reading center helped participants obtain copies of their images upon request if it proved difficult from the primary source, the site where the CT exam is performed. In addition, if requested by local physicians, cases were discussed and consulted. We did not collect data from follow-up and results of the workup of the incidental findings.

1 Significant Alerts

Alerts of potential and established significance were aortic aneurysms, dense aortic valve calcifications (aortic stenosis), lung masses (>3 cm), pneumonia, pneumothorax, and large pericardial effusions. These were communicated to field center PIs, or designee, directly:

(a) Aortic diameter >45 mm – aortic aneurysm screening is the only cardiovascular imaging modality ever shown to improve outcomes (Ashton et al. 2002). While this was an abdominal aortic aneurysm in the MAAS study, one can extrapolate that similar benefit may be obtained by evaluating ascending and descending thoracic aortic diameters.

(b) Aortic valve calcification score>500 has been shown to be associated with aortic stenosis, and follow-up echocardiography can be recommended for participants (Shavelle et al. 2003). This finding was exceptionally low in MESA to date but will slowly increase as the population continues to age. Estimated prevalence is <1 %. Figure 1 shows an example of incidental finding of aortic valve calcification.
(c) Other findings include lung masses (>30 mm), lobar pneumonia, pneumothorax, and large pericardial or pleural effusions, along with unusual findings deemed significant by the reading center.
(d) Nodules (noncalcified densities in the lung<30 mm). At the time of the study, there was no data to suggest that intervention on small nodules provides benefit, and some data suggest that there may be harm reporting asymptomatic nodules (cost, anxiety, follow-up tests, morbidity, and mortality). Given the average risk of the MESA population, the CT Committee agreed on a threshold of 8 mm. This modified the Fleischner Society guidelines, given the "intermediate risk" of the study population (risk for lung cancer, based on family history of lung cancer and smoking history) (MacMahon et al. 2005). Scans with nodules >8 mm in size prompted an evaluation of older scans for comparison. Nodules were not reported if unchanged from prior MESA scans (if available), as these were considered benign. Only solid nodules were considered. Nodule size was collected systematically in exam 1 and all nodules (including 1–2 mm) were reported. Figure 2 shows an incidental finding of a pulmonary nodule in the right lower lobe.
(e) Dense (non-cystic) lesions in the liver, spleen, and kidneys were reported.

In this way, we could focus on the primary reason for the study being performed, assessment of coronary, valve, and aortic findings, without unduly raising angst among participants about small lung nodules, which are quite ubiquitous in this population and almost universally benign, especially in a younger, largely nonsmoking population (Budoff et al. 2006; Budoff and Gopal 2007; Alfakih and Budoff 2011).

References

Agatston AS et al (1990) Quantification of coronary artery calcium using ultrafast computed tomography. J Am Coll Cardiol 15(4):827–832

Alfakih K, Budoff M (2011) Multi-detector computed tomography coronary angiography: the incidental lung findings. J R Soc Med 104(2):50–51

Ashton HA et al (2002) The Multicentre Aneurysm Screening Study (MASS) into the effect of abdominal aortic aneurysm screening on mortality in men: a randomised controlled trial. Lancet 360(9345):1531–1539

Bild DE et al (2002) Multi-Ethnic Study of Atherosclerosis: objectives and design. Am J Epidemiol 156(9): 871–881

Budoff MJ, Gopal A (2007) Incidental findings on cardiac computed tomography. Should we look? J Cardiovasc Comput Tomogr 1(2):97–105

Budoff MJ, Fischer H, Gopal A (2006) Incidental findings with cardiac CT evaluation: should we read beyond the heart? Catheter Cardiovasc Interv 68(6):965–973

Budoff MJ et al (2013a) Progression of coronary calcium and incident coronary heart disease events: MESA (Multi-Ethnic Study of Atherosclerosis). J Am Coll Cardiol 61(12):1231–1239

Budoff MJ et al (2013b) A comparison of outcomes with coronary artery calcium scanning in unselected populations: the Multi-Ethnic Study of Atherosclerosis (MESA) and Heinz Nixdorf RECALL study (HNR). J Cardiovasc Comput Tomogr 7(3):182–191

Carr JJ et al (2005) Calcified coronary artery plaque measurement with cardiac CT in population-based studies: standardized protocol of Multi-Ethnic Study of Atherosclerosis (MESA) and Coronary Artery Risk Development in Young Adults (CARDIA) study. Radiology 234(1):35–43

Detrano RC et al (2005) Coronary calcium measurements: effect of CT scanner type and calcium measure on rescan reproducibility--MESA study. Radiology 236(2):477–484

MacMahon H et al (2005) Guidelines for management of small pulmonary nodules detected on CT scans: a statement from the Fleischner Society. Radiology 237(2):395–400

Shavelle DM et al (2003) Usefulness of aortic valve calcium scores by electron beam computed tomography as a marker for aortic stenosis. Am J Cardiol 92(3): 349–353

Incidental Findings and Their Handling in the Swedish CArdioPulmonary bioImage Study (SCAPIS)

Åse Johnsson, Oskar Angerås, Anders Blomberg, David Erlinge, Agneta Flinck, Christer Janson, Hanna Markstad, Jonas Persson, Lennart Persson, Eva Swahn, Kjell Toren, Jenny Vikgren, Mats G. Hansson, and Göran Bergström

Contents

1 **Introduction** ... 92

2 **Computed Tomography Imaging** ... 93
2.1 Preparation of Subjects ... 94
2.2 CT Examination ... 94

3 **Pulmonary Nodules** ... 94
3.1 Guidelines for Follow-Up of Pulmonary Nodules ... 94
3.2 Handling of Incidental Pulmonary Nodules in the Pilot Trial ... 95
3.3 Handling of Incidental Pulmonary Nodules in the Main Trial ... 96

4 **Asymptomatic Coronary Artery Stenosis** ... 96
4.1 Guidelines for Follow-Up of Coronary Artery Stenosis ... 96
4.2 Challenges with Coronary Calcifications ... 97
4.3 Handling of Asymptomatic Coronary Stenosis in the Pilot Trial and in the Main Trial ... 97

5 **Ethics** ... 98

6 **Summary** ... 99

References ... 99

Å. Johnsson • A. Flinck • J. Vikgren
Department of Radiology, Sahlgrenska University Hospital, Gothenburg, Sweden

Department of Radiology, University of Gothenburg, Gothenburg, Sweden

O. Angerås
Department of Molecular and Clinical Medicine, University of Gothenburg, Gothenburg, Sweden

Department of Cardiology, Sahlgrenska University Hospital, Gothenburg, Sweden

A. Blomberg
Department of Public Health and Clinical Medicine, Division of Medicine/Respiratory Medicine, Umeå University, Umeå, Sweden

D. Erlinge
Department of Cardiology, Clinical Sciences, Lund University, Lund, Sweden

C. Janson
Department of Medical Sciences: Respiratory, Allergy and Sleep Research, Uppsala University, Uppsala, Sweden

H. Markstad
Department of Diagnostic Radiology, Lund University and Skåne University Hospital, Lund, Sweden

J. Persson
Division of Cardiovascular Medicine, Department of Clinical Sciences, Danderyd Hospital, Karolinska Institutet, Stockholm, Sweden

L. Persson • E. Swahn
Department of Medical and Health Sciences, Linköping University, Linköping, Sweden

K. Toren
Section of Occupational and Environmental Medicine, Institute of Medicine, University of Gothenburg, Gothenburg, Sweden

Med Radiol Diagn Imaging (2016)
DOI 10.1007/174_2016_52, © Springer International Publishing Switzerland
Published Online: 29 Mar 2016

M.G. Hansson
Department of Public Health and Caring Sciences, Centre for Research Ethics and Bioethics, Uppsala University, Uppsala, Sweden

G. Bergström (✉)
Department of Radiology, Sahlgrenska University Hospital, Gothenburg, Sweden

Department of Clinical Physiology, Sahlgrenska University Hospital, Gothenburg, Sweden

The Wallenberg Laboratory for Cardiovascular and Metabolic Research, Sahlgrenska University Hospital, Gothenburg, SE 413 45, Sweden
e-mail: Goran.bergstrom@hjl.gu.se

Abstract

The Swedish CArdioPulmonary bioImage Study (SCAPIS) combines the use of new imaging technologies, large-scale proteomics/metabolomics/genomics, and epidemiological analyses to extensively characterize a Swedish cohort of 30,000 men and women aged between 50 and 64 years. Its main aims are to improve risk prediction and to optimize our ability to study mechanisms of cardiopulmonary diseases. SCAPIS is currently recruiting at six sites in Sweden, and a pilot study was conducted in 2012 to test the feasibility of the comprehensive study protocol. In the planning phase, it was recognized that the detailed phenotyping used in SCAPIS would identify a large number of clinical findings in need of medical attention. This was confirmed by evaluation of results from the pilot study. Here we focus on pulmonary nodules and asymptomatic coronary artery stenosis. These clinical features were observed in a large number of participants, and the clinical handing and prognosis related to these observations are unclear. They thus posed great challenges for the study in their practical and ethical handling. This chapter describes how we developed procedures to handle these findings based on existing evidence and expert consensus as well as deliberations on ethical issues.

1 Introduction

The overall aim of the Swedish CArdioPulmonary bioImage Study (SCAPIS) is to extensively phenotype a Swedish cohort of 30,000 individuals (ages 50–64 years) and use the acquired information to improve risk stratification and to optimize conditions to characterize the mechanisms behind myocardial infarction (MI), stroke, and chronic obstructive pulmonary disease (COPD) and analyze the interaction between the cardiovascular diseases and COPD. SCAPIS was initiated in response to the recent changes in risk factor patterns for MI, stroke, and COPD (Capewell and Buchan 2012; GOLD 2015; Rosengren 2009), and aims to gain novel and updated information that is relevant in today's environment to identify and treat individuals with these diseases.

SCAPIS is currently recruiting subjects at six sites in Sweden and examinations are ongoing. A pilot trial of 1111 subjects was completed in 2012. Collection of baseline data in the main study was started in 2014 and will, according to plan, be completed by the end of 2018. A detailed description of the study protocol has recently been published (Bergstrom et al. 2015). Participants are randomly invited from the Swedish population registry and extensively phenotyped using validated questionnaires and a detailed examination as outlined in Fig. 1. The participation rate is around 50 %.

Imaging in SCAPIS focuses on cardiac, vascular, pulmonary, and metabolic profiling. Computed tomography (CT) is used to detect fat deposits in and around different organs. Multidetector CT (MDCT) of the lungs is used to detect and stage early signs of pulmonary disease, including emphysema and airway wall thickening. Atherosclerosis in the carotid arteries is assessed by ultrasound and, in participants with moderate-to-large plaques, magnetic resonance imaging (MRI). Coronary CT angiography (CCTA) is performed to detect plaques in the coronary arteries.

SCAPIS aims to combine these advanced imaging techniques with large-scale genotyping and recent developments in metabolomics and

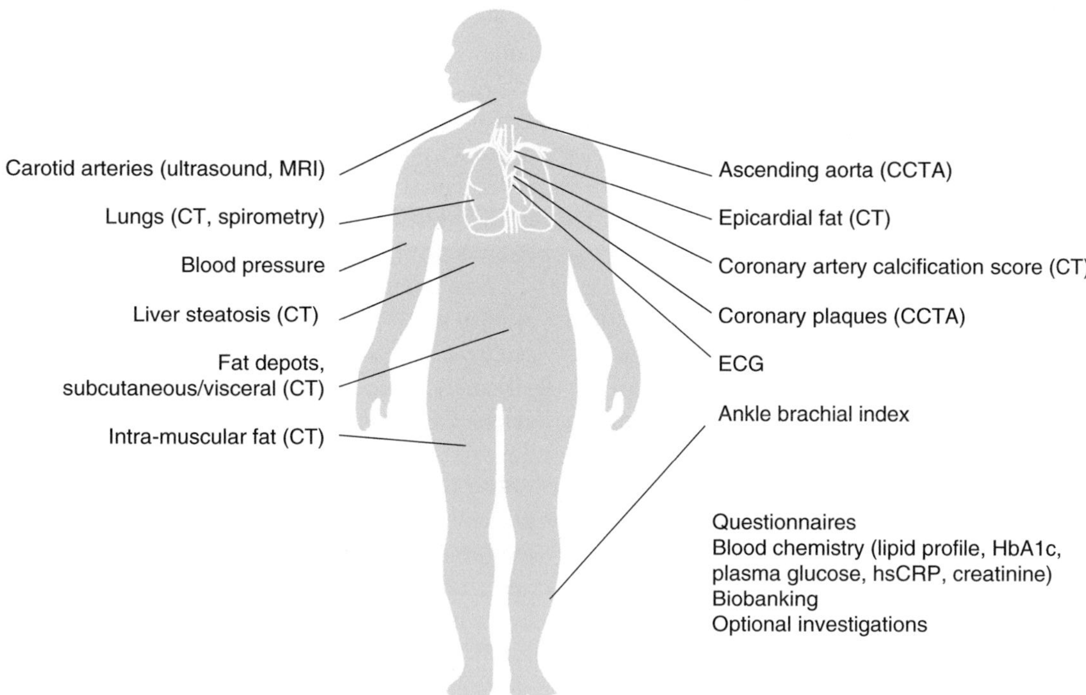

Fig. 1 Overview of the information collected from the subjects in SCAPIS. *MRI* magnetic resonance imaging, *CT* computed tomography, *CCTA* coronary computed tomography angiography, *ECG* electrocardiogram, *HbA1c* glycated hemoglobin, *hsCRP* high-sensitivity C-reactive protein (Adapted from Bergström et al. (2015).)

proteomics to build a unique data, blood and image bank, which will significantly contribute to improvements in the prediction of prognosis, prevention, and treatment of MI, stroke, and COPD. However, an inevitable consequence of exposing a large number of subjects to an extensive imaging protocol is that a considerable number of both expected and unexpected clinical findings will be identified. One of the main aims of the pilot study was to assess the volume and type of clinical findings that would arise and to develop a clinical workflow to handle them. Emphasis was put on addressing the ethical issues that inevitably would arise in either informing or choosing not to inform the subjects. Early on, the study organization decided that we had an ethical obligation to inform the subjects of all clinical findings that at the time of the examination were of relevance for the present or future health of a subject. In contrast, participants will not be individually informed on results arising as a result of future research.

Evaluation of the pilot study confirmed that a substantial number of clinical findings were identified in the clinically mostly healthy volunteers. Here we focus on our handling of pulmonary nodules and asymptomatic coronary artery stenosis found after imaging with CT – clinical features that were observed in a large number of participants and that posed great challenges for SCAPIS in their practical and ethical handling.

2 Computed Tomography Imaging

The following protocols were used for pulmonary and cardiac imaging in SCAPIS. The protocols can be found and were originally published as a supplemental file in Bergström et al. 2015. All computed tomography (CT) scanning is performed on a Somatom Definition Flash (Siemens Healthcare, Forchheim, West Germany) with a stellar detector. Care Dose 4D, Care kV, and

SAFIRE are used for dose optimization in some protocols. All sites are equipped with similar scanners and, in agreement with the vendor, no software or hardware updates are allowed during the study period.

2.1 Preparation of Subjects

Before undergoing a scan, subjects only eat light meals and avoid beverages containing stimulants (e.g., caffeine). Two hours before a scan, the participants are given a standardized meal (Modifast, Nutriton & Santé) calculated based on body mass index to achieve a stable metabolic state.

2.2 CT Examination

To plan the examination, topograms are performed in a lateral view of the thorax (scan length 512 mm) and an anterior-posterior view starting at the chin ending below the knee (scan length 1536 mm). For scan parameter details and protocol parameters, see Bergström et al. 2015.

2.2.1 Lung Images

Lung images are acquired using spiral scanning.

2.2.2 Cardiac Imaging: Coronary Artery Calcium Score (CACS) and Coronary CT Angiography (CCTA)

All cardiac imaging is ECG triggered. Renal function is assessed and potential contraindications identified to exclude subjects for whom contrast media administration could pose a risk.

Unless contraindicated, a β-blocker (metoprolol) is administered to the subjects to reduce heart rate to below 60 beats/min without too much reduction in blood pressure. This is done either 1.5 h before the scan by oral administration of 25–50 mg metoprolol and/or directly at the scan using intravenous administration of 2.5–15.0 mg metoprolol dependent on heart rate and blood pressure. In addition, subjects with a systolic blood pressure >110 mmHg are given two doses of sublingual glyceryl nitrate (4 mg/dose, GmbH & Co, KG).

For CCTA, the contrast media iohexol is administered (Omnipaque, GE Healthcare, 350 mgI/mL). The individual dose is 325 mg I/kg body weight, and the injection time is 12 s. To plan the contrast media delay time for the CCTA, a sequential scan covering 10 mm is performed using a test bolus of 10 ml contrast media (scan delay 8 s).

Two different CACS protocols are available. A flash spiral protocol is used for subjects with a body weight ≤90 kg and a regular heart rate. For all others, a sequential protocol is used. Five different CCTA protocols are used; the choice is determined according to heart rate, the regularity of the heart rate, and body weight. CCTA 1 is chosen if there are no calcifications on CACS, the subject has a regular heart rate ≤60 beats/min and a body weight ≤85 kg. CCTA 2 is chosen if heart rate is relatively stable (≤75 beats/min) and if the CT system can deliver a sufficient radiation dose for desired image quality. This is mainly related to the size of the subject. CCTA 3 is chosen if heart rate is relatively stable (>75 beats/min), and the CT system can deliver a sufficient radiation dose for the desired image quality. CCTA 4a and 4b are chosen when the heart rate is relatively stable, but radiation dose in relation to the size of the subject needs to be increased to reach an optimal image quality. It is done by using either a sequential technique with increased rotation time (0.33 s) or a spiral technique using both x-ray tubes. For the spiral technique, the pitch is chosen according to heart rate. CCTA 5 is chosen if the subject has an irregular heartbeat (e.g., atrial fibrillation or if the electrocardiogram indicates a variance of heart rate exceeding 4 beats/min). The protocol uses a spiral technique, and the pitch is chosen according to heart rate.

3 Pulmonary Nodules

3.1 Guidelines for Follow-Up of Pulmonary Nodules

A pulmonary nodule identified by CT is defined as a rounded or irregular opacity that measures up to 3 cm in diameter and that may be solid, part-solid, or non-solid (also known as a ground-glass nodule) (Hansell et al. 2008). Before the widespread use of CT, the accepted standard of care was to regard all non-calcified pulmonary nodules as potentially malignant lesions until proven stable over a period of 2 years (Tan et al. 2003). With increasing evidence in the scientific literature indicating that very few small nodules (<4–5 mm) would prove to be malignant over a 2-year period, the Fleischner Society proposed new guidelines in 2005 (MacMahon et al. 2005). These recommendations state: no follow-up for low-risk patients with nodules ≤4 mm; 1–3 follow-up CT scans for up to 2 years (depending on nodule size and patient risk factors) for solid nodules measuring 4–8 mm (longer follow-up time for ground-glass and part-solid lesions); and that further investigations such as positron emission tomography, percutaneous needle biopsy, or thoracoscopic resection for nodules >8 mm could be considered (MacMahon et al. 2005). A recent addition to these guidelines stated that non-solid lesions >5 mm and part-solid lesions should have an initial follow-up with CT at 3 months, with yearly follow-up for up to 3 years if the nodule is unchanged or biopsy or resection if the solid part measures ≥5 mm at the 3-month follow-up (Naidich et al. 2013). There is currently no lung cancer screening program in Sweden, but recently published national guidelines (Cancercentrum 2015), published after the pilot SCAPIS adhere to the previously mentioned recommendations regarding the handling of incidentally detected pulmonary nodules (MacMahon et al. 2005; Naidich et al. 2013).

In addition to nodule size, morphological characteristics of the nodule should be evaluated. Pseudocavitation, air bronchograms, cavitation, spiculation, non-solid components, and punctate and eccentric calcification are considered as features of a malignant nodule (Edey and Hansell 2009). Central, diffuse, or laminated calcification suggests a benign lesion, and the combination of fat and calcification indicates a hamartoma. It is also important to recognize benign perifissural nodules to reduce the number of follow-up examinations required for the workup of suspicious nodules (de Hoop et al. 2012).

3.2 Handling of Incidental Pulmonary Nodules in the Pilot Trial

The recommended follow-up CT examinations aim at detecting nodule growth, which is a strong lung cancer predictor (Gould et al. 2013). Both the inclusion of nodules into follow-up schemes and the detection of nodule growth are highly dependent on measurement accuracy, where the variability of two-dimensional measurements and challenges in sometimes segmenting reliable 3D volumes are well-known problems (Nair et al. 2012). The detection rates of small pulmonary nodules are influenced by a number of factors. The reconstructed slice thickness of the CT scan is one of the most important technical parameters, and the use of maximum intensity projection (MIP), volume-rendered slabs, or computer-assisted detection improves nodule detection when compared with evaluation of standard axial images (Edey and Hansell 2009).

In the pilot SCAPIS, the radiologists evaluated the participant's chest CT examinations by reviewing submillimeter as well as thicker MIP slices with the purpose of improving the nodule detection rate. Detected nodules were morphologically characterized, and two-dimensional measurements were performed at a standardized small display field of view to reduce measurement variability. Solid nodules measuring ≤4 mm were reported only in the electronic case reporting file (eCRF) because of the low anticipated risk of a malignant lesion. All participants with nodules ≥5 mm, where definite benign characteristics could not be established, were referred to the pulmonary medicine department. For participants with solid nodules measuring ≥10 mm, further workup was suggested, whereas participants with solid nodules measuring 5–9 mm had a recommendation of CT surveillance at 6, 12, and 24 months. The limit of 10 mm was chosen based on awareness of measurement variability and in accordance with the clinical routine in the west region of Sweden at the time of the study. Follow-up was also recommended for participants with part-solid and non-solid nodules measuring 5–10 mm.

In total, around 40 % of the 1111 participants in the pilot SCAPIS presented with pulmonary nodules, around 11 % of the population were referred to the pulmonary medicine department, and CT surveillance was recommended for around 10 %. The majority of the participants completed their follow-up CT examinations and, as expected, very few nodules exhibited detectable growth even when nodule volumes were measured.

3.3 Handling of Incidental Pulmonary Nodules in the Main Trial

The health-care resources required to follow-up the incidentally detected nodules in the pilot SCAPIS became a major concern and threatened the feasibility of the full-scale SCAPIS. In September 2013, the lung expert group of SCAPIS met with representatives from the NELSON trial and discussed at that timepoint unpublished data, which was later published by Horeweg et al. (2014). As a result of this meeting, SCAPIS decided to implement the following: A finding of a solid nodule with a volume <100 mm^3 should only be reported in the eCRF. This decision was based on results from the NELSON trial showing that lung cancer probability did not significantly differ between participants who had nodules measuring <100 mm^3 and those who had no detected nodules. Participants with a solid nodule measuring ≥300 mm^3 should be referred to pulmonary medicine specialists for additional workup, as this finding has been shown to indicate a participant at high risk of developing lung cancer (Horeweg et al. 2014). Participants with solid nodules measuring 100–299 mm^3 should be scheduled for a follow-up CT scan at 3 months, and smokers should have an additional follow-up CT scan at 24 months.

In the first year of SCAPIS at the Gothenburg site (n = 1719), the revised strategy compared with the pilot trial has reduced the number of participants referred to CT surveillance and direct clinical workup down to around 7 % and 2 %, respectively (Note: data on solid nodules only). It was also decided that the determination of nodule growth in the follow-up CT scans should be based on volumetric analysis and volume doubling time as suggested from the analysis of data from the NELSON trial (Horeweg et al. 2014).

Participants identified with non-solid and part-solid nodules are followed up in SCAPIS in accordance with the recently published Swedish national recommendation for such nodules: an initial follow-up with CT at 3 months for nodules ≥5 mm, with yearly follow-up CT surveillance for up to 36 months or clinical work-up depending on nodule characteristics (Cancercentrum 2015).

Recently, the cost-effectiveness of follow-up of incidentally detected pulmonary nodules on CT has been questioned (Goehler et al. 2014). Although nodule follow-up programs are expected to result in a small reduction in lung cancer mortality, the cost is substantial per quality-adjusted life-year, especially in non-smokers (Goehler et al. 2014).

4 Asymptomatic Coronary Artery Stenosis

4.1 Guidelines for Follow-Up of Coronary Artery Stenosis

In the current European Society of Cardiology (ESC) guidelines, a patient with documented coronary artery disease (CAD) is categorized as having a >10 % risk for cardiovascular death within 10 years (Perk et al. 2012). Documented CAD is defined as a positive invasive or non-invasive test, e.g., invasive coronary angiography (ICA) or nuclear imaging, or previous CAD, peripheral artery disease, or ischemic stroke.

In SCAPIS, CCTA is used to investigate plaques in coronary arteries and will therefore uncover cases of obstructive CAD. However, the ESC guidelines do not explicitly refer to CCTA-identified CAD in a sample of randomly selected mostly healthy subjects and are therefore difficult to directly apply to the SCAPIS population. Furthermore, because CCTA has previously not been used in such a large cohort of mostly healthy, asymptomatic subjects randomly invited to an examination, there is almost a complete lack of information on prognosis and no valid guidelines exist on which treatment to recommend and who should be further evaluated.

Several studies have shown an association between CCTA-identified CAD, both non-obstructive and obstructive, and mortality (Ostrom et al. 2008; Hadamitzky et al. 2009; Abdulla et al. 2011; Chow et al. 2011). CONFIRM (Coronary CT Angiography Evaluation for Clinical Outcomes: An International Multicenter Registry) recently published a follow-up of 7950 patients without chest pain and reported that the 2.5 year mortality rate was 4.1 % in patients with obstructive CAD and 1.7 % in patients without obstructive CAD (Cho et al. 2012). Patients with high-risk CAD (defined as left main stenosis >50 % or 3-vessel disease) have worse prognosis regardless of whether the patient is symptomatic or not (Chow et al. 2011; Cho et al. 2012).

4.2 Challenges with Coronary Calcifications

Plaques with large calcifications are a challenge to CCTA and tend to cause an artifact commonly called calcium blooming, which can result in overestimating the degree of obstruction caused by the plaque or in some cases prevent assessment of the plaque (Kroft et al. 2007; Dey et al. 2008). Calcium blooming is one explanation for why the positive predictive value of CCTA is low compared with invasive coronary angiography (ICA) (Husmann et al. 2008).

The degree of coronary calcification can also be assessed by calculating the calcium score using CT (Agatston et al. 1990). Calcium score predicts risk of mortality in asymptomatic patients independently of traditional risk scores, e.g., Framingham risk score (Budoff et al. 2007). Calcium score has an independent predictive value for mortality and performs best in patients with intermediate risk of cardiovascular events (Nakanishi et al. 2015), but the association in high-risk patients is also strong (Shaw et al. 2006; Raggi et al. 2004). In general, a calcium score of zero is associated with low risk, between 100 and 400 intermediate risk and >400 with high risk (Budoff et al. 2007; Erbel et al. 2010; Hou et al. 2012).

4.3 Handling of Asymptomatic Coronary Stenosis in the Pilot Trial and in the Main Trial

Because increasing evidence indicates an association between obstructive CAD (>50 %) on CCTA or high calcium score (>400) with worse outcome, the SCAPIS expert group found it reasonable to include these findings in the definition of documented CAD. In the pilot trial of SCAPIS, approximately 15 % of the subjects without prevalent CAD or signs of chest pain from the Rose questionnaire (Rose 1962; Hemingway et al. 2008) presented with either a ≥50 % stenosis in any coronary artery, extensive calcium blooming or a calcium score >400 suggesting a high risk.

There was considerable discussion within the SCAPIS expert group in cardiology on how to best treat these individuals, which resulted in the development of an algorithm to handle CCTA findings (Table 1). The algorithm was first tested in the pilot trial and later slightly modified for use in the full trial.

All patients with obstructive CAD (defined as >50 % diameter obstruction of any coronary artery on CCTA) are recommended lifestyle changes (smoking cessation and regular physical activity) and medical prevention to reach the following goals: body mass index <25 kg/m^2, waist circumference <94 cm (men) or <80 cm (women), blood pressure <140/90 mmHg, total cholesterol <4.5 mmol/L, LDL cholesterol <2.5 mmol/L, and, for those with diabetes, fasting glycemia <7.0 mmol/L and HbA1C<48 mmol/mol. The use of aspirin to prevent major cardiovascular events in asymptomatic patients is not recommended according to the ESC guidelines (Perk et al. 2012). Asymptomatic patients are recommended ICA when high-risk CAD is suspected, i.e., stenosis in left main stem, proximal left anterior descending coronary artery, or in all three major coronary

Table 1 Algorithm for managing CCTA findings in SCAPIS

	Condition	Action	Follow-up responsibility
1	>50 % stenosis of the left main stem, proximal LAD, or in all three coronary arteries (regardless of symptoms)	Angio and lifestyle changes plus medical intervention according to risk algorithm	Appropriate action for follow-up is made by the responsible research physician in cooperation with local cardiological expertise
2	>50 % stenosis in 1–2 larger coronary arteries (>2.5 mm) and symptomatic	Angio and lifestyle changes plus medical intervention according to risk algorithm	Appropriate action for follow-up is made by the responsible research physician in cooperation with local cardiological expertise
3	>50 % stenosis in 1–2 larger coronary arteries and asymptomatic	Lifestyle changes and medical intervention according to risk algorithm	Research physician (or equivalent) refers to primary care according to standard referral template
4	Calcium blooming prevents assessment of the degree of stenosis in the left main stem or proximal LAD = case for discussion Calcium score > 400 in subjects not having undergone CTA = case for discussion	Angio and/or lifestyle changes and medical intervention according to risk algorithm	Appropriate action for follow-up is made by the responsible research physician in cooperation with local cardiological expertise
5	Calcium blooming prevents assessment of the degree of stenosis in other blood vessels	Lifestyle changes and medical intervention according to risk algorithm	Research physician (or equivalent) refers to primary care according to standard referral template

Optimal medical treatment is given according to a risk algorithm based on the ESC recommendations for risk factor intervention in established CAD (Perk et al. 2012)

arteries. Participants in whom calcium blooming prevents assessment of the degree of obstruction in proximal arteries or have a calcium score >400 but are not able to undergo CCTA are subject to an individualized risk estimation by a cardiologist before ICA is recommended.

Because the positive predictive value of CCTA is relatively low, it is important to confirm the CAD visualized by CCTA using ICA. We do not have firm study data on this as yet, but a substantial number of overestimated coronary obstructions from CCTA have been reported. It is also important to determine that the stenosis visualized causes ischemia and the expert group recommends that intermediate lesions are examined by fractional flow reserve (FFR) measurement before decision on revascularization (Tonino et al. 2009). The method of revascularization is at the discretion of the interventionist and in discussion with the subject.

5 Ethics

The management of incidental findings within SCAPIS is based on a widely accepted ethical framework (Wolf et al. 2012; Wolf et al. 2008). The central requirements of this framework are that: (i) each research project for which there is reason to expect findings that are not directly related to the aims of the study should clarify the criteria for evaluating such findings and define a list of manageable findings; (ii) then analyze a particular finding and decide whether it belongs to the list; and (iii) contact the subject and provide information in a way that is sensitive to the implications of the finding and the particular need of a given subject. This should be done if a finding is: (i) analytically valid; (ii) associated with an established and substantial risk of a serious health condition; and (iii) clinically actionable, e.g., in terms of treatment and prevention.

Within the ethics literature, the arguments for disclosure may be summarized as follows (Viberg et al. 2014):

(i) Disclosure may be beneficial for the individual participant while minimizing harm.
(ii) Disclosure promotes autonomy. If individual participants get important information in time, they can change their lives and therefore be more autonomous; by knowing, individuals can take control of their life and direct it as they wish. Respect for persons includes respect for participants' self-determination and therefore also for their need to have information relevant to their health and well-being.
(iii) Reciprocity requires disclosure. Reciprocity between researchers and participants can be maintained by giving participants something in return for their decision to participate (in this case, individual research results). It has been emphasized that participants' contribution to research cannot be assumed to be purely altruistic with no expectations of some personal gain, including knowledge, in return.
(iv) Return of incidental findings accords with participants' wishes. Empirical surveys show that many want to receive individual results (Murphy et al. 2008; Meulenkamp et al. 2010).

Against this, it has been argued that:

(i) The relationship between a researcher and a research subject does not create a duty in the same sense as a doctor would have a duty to his or her own patient because they do not have the same close relationship and researchers may not be trained in the necessary counseling skills.
(ii) Disclosure can be harmful to individual participants, creating anxiety and distress, without much benefit in terms of treatment or prevention to offer.
(iii) Disclosure may also be harmful to research and jeopardize the scientific validity of the study because of changes in behavior or selective dropouts.

SCAPIS has tried to balance the advantages and disadvantages of disclosure of incidental findings in a management policy suggesting that results should be disclosed if they can enhance treatment, concern a material risk, have clinical utility, and/or are life saving. At the same time, this imposes a great responsibility on those providing the information because of its characteristic feature of being based on risk estimates, sometimes of unclear predictive value (Viberg et al. 2015). To further address these issues, SCAPIS has initiated two research projects, supported by the Swedish Heart Lung Foundation, to examine the perceptions and effects of risk communication in association with the trial.

6 Summary

In SCAPIS, pulmonary nodules and asymptomatic coronary artery stenosis will be observed in a large number of participants and present great challenges for the study in their practical and ethical handling. In the pilot trial, extensive follow-up of pulmonary nodules was a logistical threat to the study. However, after critical appraisal of available evidence, a revised plan for follow-up was developed based on volumetric analysis and volume doubling time. The focus of this revised plan is to follow-up individuals at greatest risk and to limit unnecessary follow-up and worry among study participants. A finding of significant CAD (>50 % obstruction or calcium score >400) in asymptomatic individuals in SCAPIS is taken seriously and is further evaluated using dedicated decision algorithms.

References

Abdulla J, Asferg C, Kofoed KF (2011) Prognostic value of absence or presence of coronary artery disease determined by 64-slice computed tomography coronary angiography a systematic review and meta-analysis. Int J Cardiovasc Imaging 27(3):413–420

Agatston AS, Janowitz WR, Hildner FJ, Zusmer NR, Viamonte M Jr, Detrano R (1990) Quantification of coronary artery calcium using ultrafast computed tomography. J Am Coll Cardiol 15(4):827–832

Bergstrom G, Berglund G, Blomberg A, Brandberg J, Engstrom G, Engvall J et al (2015) The Swedish CArdioPulmonary BioImage Study: objectives and design. J Intern Med 278(6):645–659

Budoff MJ, Shaw LJ, Liu ST, Weinstein SR, Mosler TP, Tseng PH et al (2007) Long-term prognosis associated with coronary calcification: observations from a registry of 25,253 patients. J Am Coll Cardiol 49(18): 1860–1870

Cancercentrum R (2015) Swedish national guidelines for lung cancer 2015 http://www.cancercentrum.se/samverkan/cancerdiagnoser/lunga-och-lungsack/vardprogram/2015

Capewell S, Buchan I (2012) Why have sustained increases in obesity and type 2 diabetes not offset declines in cardiovascular mortality over recent decades in Western countries? Nutr Metab Cardiovasc Dis NMCD 22(4):307–311

Cho I, Chang HJ, Sung JM, Pencina MJ, Lin FY, Dunning AM et al (2012) Coronary computed tomographic angiography and risk of all-cause mortality and nonfatal myocardial infarction in subjects without chest pain syndrome from the CONFIRM Registry (coronary CT angiography evaluation for clinical outcomes: an international multicenter registry). Circulation 126(3):304–313

Chow BJ, Small G, Yam Y, Chen L, Achenbach S, Al-Mallah M et al (2011) Incremental prognostic value of cardiac computed tomography in coronary artery disease using CONFIRM: COroNary computed tomography angiography evaluation for clinical outcomes: an InteRnational Multicenter registry. Circ Cardiovasc Imaging 4(5):463–472

de Hoop B, van Ginneken B, Gietema H, Prokop M (2012) Pulmonary perifissural nodules on CT scans: rapid growth is not a predictor of malignancy. Radiology 265(2):611–616

Dey D, Lee CJ, Ohba M, Gutstein A, Slomka PJ, Cheng V et al (2008) Image quality and artifacts in coronary CT angiography with dual-source CT: initial clinical experience. J Cardiovasc Comput Tomogr 2(2):105–114

Edey AJ, Hansell DM (2009) Incidentally detected small pulmonary nodules on CT. Clin Radiol 64(9): 872–884

Erbel R, Mohlenkamp S, Moebus S, Schmermund A, Lehmann N, Stang A et al (2010) Coronary risk stratification, discrimination, and reclassification improvement based on quantification of subclinical coronary atherosclerosis: the Heinz Nixdorf Recall study. J Am Coll Cardiol 56(17):1397–1406

GOLD (2015) Global strategy for the diagnosis, management, and prevention of COPD. http://www.goldcopd.org/uploads/users/files/GOLD_Report_2015.pdf.

Goehler A, McMahon PM, Lumish HS, Wu CC, Munshi V, Gilmore M et al (2014) Cost-effectiveness of follow-up of pulmonary nodules incidentally detected on cardiac computed tomographic angiography in patients with suspected coronary artery disease. Circulation 130(8):668–675

Gould MK, Donington J, Lynch WR, Mazzone PJ, Midthun DE, Naidich DP et al (2013) Evaluation of individuals with pulmonary nodules: when is it lung cancer? Diagnosis and management of lung cancer, 3rd ed: American College of Chest Physicians evidence-based clinical practice guidelines. Chest 143(5 Suppl):e93S–e120S

Hadamitzky M, Freissmuth B, Meyer T, Hein F, Kastrati A, Martinoff S et al (2009) Prognostic value of coronary computed tomographic angiography for prediction of cardiac events in patients with suspected coronary artery disease. JACC Cardiovasc Imaging 2(4):404–411

Hansell DM, Bankier AA, MacMahon H, McLoud TC, Muller NL, Remy J (2008) Fleischner Society: glossary of terms for thoracic imaging. Radiology 246(3):697–722

Hemingway H, Langenberg C, Damant J, Frost C, Pyorala K, Barrett-Connor E (2008) Prevalence of angina in women versus men: a systematic review and meta-analysis of international variations across 31 countries. Circulation 117(12):1526–1536

Horeweg N, van Rosmalen J, Heuvelmans MA, van der Aalst CM, Vliegenthart R, Scholten ET et al (2014) Lung cancer probability in patients with CT-detected pulmonary nodules: a prespecified analysis of data from the NELSON trial of low-dose CT screening. Lancet Oncol 15(12):1332–1341

Hou ZH, Lu B, Gao Y, Jiang SL, Wang Y, Li W et al (2012) Prognostic value of coronary CT angiography and calcium score for major adverse cardiac events in outpatients. JACC Cardiovasc Imaging 5(10):990–999

Husmann L, Schepis T, Scheffel H, Gaemperli O, Leschka S, Valenta I et al (2008) Comparison of diagnostic accuracy of 64-slice computed tomography coronary angiography in patients with low, intermediate, and high cardiovascular risk. Acad Radiol 15(4):452–461

Kroft LJM, de Roos A, Geleijns J (2007) Artifacts in ECG-synchronized MDCT coronary angiography. Am J Roentgenol 189(3):581–591

MacMahon H, Austin JH, Gamsu G, Herold CJ, Jett JR, Naidich DP et al (2005) Guidelines for management of small pulmonary nodules detected on CT scans: a statement from the Fleischner Society. Radiology 237(2):395–400

Meulenkamp TM, Gevers SK, Bovenberg JA, Koppelman GH, van Hylckama Vlieg A, Smets EM (2010) Communication of biobanks' research results: what do (potential) participants want? Am J Med Genet A 152A(10):2482–2492

Murphy J, Scott J, Kaufman D, Geller G, LeRoy L, Hudson K (2008) Public expectations for return of results from large-cohort genetic research. Am J Bioeth 8(11):36–43

Naidich DP, Bankier AA, MacMahon H, Schaefer-Prokop CM, Pistolesi M, Goo JM et al (2013) Recommendations for the management of subsolid pulmonary nodules detected at CT: a statement from the Fleischner Society. Radiology 266(1):304–317

Nair A, Baldwin DR, Field JK, Hansell DM, Devaraj A (2012) Measurement methods and algorithms for the management of solid nodules. J Thorac Imaging 27(4):230–239

Nakanishi R, Li D, Blaha MJ, Whelton SP, Darabian S, Flores FR et al (2015) All-cause mortality by age and gender based on coronary artery calcium scores. Eur Heart J Cardiovasc Imaging Dec 24. pii: jev328. [Epub ahead of print]

Ostrom MP, Gopal A, Ahmadi N, Nasir K, Yang E, Kakadiaris I et al (2008) Mortality incidence and the severity of coronary atherosclerosis assessed by computed tomography angiography. J Am Coll Cardiol 52(16):1335–1343

Perk J, De Backer G, Gohlke H, Graham I, Reiner Z, Verschuren M et al (2012) European Guidelines on cardiovascular disease prevention in clinical practice (version 2012). The Fifth Joint Task Force of the European Society of Cardiology and Other Societies on Cardiovascular Disease Prevention in Clinical Practice (constituted by representatives of nine societies and by invited experts). Eur Heart J 33(13):1635–1701

Raggi P, Shaw LJ, Berman DS, Callister TQ (2004) Prognostic value of coronary artery calcium screening in subjects with and without diabetes. J Am Coll Cardiol 43(9):1663–1669

Rose GA (1962) The diagnosis of ischaemic heart pain and intermittent claudication in field surveys. Bull World Health Organ 27:645–658

Rosengren A (2009) Declining cardiovascular mortality and increasing obesity: a paradox. Can Med Assoc J 181(3-4):127–128

Shaw LJ, Raggi P, Callister TQ, Berman DS (2006) Prognostic value of coronary artery calcium screening in asymptomatic smokers and non-smokers. Eur Heart J 27(8):968–975

Tan BB, Flaherty KR, Kazerooni EA, Iannettoni MD, American College of Chest P (2003) The solitary pulmonary nodule. Chest 123(1 Suppl):89S–96S

Tonino PA, De Bruyne B, Pijls NH, Siebert U, Ikeno F, Van't Veer M et al (2009) Fractional flow reserve versus angiography for guiding percutaneous coronary intervention. N Engl J Med 360(3):213–224

Viberg J, Hansson MG, Langenskiold S, Segerdahl P (2014) Incidental findings: the time is not yet ripe for a policy for biobanks. Eur J Hum Genet 22(4): 437–441

Viberg J, Segerdahl P, Langenskiold S, Hansson MG (2015) Freedom of choice about incidental findings can frustrate participants' true preferences. Bioethics 30(3):203–209

Wolf SM, Lawrenz FP, Nelson CA, Kahn JP, Cho MK, Clayton EW et al (2008) Managing incidental findings in human subjects research: analysis and recommendations. J Law Med Ethics 36(2):219–248, 1

Wolf SM, Crock BN, Van Ness B, Lawrenz F, Kahn JP, Beskow LM et al (2012) Managing incidental findings and research results in genomic research involving biobanks and archived data sets. Genet Med 14(4): 361–384

Part IV

Differences Between IF in Population Based Imaging and Patients

Management of Incidental Findings in Patients

Katharina Müller-Peltzer, Melvin D' Anastasi and Wieland Sommer

Contents

1 **Pulmonary Incidental Findings** 106
1.1 Small Pulmonary Nodules 106
1.2 Subsolid Pulmonary Nodules 106
1.3 Pulmonary Perifissural Nodules 107

2 **Abdominal Incidental Findings** 107
2.1 Cystic Renal Mass 107
2.2 Liver Mass 108
2.3 Adrenal Mass 108
2.4 Adnexal Findings 109

3 **Summary** 110

References 110

K. Müller-Peltzer, MD (✉) • M. D'Anastasi, MD
W. Sommer, MD
Institute of Clinical Radiology, Ludwig-Maximilians-University Hospital, Munich, Bavaria, Germany

There are major differences how to deal with incidental findings in study participants and patients. While a study participant might see himself as part of a research project, he is less likely to expect diagnoses from cross-sectional imaging examinations. In contrast, a patient in a clinical setting undergoes imaging examinations for a particular reason, that is, to exclude, confirm, or follow up a certain diagnosis. Therefore, the patient expects a particular – positive or negative – report related to the original clinical question. Additional findings not related to the initial indication for the examination are generally reported. These incidental findings need to be handled carefully both by the reporting radiologist and by the physician in charge. Well-considered recommendations given by the radiologist are the most important part of handling incidental findings responsibly. Depending on certain parameters, such as the chosen modality or the image quality, differentiating between "normal" and "pathological" becomes a real challenge for several incidental findings. The reporting radiologist has to decide how to report and assess those incidental findings. By now, there are several recommendations by different societies and committees that can help radiologists in the assessment of incidental findings. In this chapter, we aim to give a brief overview of the most helpful recommendations, which refer to the most frequently occurring incidental findings on thoracic and abdominal CT or MRI.

Med Radiol Diagn Imaging (2017)
DOI 10.1007/174_2016_78, © Springer International Publishing Switzerland
Published Online: 03 Feb 2017

1 Pulmonary Incidental Findings

For the assessment of pulmonary nodules, the guidelines of the Fleischner Society are well established. Their recommendations for solid and subsolid lung nodules can help the radiologist in classifying a finding as (most likely) benign and advising follow-up examinations.

1.1 Small Pulmonary Nodules

Small pulmonary nodules are very common findings. They can be detected in scans that involve the whole chest, for example, a trauma scan after a car crash, as well as in scans that only show parts of the lung parenchyma such as a contrast-enhanced CT scan of the supra-aortic arteries. The likelihood increases with the age of the patient collective, and is higher in smokers than in nonsmokers. With current modern scanners, detecting even the smallest nodules with 1–2 mm in diameter has become routine. Since only a slight percentage of incidentally detected, small pulmonary nodules will be malignant, controlling all of them several times is not feasible. Therefore, the Fleischner Society published a position paper in 2005 (MacMahon et al. 2005). This paper should provide practical guidelines for the management of incidentally detected, small pulmonary nodules. The given recommendations apply to adult patients (>35 years) without any known or suspected malignant disease and without fever. The guidelines are based on several follow-up studies evaluating the risk of having or developing lung cancer when a small pulmonary nodule is found. For this assessment, several characteristics of incidental, small pulmonary nodules need to be taken into consideration, such as nodule size, growth rate, and risk factors: the larger the nodule the more likely it is malignant, and follow-ups need to be more frequent. Growth rates of lung nodules differ between ground-glass opacities, ground-glass opacities with a solid component, and solid nodules, with solid nodules showing the shortest mean volume-doubling time. Furthermore, the relative risk for developing lung carcinoma is an important parameter, with smoking being the most important risk factor. For example, the Fleischner Society follow-up and management recommendations for incidentally detected, small pulmonary nodules say that no follow-up is needed for a nodule smaller than 4 mm in a patient with a minimal or absent history of smoking and of other known risk factors. If a nodule of the same size is found in a patient with a history of smoking or with other known risk factors, a follow-up CT after 12 months is recommended. If the nodule size is unchanged, no further scans are required. But, it needs to be considered that a ground-glass or partly solid nodule may require a longer follow-up to exclude indolent adenocarcinoma due to a longer mean volume-doubling time of nonsolid nodules (MacMahon et al. 2005). Equivalent recommendations are given for nodules with a size between 4 and 6 mm, 6 and 8 mm, and for those larger than 8 mm (for further details, please see the table "Recommendations for follow-up and management of nodules smaller than 8 mm detected incidentally at non-screening CT" (MacMahon et al. 2005)).

1.2 Subsolid Pulmonary Nodules

The recommendations mentioned above already cover a significant proportion of the different types of incidentally detected lung nodules. However, these guidelines lack a detailed consideration of subsolid lung nodules. Therefore, the Fleischner Society provided additional recommendations for the management of subsolid pulmonary nodules in 2012 (Naidich et al. 2013). The term "subsolid" in this paper encompasses the entity of "pure ground-glass nodules" (pure GGN) where no solid component is present and the "part-solid ground-glass nodules" (part-solid GGN) that include a solid component. An important difference between the guidelines from 2005 and the additional recommendations from 2012 is that there is no low-risk/high-risk distinction between smokers and nonsmokers. The main characteristics are the overall size of the lesion(s) and the size of the solid component, if present.

For image acquisition and quality, contiguous thin sections (1 mm) reconstructed with narrow and/or mediastinal windows are recommended to evaluate the solid component. Additionally, wide and/or lung windows will be needed to evaluate the nonsolid component of nodules. The authors further advise the use of a consistent low-dose technique.This is of particular importance in cases for which prolonged follow-up scans are recommended as well as in younger patients. If several scans are available over time, it is important to always compare with the original baseline study to detect subtle changes in growth (Naidich et al. 2013). For example, a solitary, pure GGN ≤5 mm would not require a follow-up CT scan according to the "Recommendations for the management of subsolid pulmonary nodules detected at CT.". Whereas a solitary, pure GGN >5 mm requires a follow-up at 3 months. If the GGN is unchanged in this scan, an annual surveillance for a minimum of 3 years is recommended. If multiple, pure GGN ≤5 mm are found, a follow-up at 2 and 4 years is recommended, and alternate causes for those multiple nodules should be considered. (For supplementary details, please see the table "Recommendations for the management of subsolid pulmonary nodules detected at CT" (Naidich et al. 2013)).

1.3 Pulmonary Perifissural Nodules

Pulmonary perifissural nodules (PFN) represent another important entity of pulmonary nodules commonly seen on chest scans. It is likely that the majority of these nodules represent lymph nodes. This can be hypothesized by their demonstrated growth rate (they can expand or regress over time), morphological features, and resected PFN. Adequate assessment of pulmonary nodules as PFN plays an important role in reducing the number of recommended follow-up scans. Within the framework of the Dutch–Belgian Randomised Lung Cancer Screening Trial (NELSON), de Hoop et al. have been evaluating PFN over time. Perifissural nodules have been categorized as typical PFN, atypical PFN, and non-PFN. A typical PFN was defined as fissure-attached, homogeneous, solid nodule with smooth margins and a triangular, lentiform, or oval shape. An atypical PFN was not fissure-attached, but perifissural, otherwise showing all features of a typical PFN. All other nodules not meeting these criteria were defined as non-PFN, including spherical or speculated nodules. In the study of de Hoop et al., none of the typical or atypical-defined PFN showed signs of malignancy in the 5.5 years of follow-up (de Hoop et al. 2012).

2 Abdominal Incidental Findings

In 2010 and 2013, ACR Incidental Findings Committee published detailed recommendations on managing incidental findings on abdominal CT and MRI. Different subcommittees compiled flowcharts and tables based on numerous reviews and original papers. The White Papers of the ACR Incidental Findings Committees I and II give a comprehensive overview over most of the abdominal incidental findings and provide helpful tools for every radiologist. Only a selection of recommendations for the most common abdominal incidental findings will be presented here.

2.1 Cystic Renal Mass

Cystic renal masses are among the most frequent incidental findings. As such, they can be partially imaged, for example, on a chest scan, or fully imaged on an abdominal MRI or CT scan or an abdominal ultrasound. The great majority of cystic renal masses can be characterized sufficiently using ultrasound or a contrast-enhanced CT. The first step in managing incidental cystic renal masses is to exclude nonneoplastic causes such as infections, for example, pyelonephritis.

It is well established to categorize cystic renal masses according to the approach of Bosniak. In this classification, the size of the lesion is subordinate to the characterization of the wall and septa if present. The management of incidental cystic renal masses should be adapted if comorbidities are present or life expectancy is limited. In these patients, observing a lesion might be a better approach than surgery. Therefore, the recommendations for managing incidental cystic renal masses differentiate between "general population" and patients with severe comorbidities or a limited life expectancy. Still, the recommendations given by the ACR Incidental Findings Committee need to be adapted individually. Depending on the patient, the image quality and the experience of the reporting radiologist, duration and frequency of controls may be changed, or a certain approach might be favoured (Berland et al. 2010; Silverman et al. 2008). (For further details, please see the table "Management recommendations for patients with incidental cystic renal masses" (Silverman et al. 2008).)

The Incidental Findings Committee elaborated a detailed flowchart with recommendations for managing incidental cystic renal masses detected on CT. Within this flowchart, green "action boxes" indicate where action is needed either in the form of follow-up imaging or in form of a surgical approach; this would be necessary in Bosniak IIF and Bosniak III or IV lesions. If a Bosniak IIF lesion reveals morphological changes in the follow-up, surgery should be considered. Morphological change is especially referring to a change in characteristic features, such as number and thickness of septations. Growth of a Bosniak IIF lesion should be reported, but is by itself not indicating malignancy. Red boxes indicate that no further follow-up is necessary as for Bosniak I and II cysts. (For further details, please see "Flowchart for incidental cystic renal mass detected on CT" (Berland et al. 2010)).

2.2 Liver Mass

Due to technical advantages, there are liver masses that can be detected on CT, MRI, and PET that in the past remained undiscovered. Especially in oncological patients, it is of vital importance to distinguish a benign incidental liver lesion from a malignant lesion. The recommendations about managing incidental liver masses detected on CT by the Incidental Findings Committee had been assessed by the appearance of the liver lesion and by the patients' risk factors to develop an important liver mass. The appearance of the lesion includes the size (<0.5 cm, 0.5–1.5 cm, and >1.5 cm), margins, attenuation, and enhancement. A low-risk patient is defined as a young patient (≤40 years) with no known malignancies, hepatic dysfunction, risk factors for hepatic malignancies, or symptoms typical for liver diseases. An average risk is attributed to a patient >40 years with no known malignancies, hepatic dysfunction, risk factors for hepatic malignancies, or symptoms typical for liver diseases. A high-risk patient has a known primary malignancy with propensity to metastasize to the liver, liver cirrhosis, or other hepatic risk factors including hepatitis, sclerosing cholangitis, hemochromatosis, hepatic dysfunction, and long-term oral contraceptive medication (Berland et al. 2010). For example, an incidental liver mass smaller than 0.5 cm in a patient with a low or average risk profile is considered benign and needs no further follow-up. An incidental liver mass of the same size in a patient with known cirrhosis or hemochromatosis, for example, requires follow-up in CT or MRI in 6 months. If this patient is a candidate for liver transplant, then follow-ups need to be more frequent. An incidental liver mass >1.5 cm with low attenuation, ill-defined margins, and an enhancement > 20 HU should be followed up in a low-risk patient and further evaluated in a patient with an average risk profile using multiphasic MRI. If such a lesion is found in a high-risk patient, biopsy is recommended. (For supplemental details, please see "Flowchart for incidental liver mass detected on CT" (Berland et al. 2010)).

2.3 Adrenal Mass

An adrenal incidentaloma is an adrenal mass ≥1 cm incidentally discovered on cross-sectional imaging. Such adrenal incidentalomas are quite common, and most frequently pathology reveals a nonhyperfunctioning adenoma. Less common benign lesions are myelolipomas, cysts, or hemorrhage. Due to the high prevalence of non-hyperfunctioning adrenal adenomas, an incidentally discovered adrenal mass is most likely to be benign, both in patients with no known malignancy and in oncology patients (Berland et al.2010). However, there are cancer entities that metastasize to the adrenal gland, including lung and breast cancer, malignant melanoma, and renal cancer (McLean et al. 2011). Furthermore, there are primary adrenal tumors such as pheochromocytomas or primary adrenocortical carcinomas. As with every incidental finding, the aim is to differentiate between benign lesions where no further evaluation is needed and potentially malignant lesions that require treatment. The detailed algorithm from the Incidental Findings Committee distinguishes between diagnostic and nondiagnostic imaging features. If an adrenal mass shows density values ≤10 Hounsfield Units on unenhanced CT, this is considered diagnostic of an adrenal adenoma; therefore, no follow-up is recommended. If the imaging features are not diagnostic, the reporting radiologist has to compare the lesion to prior imaging, if available. Size, imaging features, growth over time, and the patient's history need to be considered. To distinguish between adenomas and metastases, a closer look at the contrast enhancement and washout following contrast administration might help. Both adenomas and metastases enhance rapidly. While adenomas show a rapid washout as well, metastases show a prolonged washout. If an unenhanced CT scan is available, the absolute percentage washout (APW) can be calculated using the formula (enhanced HU – 15-min delayed HU)/(enhanced HU – unenhanced HU) × 100. An APW value ≥60 % is diagnostic of an adenoma. If no unenhanced CT scan is available, the relative percentage washout (RPW) can be calculated, and the formula needed is (enhanced HU – 15-min delayed HU)/enhanced HU × 100. Using this formula, a RPW value >40 % is diagnostic of an adenoma (Berland et al. 2010). Following the "Flowchart for incidental adrenal mass detected on CT or MR" might help the reporting radiologist to give a well-considered recommendation. The management recommendation might have to be adapted according to patient wishes, imaging quality, or the experience level of the reporting radiologist (Berland et al.2010).

2.4 Adnexal Findings

The following recommendations given by the ACR Incidental Findings Committee II on Adnexal Findings address incidental findings detected on cross-sectional imaging (CT or MRI) in nonpregnant, postmenarchal patients with no known or suspected adnexal disorder. In contrast to a gynecological ultrasound, it is not common to document the date of the patient's last menstrual period prior to a CT or MRI scan. Though, knowing the date of the last menstrual period might help the reporting radiologist to interpret adnexal findings in premenopausal patients. If the onset of menopause in patients around or older than 50 years is unknown, 50 years can be used as an arbitrary designation for the age of menopause. Postmenopause can be divided into early postmenopause within 5 years after the final menstrual period and the late postmenopause >5 years from the last menstruation. This division might help to evaluate incidental adnexal findings in postmenopausal women.

When follicles are counted as cysts, incidental adnexal cysts are almost ubiquitous in premenopausal women and quite common in postmenopausal women. Adnexal cysts are categorized by their morphology into benign-appearing and probably benign cysts. A benign-appearing cyst is an oval or round unilocular mass of uniform fluid signal and attenuation. It has a regular shaped or imperceptible wall and shows no solid areas or mural nodules. The maximum diameter is <10 cm. If the patient is premenopausal, the cyst can contain layering hemorrhage. A probably benign cyst shows angulated margins, and the shape is neither round nor oval. Furthermore, a cyst is defined as probably benign if a portion of the cyst is poorly imaged (e.g., due to metal streak artifacts) or the image has a reduced signal-to-noise ratio (due to technical parameters or to an unenhanced scan). Additionally, it is useful to differentiate whether the cysts are detected in premenopausal or postmenopausal women (Patel et al.2013).

2.4.1 Adnexal Cysts in Premenopausal Women

Because nonneoplastic, physiological cysts in premenopausal women are very common, a benign-appearing or probably benign cyst with a maximum diameter ≤3 cm should be considered normal. Evaluating the morphology of a cyst with a maximum diameter >3 cm in CT or MRI should permit a statement which category the cyst belongs to: benign-appearing or probably benign. An incidental, benign-appearing, asymptomatic cyst with a maximum diameter ≤5 cm will not need further evaluation. Short-interval follow-up with ultrasound is recommended for benign-appearing cysts >5 cm and probably benign cysts >3 cm, because small mural nodules might not be detectable in primary CT or MRI. The recommended interval is 6–12 weeks; during this time, the cyst may decrease in size or resolve. If the cyst persists, the ultrasound will help to evaluate possible small mural nodules, which are seen in some borderline malignancies.

2.4.2 Adnexal Cysts in Postmenopausal Women

Simple cysts are quite common in women in early and late postmenopause. The majority of these cysts are <3 cm, and a malignant cyst is very rare. The pathogenesis of those nonmalignant cysts includes paraovarian or paratubal cysts as well as cystadenomas and cystadenofibromas. It is recommended that incidental, adnexal cysts with a maximum diameter ≤1 cm in early or late postmenopausal women should be considered benign unless there are suspicious imaging features of metastatic ovarian cancer. In early postmenopause follow-up, ultrasound in 6–12 months is recommended for benign-appearing cysts >3 and ≤5 cm; a direct ultrasound evaluation is recommended for cysts >5 cm. A benign-appearing cyst >3 cm in late postmenopause should be evaluated promptly with ultrasound. Direct evaluation with ultrasound is further recommended for probably benign cysts >3 cm in early postmenopause and >1 cm in late postmenopause.

For additional details, please see "Incidental adnexal cystic mass flowchart" (Patel et al. 2013).

3 Summary

Managing incidental findings in patients is a daily task for every practicing radiologist. Thus, it is crucial to give well-considered recommendations on whether and how to follow up incidental findings. Patient's comorbidities, imaging quality, experience in reporting, as well as psychological stress for the patient and resulting costs for the health care system, are factors that need to be taken into consideration. The Fleischner Society and the ACR Incidental Findings Committee I and II published helpful recommendations over the last few years regarding thoracic and abdominal incidental findings. These recommendations provide useful guidance, but may need to be adapted to every individual case.

References

Berland LL, Silverman SG, Gore RM, Mayo-Smith WW, Megibow AJ, Yee J et al (2010) Managing incidental findings on abdominal CT: white paper of the ACR incidental findings committee. J Am CollRadiol 7(10):754–773. Epub 2010/10/05. doi:10.1016/j.jacr.2010.06.013. PubMed PMID: 20889105

de Hoop B, van Ginneken B, Gietema H, Prokop M (2012) Pulmonary perifissural nodules on CT scans: rapid growth is not a predictor of malignancy. Radiology 265(2):611–616. Epub 2012/08/30. doi: 10.1148/radiol.12112351. PubMed PMID: 22929331

MacMahon H, Austin JH, Gamsu G, Herold CJ, Jett JR, Naidich DP et al (2005) Guidelines for management of small pulmonary nodules detected on CT scans: a statement from the Fleischner Society. Radiology 237(2):395–400. Epub 2005/10/26. doi:10.1148/radiol.2372041887. PubMedPMID: 16244247

McLean K, Lilienfeld H, Caracciolo JT, Hoffe S, Tourtelot JB, Carter WB (2011) Management of isolated Adrenal Lesions in Cancer Patients. Cancer Control J Moffitt Cancer Center 18(2):113–126. Epub 2011/04/01. PubMed PMID: 21451454

Naidich DP, Bankier AA, MacMahon H, Schaefer-Prokop CM, Pistolesi M, Goo JM et al (2013) Recommendations for the management of subsolid pulmonary nodules detected at CT: a statement from the Fleischner Society. Radiology 266(1):304–317. Epub 2012/10/17. doi:10.1148/radiol.12120628. PubMed PMID: 23070270

Patel MD, Ascher SM, Paspulati RM, Shanbhogue AK, Siegelman ES, Stein MW et al (2013) Managing incidental findings on abdominal and pelvic CT and MRI, part 1: white paper of the ACR Incidental Findings Committee II on adnexal findings. J Am CollRadiol 10(9):675–681. Epub 2013/09/07. doi:10.1016/j.jacr.2013.05.023. PubMed PMID: 24007607

Silverman SG, Israel GM, Herts BR, Richie JP (2008) Management of the incidental renal mass. Radiology 249(1):16–31. Epub 2008/09/18. doi:10.1148/radiol.2491070783. PubMed PMID: 18796665

Classification of Incidental Findings

Lale Umutlu

Contents

1 **Introduction** 113

2 **Classification of Incidental Findings in a Research Setting** 114

3 **Classification of Incidental Findings in a Clinical Setting** 118

References 125

L. Umutlu
University Hospital Essen, Department of Diagnostic and Interventional Radiology and Neuroradiology, Hufelandstr. 55, 45122 Essen, Germany
e-mail: Lale.Umutlu@uk-essen.de

1 Introduction

Cross-sectional imaging, by means of CT and MR imaging, has evolved to play a major part in patient management as well for investigations on population based cohorts. Due to continuous improvements in scanner and sequence technology, cross-sectional imaging has steadily advanced to provide excellent spatiotemporal resolution imaging, enabling the detection of complex disease processes as well as subclinical disease states (Bamberg et al. 2015). Apart from aiding to assess the target structures and sought medical issues, the increased application of cross-sectional imaging methods has resulted in an increased detection of incidental findings (IF). While some studies indicate that a high number of IFs derived from research studies result in important clinical benefits, such as earlier diagnosis to a small but significant minority of participants (Orme et al. 2010; Espinoza et al. 2014), the American College of Radiology pleads caution on the potential cascade of additional (noninvasive and invasive) investigations, anxiety and morbidity caused by the discovery of IFs (Berland et al. 2010). Hence, guidance on IF categorization and management is indispensable, yet difficult to allocate. While most population-based screening studies provide dedicated guidelines for IF management, the lack of clear-cut recommendations for IF management in the clinical setting results in high variations in practice among reporting radiologists.

Med Radiol Diagn Imaging (2016)
DOI 10.1007/174_2016_79, © Springer International Publishing Switzerland
Published Online: 26 Nov 2016

2 Classification of Incidental Findings in a Research Setting

The increasing application of imaging in population-based cohorts has helped to provide unbiased data to estimate the prevalence of certain diseases as well as to further understand complex disease processes, as well as the identification of novel imaging biomarkers (Schmermund et al. 2002; Bamberg et al. 2015). Numerous multicenter population-based studies have demonstrated the highly valuable integration of imaging and nonimaging modalities for risk assessment and prediction of diseases, such as cardiac events, investigated in the Heinz Nixdorf Recall Study (Erbel et al. 2010). While research imaging is designed to address specific questions regarding the population-based study set-up, its primary function is not a diagnostic test for clinical conditions, potentially lacking the standard of clinical diagnostic imaging (The Royal College of Radiologists 2011). A systematic review and meta-analysis on 16 population-based studies totaling 19,559 participants underlined the significant difference of IF detection rates due to the application of high-resolution versus low-resolution sequences in brain MRI, resulting in differing IF detection rates of 4.3 % (high-resolution) versus 1.7 % (low-resolution) (Morris et al. 2009). Furthermore, apart from the study protocols for research imaging being designed for epidemiologic use with specific protocol parameters, population-based cohort studies are accompanied by the additional defiance of the readers' blindness to information regarding the clinical status of the participants as well as the participants' associated risk for development of significant diseases (Bamberg et al. 2015). Apart from its important value to improved understanding of certain diseases, the wider use of research imaging has also led to an increased detection of incidental imaging findings of potentially unclear clinical relevance to the participant, raising awareness for the need for clarity and uniformity of IF categorization and management. Hence, there is a valid demand for the implementation of standardized protocols and guidelines for the correct handling of incidental findings in research to ensure that research procedures mirror the best interests of participants (Espinoza et al. 2014). These kind of universal agreements should take account ethical principles of medicine and consider the level of duty of care of a researcher to the research participant in regard of potentially harmful incidental findings, while preserve feasibility and practicability within the resourcing, workload and financial constraints of research studies.

Up to current status, there are no standardized guidelines established to cover all population-based research studies, instead most research trials determine study-based classifications and guidelines for IF management in accordance with appropriate ethical standards. While all guidelines are consent on the graduation of IFs according to their clinical relevance, there still is a wide diversity on the dedicated classification systems, modified in accordance with the investigated body region as well as age, gender, and body-mass-index of the studied cohort (Furtado et al. 2005; Orme et al. 2010). Well-accepted overall recommendations on IF classifications and indications on management, suggested by the Royal College of Radiologists (2011) and published by Wolf et al., comprise genetic- as well as imaging-based research studies (Wolf et al. 2008). These recommendations classify relevant imaging incidental findings into three categories:

Category 1: Strong net benefit, disclosure to participant suggested

- (a) Information revealing a condition likely to be life-threatening
- (b) Information revealing a condition likely to be grave that can be avoided or ameliorated

Category 2: Possible net benefit, may be disclosed to participant

- (c) Information revealing a nonfatal condition that is likely to be grave or serious but that cannot be avoided or ameliorated, when a research participant is likely to deem that information important

Category 3: Unlikely benefit, no disclosure to participant suggested

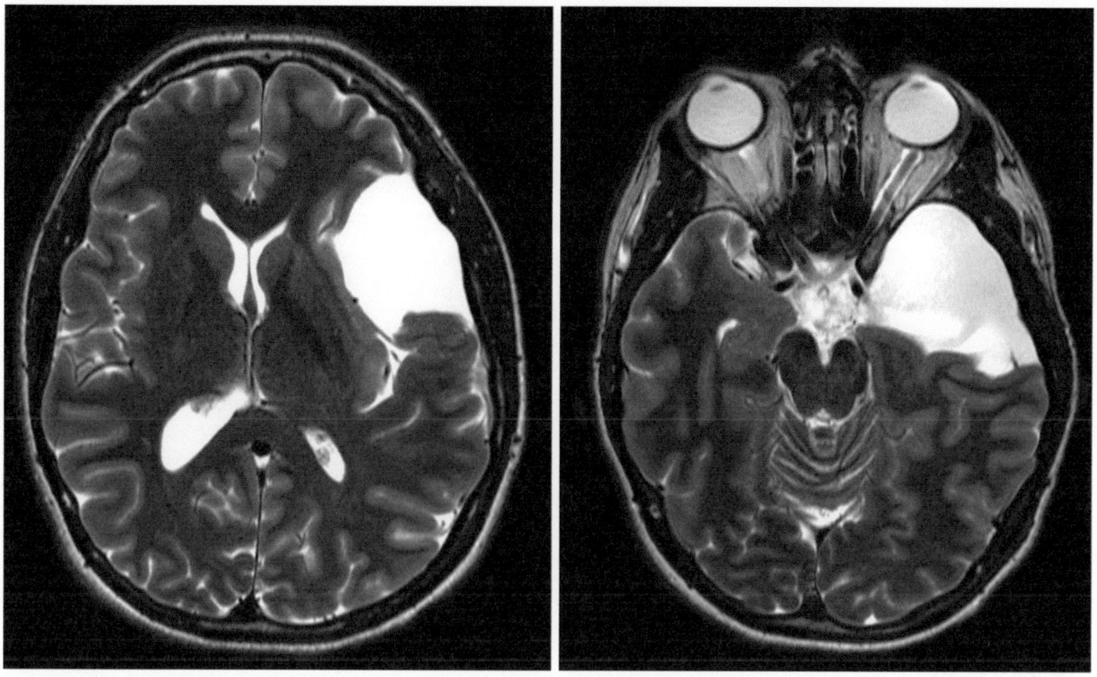

Fig. 1 Mega-arachnoid cyst in the left frontobasal lobe in a 38-year-old patient detected during an MR scan performed for exclusion of metastases of an extracranial primary

(d) Information revealing a condition that is not likely to be of serious health or reproductive importance
(e) Information whose likely heath or reproductive importance cannot be ascertained

More dedicated classification systems, subdivided into brain and body imaging and comprising imaging examples, will be given in the following section.

Brain imaging

While CT of the brain is typically performed in a clinical setting due to the utilization of ionizing radiation, MR imaging is commonly the diagnostic method of choice for screening purposes (Boutet et al 2016). Incidental brain findings include potentially symptomatic or treatable abnormalities such as neoplasms, cysts, structural vascular abnormalities or inflammatory lesions as well as potential markers of cerebrovascular disease such as white matter lesions or silent brain infarcts (Morris et al. 2009). While the classification of brain IFs remains comparable in accordance with the clinical significance in a majority of the studies, the overall prevalence and type of IFs may vary significantly according to the enrolled study population. Up to 20–50 % of IFs are known to be reported in adult research cohorts, with 2–8 % of the IFs being potentially clinically relevant, requiring follow-up (Malova et al. 2016). The reported IF incidence in children is shown to range from 7 to 36 % with even lower mean rates in preterm infants (10.1 %) (Malova et al. 2016). In addition to the different prevalence rates of IFs, the types of IFs are shown to significantly differ as well, revealing an increasing prevalence with age for white matter hyperintensities, silent brain infarcts, as well as neoplastic findings (Morris et al. 2009). Some of the most common IFs in brain MR imaging studies on the elderly include arachnoid cysts, aneurysms, meningiomas, cavernous malformations, or low-grade glioma (in descending prevalence) (The Royal College of Radiologists 2011). In a study on healthy young men with a mean age of 20.5 years (age range 17–35 years), the most common incidental findings were shown to be arachnoid cysts (Fig. 1) as well as Chiari I-malformation and dystope cere-

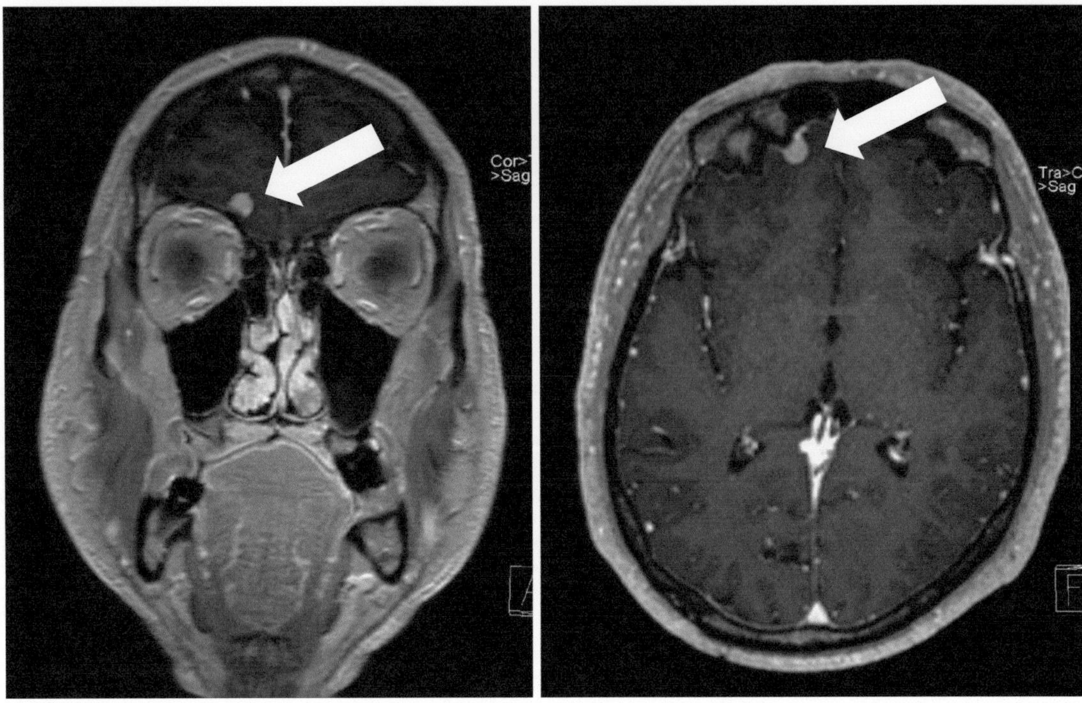

Fig. 2 An incidental finding of minor significance, by means of a very small meningeoma in the right frontal lobe

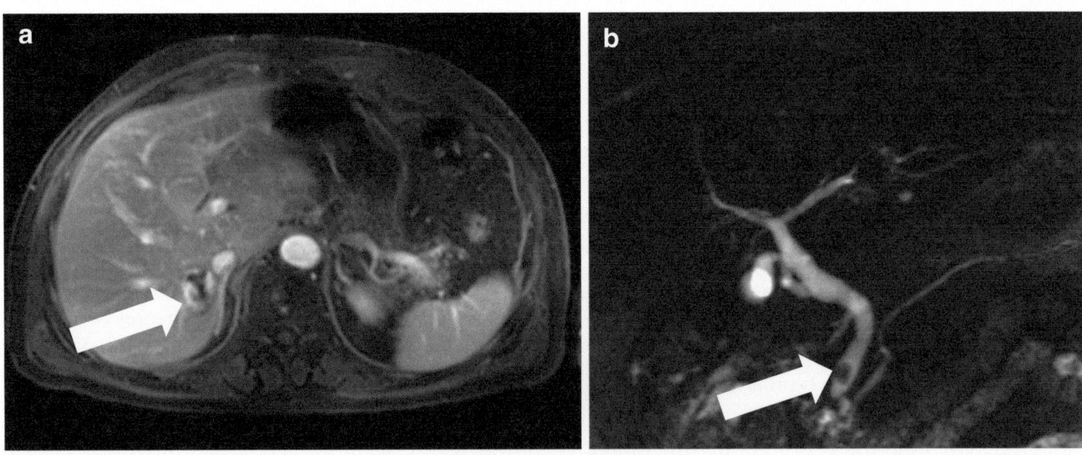

Fig. 3 Liver MR scan performed for further characterization of a CT-detected lesion in liver segment 7 (haemangioma marked with *arrow* in **a**). Incidental finding of moderate significance in the same patient, by means of a gall stone in the common bile duct (*arrow* **b**)

bellar tonsils (43 each out of a total of 166 abnormal findings) (Weber et al. 2006). As for tumor-type IFs, meningioma (Fig. 2) is the most common of all the incidental intracranial tumors, making up to 33 % of incidental tumors found at autopsy (Eskandary et al. 2005). With regard to vascular IFs, intracranial aneurysms (Fig. 3) are considered the most common incidental findings. Based on recent data derived from the population-based Rotterdam study, intracranial aneurysms were present in 134 out of the 5800 enrolled subjects (2.3 %), followed by 37 incidentally detected cavernous angiomas, dural fistulas, and arteriovenous malformations (Bos et al. 2016). While the detection of most incidental findings may be of little clinical significance, intracranial aneurysms bear the potential of acute bleeding, hence, demanding a clinical diagnostic work-up (contrast-enhanced CT or MR angiography and/or digital subtraction angiography). Of the abovenamed incidental aneurysms, 118 participants were enrolled in follow-up imaging and 16 were referred to a neurologist based on the size and location criteria of the aneurysms (as stated in the study protocol). Clinical management involved a wait-and-see policy in the vast majority of the participants, as well as endovascular treatment and surgery in a total of five subjects (Bos et al. 2016).

In terms of classification of IFs, the majority of studies are consent on the graduation of IFs according to their clinical relevance, mainly into three to four categories. Most studies stratify the incidental findings into three categories as follows (Teuber et al. 2016):

Category 1: Normal findings/Incidental finding without clinical significance, including anatomical variations within the normal range (cavum septi pellucidi), known pathologies or (common) findings without prognostic relevance (e.g., developmental venous anomalies)

Category 2: Incidental finding that requires further radiological or medical evaluation, for exampe, additional sequences or contrast-enhanced examinations (suspected neoplastic lesions)

Category 3: Incidental findings that require immediate medical referral (space-occupying lesion, suspected acute hemorrhagic stroke)

Some classification system put further emphasis on the timing of referral according to clinical relevance (Katzman et al. 1999):

Category 1: No referral necessary, normal or findings common in asymptomatic subjects (e.g., sinusitis)

Category 2: *Routine* referral; findings not requiring immediate or urgent medical evaluation, but should be reported to the referring physician (e.g., old infarction)

Category 3: *Urgent* referral required within weeks of study for any abnormality that will need further yet nonemergent evaluation (e.g., low-grade astrocytoma)

Category 4: *Immediate* referral required (e.g., subacute subdural hematoma)

The type of disclosure of the IF to the participant depends on its clinical relevance, differentiating between direct (phone) contact to the participant within a 24 h period in case of urgent IFs and a standardized letter within 10 days for reportable, yet not actionable IFs (Bamberg et al. 2015).

Body imaging

Similar to brain imaging, there is no universal classification system for incidental findings in body imaging either, leaving the dedicated classification of the IFs to study-based guidelines and ethical standards. Nevertheless, similar to brain imaging, there is a universal consent on graduation of the incidental findings according to their clinical relevance. One rather general classification system, that is, recommended by the Royal College of Radiologists, subdivides the common IFs on body imaging into three major categories according to their potential implications for medical management (The Royal College of Radiologists 2011):

Category 1: Major significance – always requiring further investigation and likely to have adverse health effects (e.g., aortic aneurysm >5 cm, aortic dissection, solid liver mass)

Category 2: Moderate significance – usually requires further investigation but health effects unclear; (e.g., gallstone in common bile duct (Fig. 3), splenomegaly, indeterminate liver lesion)

Category 3: Minor significance – rarely requires further investigation and unlikely to have adverse health effects (e.g., left-sided inferior vena cava, gallstones in gallbladder).

While this general classification system covers a majority of the most common IFs on body imaging, it provides rather little guidance on IF management, in terms of timing and type (letter, phone call) of disclosure of the IFs to the participants. Hence, to ensure correct IF and disclosure handling, most population-based studies on body imaging provide more detailed IF management guidelines.

In the National German cohort study, an expert panel categorized potential incidental findings into three groups, comprising "actionable," "reportable," and "nonreportable" IFs in accordance with clinical guidelines, recent research results and ethical considerations.

1. Actionable results are defined as incidental findings that bear a high likelihood to affect the participants' well-being within a short time and require urgent medical treatment. This group of IFs comprises, for example, pneumothoraces, aortic dissection. After detecting and reporting the IF, the reader is required to seek for direct participant contact and further guidance of clinical work-up (Fig. 4).
2. Reportable results involve findings that are associated with a reasonably high likelihood to alter the participants' well-being, such as aortic aneurysms with a diameter >5 cm or an abdominal mass >3 cm. In case of a "reportable result," the participant is informed via standardized letter within a time period of <10 working days.
3. All other IFs are categorized as nonreportable results without known clinical relevance, including renal cysts, gall bladder stones, etc. (Fig. 5) (Bamberg et al. 2015).

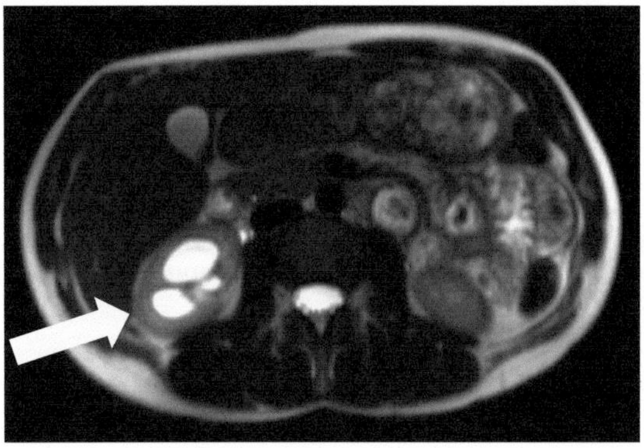

Fig. 4 Urinary congestion of the right kidney in a participant of a population-based cohort study. Immediate IF disclosure to the participant is required

3 Classification of Incidental Findings in a Clinical Setting

Within the last decades, imaging itself, and particularly cross-sectional imaging, has evolved to become an inevitable part of patient management, including assessment of acute and chronic benign diseases as well as staging, therapy monitoring, and aftercare of malignant diseases. While the aim of imaging in the clinical setting is set to address to sought the reason the study was ordered, the growing number of imaging examinations, particularly cross-sectional scans performed per patient, results in an increasing number of incidental findings. While IF classification and management is fairly settled in a research setting due to imposed study-based guidelines, the management of IFs detected in

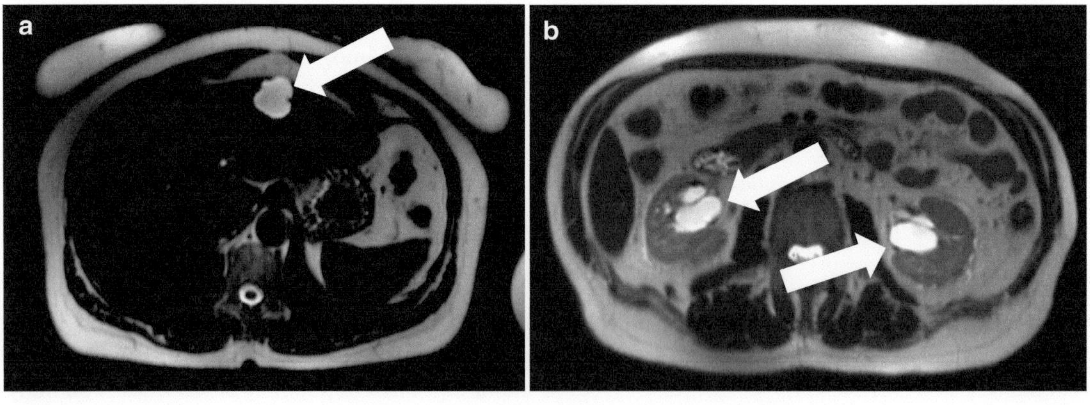

Fig. 5 Nonreportable IFs in two different participants of a population-based cohort study. The *arrows* mark a liver cyst (**a**) and bilateral parapelvin renal cysts (**b**)

clinical imaging is not guided by clear-cut recommendations, causing high variations in practice among reporting radiologists. An important difference between IFs detected in the clinical setting and IFs detected in a research environment, which may significantly influence patient management and is also reflected in most IF recommendations, is caused by the readers' knowledge of patient history, previous imaging studies, and potential comorbidities. Furthermore, in contrary to the predominantly MR-based research imaging studies, CT imaging plays an important role in clinical patient care, imposing a platform for other types of incidental findings that may not be detected by MRI, such as subsolid pulmonary nodules or atherosclerotic calcifications. In a systematic review by Lumbreras et al., the mean frequency of incidental findings was found to be as high as 23.6 % with an increased frequency of IFs in studies involving CT technology (mean 31.1 %) (Lumbreras et al. 2010). In a publication by Barrett et al., the reviewers analyzed the prevalence of incidental findings in trauma patients detected by computed tomography imaging, classifying the incidental findings into two categories: type 1 findings comprise findings that are potentially serious results and that demand further evaluation and close follow-up; type 2 findings comprise findings that require informing the patient but do not necessitate further follow-up. A third group of IFs comprise findings of little clinical consequence and did not necessitate patient notice, such as sinus mucuous retention cysts (Barrett et al. 2009). The analysis revealed a significant number of trauma patients diagnosed with potentially serious incidental findings, including 32.0 % of type 1 findings and 51.2 % of type 2 findings with the female sex showing a higher association to type 1 findings. While abdominal atherosclerosis (9.0 %), pulmonary nodules (7.4 %), and thoracic/mediastinal lymphadenopathy (5.6 %) constituted the most frequent type 1 IFs, a total of 631 incidental findings were considered suspicious of neoplastic foci (Barrett et al. 2009). Renal cysts, interstitial lung diseases, hepatic cysts, diverticulosis /-it is, and fatty liver were stated among the top five type 2 IFs, requiring patient information, yet no further follow-up investigations as proposed by the study protocol.

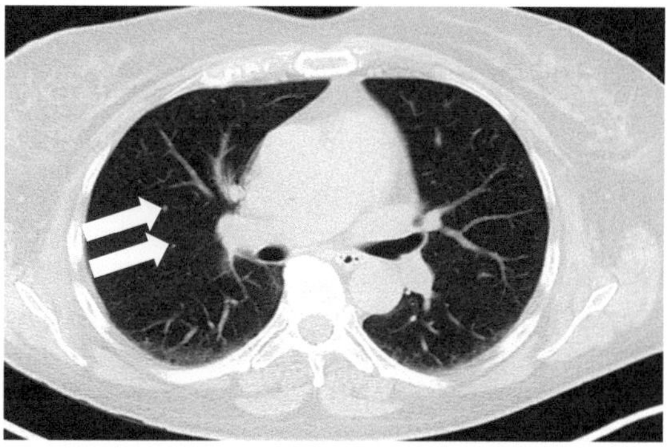

Fig. 6 Two pulmonary nodules (<4 mm) detected in a 52-year-old patient with no history of smoking or other risk factors. According to the Fleischner criteria no follow-up is needed

Numerous guidelines, mostly dedicated to organ-specific lesions such as the Fleischner classification for pulmonary nodules (Fig. 6), have been published over the years (MacMahon et al. 2005; Naidich et al. 2013). To provide a more comprehensive overview and management guidance, the American College of Radiology released conjoint recommendations, comprising pulmonary and abdominopelvic IFs as well as vascular findings (Berland et al. 2010; Heller et al. 2013; Khosa et al. 2013; Patel et al. 2013; Sebastian et al. 2013), including solid and subsolid pulmonary nodules, adrenal lesions, pancreatic cystic lesions, liver and renal lesions, splenic lesions, lymph nodes, as well as IFs of the biliary tract.

Examplatory organ-specific classification systems will be shown in the following section.

Lung

Incidental pulmonary nodules are encountered commonly in chest radiography and even more so in cross-sectional imaging due to its higher resolution and improved lesion-to-lung contrast. The incidental detection rates have been noted as low as 0.09– 0.2 % of all chest radiographs (Albert and Russel 2009) and as high as 31 %, for example, in a cohort study of patients undergoing CT scans for coronary calcium scoring (Burt et al. 2008). Overall, the estimated prevalence of solitary pulmonary nodules in the literature ranges from 8 to 51 % (Albert and Russel 2009). A solitary pulmonary nodule (SPN) is defined as a well-circumscribed, radiographic opacity measuring less than or equal to 30 mm in diameter, surrounded completely by aerated lung, and is not associated with adenopathy or atelectasis (Albert and Russel 2009; Gould et al. 2007). The differential diagnosis for pulmonary nodules comprises benign and malignant causes and demands further correlation regarding its radiologic features, patient history, as well as patient risk factors for cancer. Radiographic criteria utilized to estimate the probability of malignancy of a pulmonary nodule comprise potential calcification, nodule size, growth rate, as well as edge characteristics (Gurney et al. 1993; Cummings et al. 1986). While a lesion size <5 mm, smooth borders, solid density, and concentric or popcorn-like calcifications are considered suggestive for benign SPN, a lesion size >10 mm, spiculated borders, as well as a doubling time ranging from 1 month to 1 year are considered suggestive for malignancy (Albert and Russel 2009). Out of the above-named radiologic features, the size of the lesion seems to show the strongest link to the probability of malignancy at the time of detection as the prevalence of malignancy is 0–1 % for nodules <5 mm, 6–28 % for nodules 5–10 mm, and 64–82 % for nodules >20 mm in diameter (Wahidi et al. 2007). For nodules more than 3 cm in diameter, 93–97 % are malignant (Siegelman et al. 1986). After careful consideration of all clinical and radiographic criteria and estimation of probability of malignancy, further patient management regarding future (noninvasive) surveillance or potential invasive evaluation should be performed in accordance with the guidelines. A widely applied guideline for management of pulmonary nodules was introduced by the Fleischner society, categorizing solid and subsolid pulmonary nodules according to their size and patients' risk for malignancy and recommending follow-up imaging or PET/biopsy, accordingly (MacMahon et al. 2005; Naidich et al. 2013).

Kidney

With renal cysts being one of the most common incidental findings in abdominal imaging, renal lesions detected on CT imaging are categorized into solid and cystic lesions, including a more dedicated classification of the cystic lesions according to Bosniak (Berland et al. 2010). The Bosniak classification is a well-accepted means of triaging renal incidentalomas, subdividing renal cysts into five groups according to their morphologic features (Curry et al. 2000):

Category 1: Benign simple cyst with thin wall without septa, calcifications, or solid components; no contrast-enhancement, water-equal density.

Category 2: Benign cyst with a few thin septa, which may contain fine calcifications or small segments of mildly thickened calcification. This includes homogenous, high-attenuation lesions less than 3 cm with sharp margins but without enhancement. Hyperdense cysts must be exophytic with at least 75 % of its wall outside the kidney to allow for appropriate assessment of margins, otherwise they are categorized as IFs.

Category 2F: Up to 5 % of these cysts are malignant and as such they require follow-up imaging, though there is no consensus recommendation on the appropriate interval of follow-up. Well-marginated cysts with a number of thin septa, with or without mild enhancement or thickening of septa. Calcifications may be present; these may be thick and nodular. There are no enhancing soft tissue components. This also includes nonenhancing high-attenuation lesions that are completely contained within the kidney and are 3 cm or larger.

Category 3: Indeterminate cystic masses with thickened irregular septa with enhancement.

Category 4: Malignant cystic masses with all the characteristics of category III lesions as well as enhancing soft tissue components independent of but adjacent to the septa.

With increasing likelihood of malignancy, category 2F cysts show a risk of malignancy of up to 5 %, category 3 cysts of 50 %, and the majority of category 4 cysts are shown to be malignant, affecting patient management regarding follow-up and/or surgical procedures accordingly.

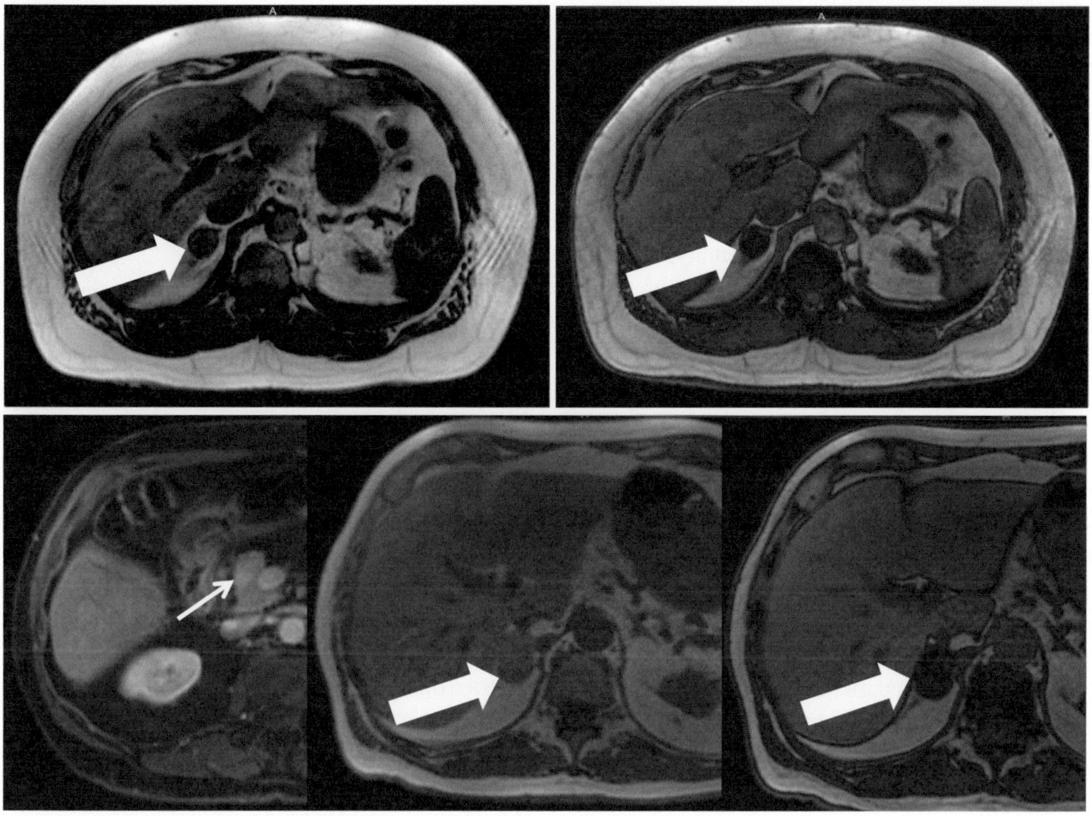

Fig. 7 The *upper row* shows In -(*left image*) and Opposed (*right image*) phase imaging of a participant in a population-based MRI study. The *arrows* point at an incidental adrenal adenoma. The images in the *bottom row* show an incidentaloma (*thick arrows* in the *middle and right image*) detected in a clinical study in a patient with a pancreatic tumor (*thin arrow left image*)

Adrenal gland

Adrenal incidentalomas are considered a disease of modern technology, as their detection as an incidental finding has significantly increased with improving technology and increasing application of cross-sectional imaging. The prevalence of adrenal incidentalomas has been reported as high as 8 % in autopsy series and 4 % in diagnostic imaging (Kapoor et al. 2008). Adrenal lesions can be categorized as primary or metastatic, benign or malignant, and functioning or nonfunctioning (Boland et al. 2008). Based on the significant association between the size of an adrenal incidentaloma and its likelihood of malignancy, adrenal masses are subdivided into two groups, by means of 1–4 cm in adrenal mass size and >4 cm. As approximately 70 % in adrenal masses >4 cm (85 % if larger than 6 cm) are known to be malignant, interventional investigations (biopsy/resection) are recommended accordingly (Berland et al. 2010). With nonfunctioning adrenal adenomas being the most common type of adrenal incidentaloma, recommendations on diagnostic procedures include CT densitometry and/or MR-based chemical shift imaging to detect a potential signal drop in Opposed-Phase-imaging, indicative for fatty adrenal tissue in adenomas (Boland et al. 2008). Recent recommendations also propose CT perfusion imaging to assess the washout kinetics of the adrenal lesions for further characterization (Boland 2011).

Furthermore, as in all clinical patient imaging studies, prior studies as well as patient history (e.g., history of lung cancer with a high likelihood of adrenal metastases; Fig. 7) should be taken into account when considering further diagnostic procedures/diagnoses.

Liver

Liver cysts are considered one of the most common incidental findings in abdominal imaging and do not need any further diagnostic work-up in the majority of the cases. In contrary, incidental liver masses, yielding a more potent risk of malignancy, require further evaluation and are categorized based on a combined analysis of size, morphologic features, as well as risk of malignancy in accordance with the patient history regarding hepatic dysfunction or known malignancy as well as age. As the patients' risk for malignancy based on prior hepatic diseases and age plays an important role for further liver IF management (apart from size and morphologic features of the lesions), the ACR recommends a separation into three groups:

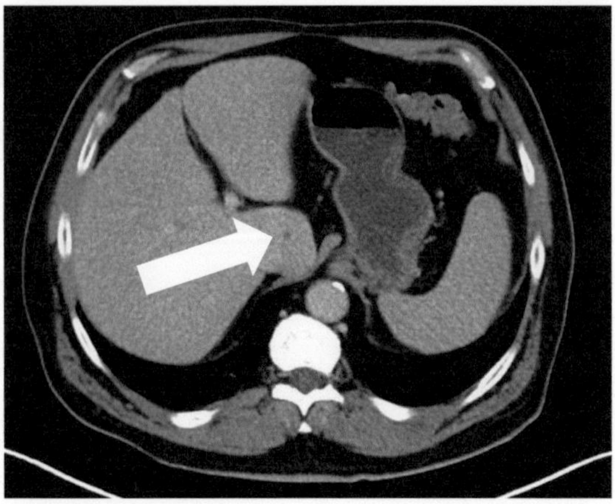

Fig. 8 Small lesion (<5 mm) detected in a low-risk individual, no follow-up needed according to ACR recommendations

1. Low risk individuals: Young patient (≤40 years old), with no known malignancy, hepatic dysfunction, hepatic malignant risk factors, or symptoms attributable to the liver.
2. Average risk individuals: Patient >40 years old, with no known malignancy, hepatic dysfunction, abnormal liver function tests, or hepatic malignant risk factors or symptoms attributable to the liver.
3. High risk individuals: Known primary malignancy with a propensity to metastasize to the liver, cirrhosis, and/or other hepatic risk factors. Hepatic risk factors include hepatitis, chronic active hepatitis, sclerosing cholangitis, primary biliary cirrhosis, hemochromatosis, hemosiderosis, oral contraceptive use, anabolic steroid use.

In terms of imaging-based classifications, the American College of Radiology recommends an initial classification of the liver IFs according their size into three subgroups: (1) <0.5 cm, (2) 0.5–1.5 cm and (3) >1.5 cm. As lesions <0.5 cm are commonly too small to be further characterized into benign or malignant lesions on CT imaging, patient management should be performed related to the patients' risk for malignancy (low and average risk individuals: no follow-up; high risk individuals: follow-up in 6 months) (Fig. 8). Lesions >0.5 cm should be further analyzed regarding their imaging characteristics (benign or malignant characteristics) as well as the patients' general risk for malignancy. A more dedicated algorithm for classification and management of liver lesions has been implemented for patients with cirrhosis or who are at risk for HCC, by means of the LI-RADS® criteria (Mitchell et al. 2015).

Spine

Incidental findings of the spine are commonly detected, regardless if the application field is dedicated to spine imaging, for example, for disk disease evaluation, or if the spine is unwittingly imaged as part of a cross-sectional cervical/thoracal or abdominal scan (Cieszanowski et al. 2014). Studies on incidental findings in dedicated lumbar spine MRI have reported mean detection rates of IFs of approximately 8.4 %, revealing mostly benign findings and associations with age and sex. In a publication by Park et al., 1268 patients' lumbar spine scans were re-investigated, yielding a total of 107 patients scans with lesion-type incidental findings, comprising fibrolipoma (3.2 %) as the most common IF, followed by Tarlov cysts (2.1 %) and vertebral hemangiomas (1.5 %) (Park et al. 2011). Naturally, age-related degenerative spine disease is one of the most common incidental findings, comprising a wide spectrum of degenerative abnormalities such as disk bulging or herniation, osteochondrosis, spondylosis deformans, spondylolysis, or spondylolisthesis. In a recent publication by Cieszanowski et al., a vast majority of the enrolled participants for whole-body screening MRI showed incidental degenerative spinal disease (86.7 % of the subjects <50 years and 98.1% of the subjects >50 years) (Cieszanowski et al. 2014). While the classification of incidental findings in a research setting is defined by the study set-up [e.g., type I: insignificant/low significance; type II: moderately or potentially significant; type III: further medical evaluation required; could cause clinical symptoms or require treatment; (Cieszanowski et al. 2014)], clinical imaging demands elaborate reporting of the radiologist to differentiate between IFs that should or should not be dedicatedly reported to prevent psychosocial distress. While clinical imaging lacks a universal classification for guidance of spinal IFs, a large number of classification systems for dedicated IFs have been established within time, comprising degenerative disk and osseous spine changes.

One classification to categorize disk degeneration was established by Pfirmann et al. Pfirmann et al. devised a widely used 5-point grading system for disk degeneration based on MR signal intensity, disk structure, distinction between nucleus and annulus, and disk height (Pfirrmann et al. 2001). Griffith et al. recently introduced a modified grading system referring to the Pfirrmann system to improve the discrimination of the severity of disk degeneration in elderly subjects (Griffith et al. 2007). While disk disease evaluation is considered one of the most common reasons to perform spine MRI, the causal relation between disk disease (e.g. protrusion) and back pain seems controversial. One of the first studies to evaluate the causal relation between abnormalities in the lumbar spine and low back bain was published in the early years of MR imaging by Jensen et al. (1994). Fifty-two percent of the enrolled 98 asymptomatic subjects in this study showed a bulge at least one level, 27 % a protrusion, and 1 % an extrusion. While the prevalence of bulges increased with ages, the findings did not show any gender-specific differences (Jensen et al. 1994). Considering the high prevalence of disk disease without associated back pain, disk disease may also be treated as an incidental finding, when the imaging is performed for other reasons than disk disease evaluation such as staging in oncologic patients. A commonly applied general classification of disk lesions subdivides the lesions into six categories:

Category 1: Normal (excluding aging changes)
Category 2: Congenital/developmental variants
Category 3: Degenerative/traumatic
- Anular tear
- Herniation:
  - Protrusion/extrusion
  - Intravertebral
- Degeneration:
  - Spondylosis deformans
  - Intervertebral osteochondrosis

Category 4: Inflammation/infection
Category 5: Neoplasia
Category 6: Morphologic variant of unknown significance

With lumbar discectomy being the most common surgical procedure performed in patients suffering from back pain and sciatica, the MSU (Michigan State University) classification was established to objectively measure lumbar disk herniation on MRI (Mysliwiec et al. 2010). The MSU classification of herniations according to size (1-2-3) and location (zone A-B-C) and correlation to appropriate clinical findings bears the potential to objectify criteria that may lead to improved surgery outcomes (Mysliwiec et al. 2010).

Even though a clear differentiation between disk-related spine disease and solely vertebrae-related spine disease is difficult to define, a number of classification systems focusing on osseous changes have been introduced over time. The Modic classification was first described and defined by Dr. Michael Modic in 1988, representing a classification for vertebral body end-plate changes on MRI (Modic et al. 1988) (Fig. 9).

- Modic type 1:
  - T1 low signal/T2 high signal
  - Represents bone marrow edema and inflammation (Fig. 10)
- Modic type 2:
  - T1 high signal/T2 iso to high signal
  - Represents normal red haemopoetic bone marrow into fatty marrow

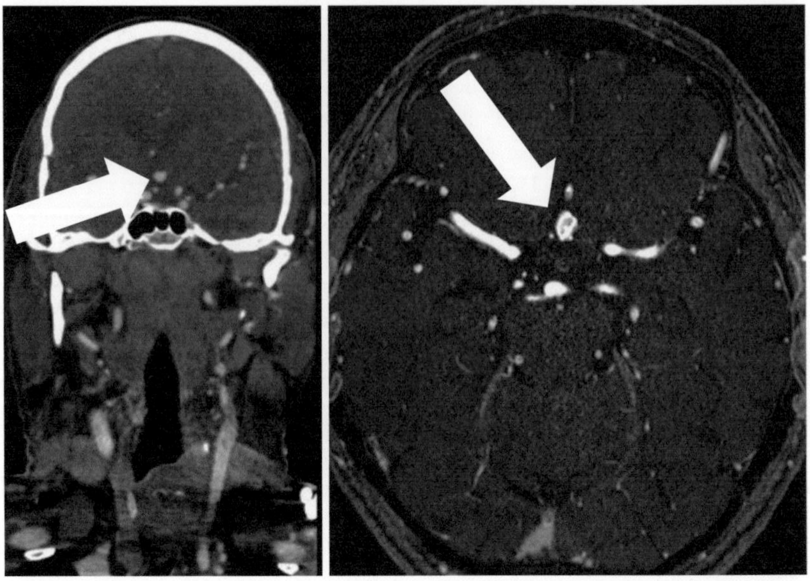

Fig. 9 Incidentally detected aneurysm of the anterior communicating artery in a 62-year-old patient (*arrows*). The initial CT angiography scan (*left*) was performed for exclusion of vessel occlusion after hemiparesis and hyposthesia. MRA was performed subsequently for verification of the IF (*right image* TOF MRA)

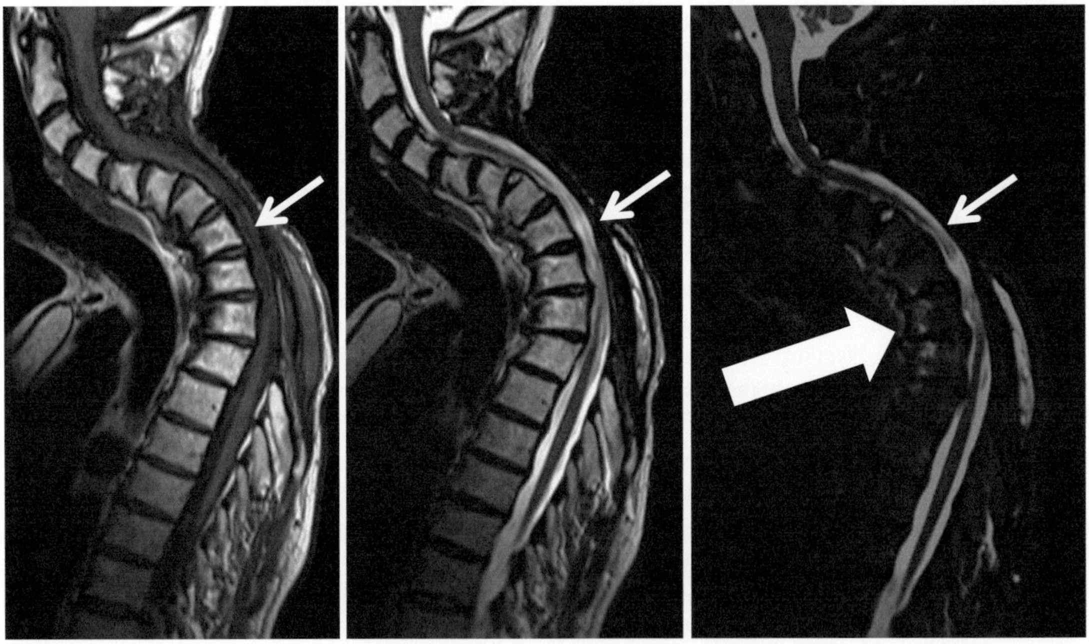

Fig. 10 T1 weighted (*left*), T2 weighted (*middle*), and STIR imaging (*right*) of the spine in a patient with known hyperkyposis (*thin arrows*). *Arrows* point at incidentally detected vertebral body end-plate changes of Modic type 1, representing bone marrow edema and inflammation

- Modic type 3:
  – T1 low signal/T2 low signal
  – Represents subchondral bony sclerosis

A commonly applied classification system for spondylolisthesis was introduced by Meyerding et al. This classification method grades spondylolisthesis according to the ratio of overhanging part of the superior vertebral body to the anteroposterior length of the adjacent inferior body into 5 grades, ranging from 0 to 25 % (grade 1) to grade 5 (spondyloloptosis: >100 %).

References

Albert RH, Russel JJ (2009) Evaluation of the solitary pulmonary nodule. Am Fam Physician 80:827–831

Bamberg F, Kauczor HU, Weckbach S, Schlett CL, Forsting M, Ladd SC, Greiser KH, Weber MA, Schulz-Menger J, Niendorf T, Pischon T, Caspers S, Amunts K, Berger K, Bülow R, Hosten N, Hegenscheid K, Kröncke T, Linseisen J, Günther M, Hirsch JG, Köhn A, Hendel T, Wichmann HE, Schmidt B, Jöckel KH, Hoffmann W, Kaaks R, Reiser MF, Völzke H, German National Cohort MRI Study Investigators (2015) Whole-body MR imaging in the German National Cohort: rationale, design, and technical background. Radiology 277(1):206–220

Barrett TW, Schierling M, Zhou C, Colfax JD, Russ S, Conatser P, Lancaster P, Wrenn K (2009) Prevalence of incidental findings in trauma patients detected by computed tomography imaging. Am J Emerg Med 4:428–435

Berland LL, Silverman SG, Gore RM, Mayo-Smith WW, Megibow AJ, Yee J, Brink JA, Baker ME, Federle MP, Foley WD, Francis IR, Herts BR, Israel GM, Krinsky G, Platt JF, Shuman WP, Taylor AJ (2010) Managing incidental findings on abdominal CT: white paper of the ACR Incidental Findings Committee. J Am Coll Radiol 7:754–773

Boland GW (2011) Adrenal imaging: why, when, what, and how? Part 3. The algorithmic approach to definitive characterization of the adrenal incidentaloma. AJR Am J Roentgenol 196:W109–W111

Boland GW, Blake MA, Hahn PF, Mayo-Smith WW (2008) Incidental adrenal lesions: principles, techniques, and algorithms for imaging characterization. Radiology 249:756–775

Bos D, Poels MM, Adams HH, Akoudad S, Cremers LG, Zonneveld HI, Hoogendam YY, Verhaaren BF, Verlinden VJ, Verbruggen JG, Peymani A, Hofman A, Krestin GP, Vincent AJ, Feelders RA, Koudstaal PJ, van der Lugt A, Ikram MA, Vernooij MW (2016) Prevalence, clinical management, and natural course of incidental findings on brain MR images: the population-based Rotterdam scan study. Radiology 23:160218. [Epub ahead of print]

Boutet C, Vassal F, Celle S, Schneider FC, Barthélémy JC, Laurent B, Barral FG, Roche F (2016) Incidental findings on brain magnetic resonance imaging in the elderly: the PROOF study. Brain Imaging Behav. [Epub ahead of print]

Burt JR, Iribarren C, Fair JM, Norton LC, Mahbouba M, Rubin GD, Hlatky MA, Go AS, Fortmann SP, Atherosclerotic Disease, Vascular Function, and Genetic Epidemiology (ADVANCE) Study (2008) Incidental findings on cardiac multidetector row computed tomography among healthy older adults: prevalence and clinical correlates. Arch Intern Med 168:756–761

Cieszanowski A, Maj E, Kulisiewicz P, Grudzinski IP, Jakoniuk-Glodala K, Chlipala-Nitek I, Kaczynski B, Rowinski O (2014) Non-contrast-enhanced whole-body magnetic resonance imaging in the general population: the incidence of abnormal findings in patients 50 years old and younger compared to older subjects. PLoS One 9(9):e107840

Cummings SR, Lillington GA, Richard RJ (1986) Estimating the probability of malignancy in solitary pulmonary nodules: a Bayesian approach. Am Rev Respir Dis 134:449–452

Curry NS, Cochran ST, Bissada NK (2000) Cystic renal masses: accurate Bosniak classification requires adequate renal CT. Am J Roentgenol 175:339–342

Erbel R, Möhlenkamp S, Moebus S, Schmermund A, Lehmann N, Stang A, Dragano N, Grönemeyer D, Seibel R, Kälsch H, Bröcker-Preuss M, Mann K, Siegrist J, Jöckel KH (2010) Coronary risk stratification, discrimination, and reclassification improvement based on quantification of subclinical coronary atherosclerosis: the Heinz Nixdorf Recall study. Heinz Nixdorf Recall Study Investigative Group. J Am Coll Cardiol. 56(17):1397–406. doi:10.1016/j.jacc.2010.06.030

Eskandary H, Sabba M, Khajehpour F, Eskandari M (2005) Incidental findings in brain computed tomography scans of 3000 head trauma patients. Surg Neurol 63:550–553

Espinoza A, Malone K, Balyakina E, Fulda KG, Cardarelli R (2014) Incidental computer tomography radiologic findings through research participation in the North Texas Healthy Heart Study. J Am Board Fam Med 27:314–320

Furtado CD, Aguirre DA, Sirlin CB, Dang D, Stamato SK, Lee P, Sani F, Brown MA, Levin DL, Casola G (2005) Whole-body CT screening: spectrum of findings and recommendations in 1192 patients. Radiology 237:385–394

Gould MK, Fletcher J, Iannettoni MD, Lynch WR, Midthun DE, Naidich DP, Ost DE, American College of Chest Physicians (2007) Evaluation of patients with pulmonary nodules: when is it lung cancer?: ACCP evidence-based clinical practice guidelines (2nd edition). Chest 132(Suppl 3):108S–130S

Griffith JF, Wang YX, Antonio GE, Choi KC, Yu A, Ahuja AT, Leung PC (2007) Modified Pfirrmann grading system for lumbar intervertebral disc degeneration. Spine (Phila Pa 1976) 32(24):E708–E712

Gurney JW, Lyddon DM, McKay JA (1993) Determining the likelihood of malignancy in solitary pulmonary nodules with Bayesian analysis. Part II: application. Radiology 186:415–422

Heller MT, Harisinghani M, Neitlich JD, Yeghiayan P, Berland LL (2013) Managing incidental findings on abdominal and pelvic CT and MRI, part 3: white paper of the ACR Incidental Findings Committee II on splenic and nodal findings. J Am Coll Radiol 10:833–839

Jensen MC, Brant-Zawadzki MN, Obuchowski N, Modic MT, Malkasian D, Ross JS (1994) Magnetic resonance imaging of the lumbar spine in people without back pain. N Engl J Med 331(2):69–73

Kapoor A, Morris T, Rebello R (2008) Guidelines for the management of the incidentally discovered adrenal mass. Radiology 249:756–775

Katzman GL, Dagher AP, Patronas NJ (1999) Incidental findings on brain magnetic resonance imaging from 1000 asymptomatic volunteers. JAMA 282:36–39

Khosa F, Krinsky G, Macari M, Yucel EK, Berland LL (2013) Managing incidental findings on abdominal and pelvic CT and MRI, part 2: white paper of the ACR Incidental Findings Committee II on vascular findings. J Am Coll Radiol 10:789–794

Lumbreras B, Donat L, Hernández-Aguado I (2010) Incidental findings in imaging diagnostic tests: a systematic review. Br J Radiol 83:276–289

MacMahon H, Austin JH, Gamsu G, Herold CJ, Jett JR, Naidich DP, Patz EF Jr, Swensen SJ, Fleischner Society (2005) Guidelines for management of small pulmonary nodules detected on CT scans: a statement from the Fleischner Society. Radiology 237:395–400

Malova M, Rossi A, Severino M, Parodi A, Morana G, Sannia A, Cama A, Ramenghi LA (2016) Incidental findings on routine brain MRI scans in preterm infants. Arch Dis Child Fetal Neonatal Ed. pii: fetalneonatal-2015-310333 [Epub ahead of print]

Mitchell DG, Bruix J, Sherman M, Sirlin CB (2015) LI-RADS (Liver Imaging Reporting and Data System): summary, discussion, and consensus of theLI-RADS Management Working Group and future directions. Hepatology 61:1056–1065

Modic MT, Steinberg PM, Ross JS, Masaryk TJ, Carter JR (1988) Degenerative disk disease: assessment of changes in vertebral body marrow with MR imaging. Radiology 166(1 Pt 1):193–199

Morris Z, Whiteley WN, Longstreth WT Jr, Weber F, Lee YC, Tsushima Y, Alphs H, Ladd SC, Warlow C, Wardlaw JM, Al-Shahi Salman R (2009) Incidental findings on brain magnetic resonance imaging: systematic review and meta-analysis. BMJ 339:b3016

Mysliwiec LW, Cholewicki J, Winkelpleck MD, Eis GP (2010) MSU Classification for herniated lumbar discs on MRI: toward developing objective criteria for surgical selection. Eur Spine J 19:1087–1093. doi:10.1007/s00586-009-1274-4

Naidich DP, Bankier AA, MacMahon H, Schaefer-Prokop CM, Pistolesi M, Goo JM, Macchiarini P, Crapo JD, Herold CJ, Austin JH, Travis WD (2013) Recommendations for the management of subsolid pulmonary nodules detected at CT: a statement from the Fleischner Society. Radiology 266:304–317

Orme NM, Fletcher JG, Siddiki HA, Harmsen WS, O'Byrne MM, Port JD, Tremaine WJ, Pitot HC, McFarland EG, Robinson ME, Koenig BA, King BF, Wolf SM (2010) Incidental findings in imaging research: evaluating incidence, benefit, and burden. Arch Intern Med 170:1525–1532

Park HJ, Jeon Y-H, Rho M-H, Lee E-J, Park N-H, Park S-I, Jo J-H (2011) Incidental findings of the lumbar spine at MRI during herniated intervertebral disk disease evaluation. AJR Am J Roentgenol 196:1151–1155

Patel MD, Ascher SM, Paspulati RM, Shanbhogue AK, Siegelman ES, Stein MW, Berland LL (2013) Managing incidental findings on abdominal and pelvic CT and MRI, part 1: white paper of the ACR Incidental Findings Committee II on adnexal findings. J Am Coll Radiol 10:675–681

Pfirrmann CW, Metzdorf A, Zanetti M et al (2001) Magnetic resonance classification of lumbar intervertebral disc degeneration. Spine 26:1873–1878

Schmermund A, Möhlenkamp S, Stang A, Grönemeyer D, Seibel R, Hirche H, Mann K, Siffert W, Lauterbach K, Siegrist J, Jöckel KH, Erbel R (2002) Assessment of clinically silent atherosclerotic disease and established and novel risk factors for predicting myocardial infarction and cardiac death in healthy middle-aged subjects: rationale and design of the Heinz Nixdorf RECALL Study. Risk Factors, Evaluation of Coronary Calcium and Lifestyle. Am Heart J 144:212–218

Sebastian S, Araujo C, Neitlich JD, Berland LL (2013) Managing incidental findings on abdominal and pelvic CT and MRI, part 4: white paper of the ACR Incidental Findings Committee II on gallbladder and biliary findings. J Am Coll Radiol 10:953–956

Siegelman SS, Khouri NF, Leo FP, Fishman EK, Braverman RM, Zerhouni EA (1986) Solitary pulmonary nodules: CT assessment. Radiology 160: 307–312

Teuber A, Sundermann B, Kugel H, Schwindt W, Heindel W, Minnerup J, Dannlowski U, Berger K, Wersching H (2016) MR imaging of the brain in large cohort studies: feasibility report of the population- and patient-based BiDirect study. Eur Radiol. [Epub ahead of print]

The Royal College of Radiologists (2011) Management of incidental findings detected during research imaging. Royal College of Radiologists, London. 60 p

Wahidi MM, Govert JA, Goudar RK, Gould MK, McCrory DC, American College of Chest Physicians (2007) Evidence for the treatment of patients with pulmonary nodules: when is it lung cancer? ACCP evidence-based clinical practice guidelines (2nd edition). Chest 132(Suppl 3):94S–107S

Weber F, Knopf H (2006) Incidental findings in magnetic resonance imaging of the brains of healthy young men. J Neurol Sci 240(1-2):81–4

Wolf SM, Lawrenz FP, Nelson CA, Kahn JP, Cho MK, Clayton EW, Fletcher JG, Georgieff MK, Hammerschmidt D, Hudson K, Illes J, Kapur V, Keane MA, Koenig BA, Leroy BS, McFarland EG, Paradise J, Parker LS, Terry SF, Van Ness B, Wilfond BS (2008) Managing incidental findings in human subjects research: analysis and recommendations. J Law Med Ethics 36:219–248

Incidental Findings on Abdominal CT

Mikael Hellström

Contents

1 **Misunderstandings About Incidental Findings/Incidentalomas** ... 128

2 **How Common Are Incidental Findings on CT of the Abdomen?** ... 129
2.1 Abdominal CT ... 129
2.2 CT Colonography ... 129

3 **How Extensively Should We Look for Incidental Findings on Abdominal CT?** ... 131

4 **Technical Factors Affecting the Detection and Characterization of Incidental Findings on Abdominal CT** ... 131

5 **Kidneys** ... 132
5.1 Solid Renal Tumors ... 132
5.2 Benign Renal Lesions ... 135
5.3 Small Lesions ... 136
5.4 Cystic Renal Lesions ... 137
5.5 Simple Cysts ... 137
5.6 Complex Cysts ... 138
5.7 Bosniak Classification ... 139
5.8 Renal Calcifications ... 140
5.9 False-Positive Renal Masses ... 140
5.10 Renal Size ... 140
5.11 Normal Variants and Malformations ... 141
5.12 Hydronephrosis ... 141

6 **Urinary Bladder and Upper Urinary Tract Tumors** ... 141

7 **Adrenals** ... 143
7.1 Shape and Size of Adrenals ... 145
7.2 Management of Adrenal Incidentalomas ... 145
7.3 Patients with a History of Extra-Adrenal Malignancy ... 146
7.4 Young Patients with Adrenal Incidentaloma ... 146

8 **Liver** ... 146
8.1 Cystic Lesions ... 146
8.2 Hemangioma ... 147
8.3 Non-cystic Benign Liver Lesions ... 148
8.4 Approach to an Incidental Liver Mass Detected on CT ... 149
8.5 Steatosis ... 150

9 **Gallbladder and Biliary Tree** ... 150

10 **Spleen** ... 151

11 **Lymph Nodes** ... 151

12 **Pancreas** ... 152
12.1 Solid Tumors ... 152
12.2 Cystic Lesions ... 152

13 **Gastrointestinal Tract** ... 153
13.1 Stomach ... 154
13.2 Small Bowel ... 154
13.3 Large Bowel ... 154
13.4 Appendix ... 155

14 **Vascular Structures** ... 155

15 **Adnexal and Uterine Lesions (Not Including Incidental Lesions in Children or Pregnant Women)** ... 156
15.1 Adnexal cysts and teratomas ... 157
15.2 Uterus ... 159

16 **Prostate** ... 160

17 **Skeletal Lesions** ... 161

The original version of this chapter was revised. Water marks and line numbers have been removed.

M. Hellström, MD, PhD
Professor, Department of Radiology, Sahlgrenska University Hospital and Sahlgrenska Academy, Gothenburg University, Gothenburg, Sweden
e-mail: mikael.hellstrom@xray.gu.se

Med Radiol Diagn Imaging (2017)
DOI 10.1007/174_2016_97, © Springer International Publishing Switzerland
Published Online: 11 Mar 2017

18 **To What Extent Are Incidental Findings Reported?** 161
19 **Why Do Radiologists Report or Not Report Incidental Findings?** 162
20 **Do the Patients Want to Know About Incidental Findings?** 162
21 **Who Should Decide Which Information to Convey to the Referring Physician and to the Patient?** 163
22 **Potential Impact of e-Medicine** 164
Conclusion 164
References 165

Abdominal CT examinations usually cover the entire abdomen and pelvis, including all organs and tissues in the intraperitoneal, retroperitoneal, extraperitoneal/pelvic spaces, as well as the extra-abdominal soft tissues, bony structures of the spine, sacrum, pelvis, and hips, and lower part of the chest including parts of the lungs and pleural spaces. The multitude of organs and tissues involved makes abdominal CT reading complex and allows for a multitude of incidental findings that may be of degenerative, neoplastic, or other etiologies. Although scanning is sometimes limited to only the "abdomen" or only the "pelvis," "abdominal CT" in this chapter refers to abdominal-pelvic CT, i.e. both compartments.

The following chapter does not intend to cover every aspect of incidental abdominal CT findings or systematically cover all abdominal organs but concentrates on some general aspects and highlights some relevant organ-specific incidental findings in adults. Incidental findings in the chest are discussed in another chapter.

1 Misunderstandings About Incidental Findings/Incidentalomas

An incidental finding, sometimes called incidentaloma, can be described as a radiological finding not intentionally searched for or an incidentally discovered mass or lesion, detected by CT or other imaging modalities, performed for an unrelated reason. The terms incidental finding and incidentaloma are therefore inappropriate when the radiological finding is related to the clinical question or to the clinical symptoms or signs that motivated the CT examination. Thus, incidentaloma and incidental finding are inappropriate terms when, for example, a tumorous lesion is identified in a patient with a history of cancer, as the lesion may represent a metastasis related to the known malignancy. The same logic applies when there is high clinical suspicion of a malignant process in a patient without known malignancy. In such a case, the organs and tissues are intentionally scrutinized for masses at any location, and therefore the finding of a lesion in, e.g., the adrenal, may not be entirely incidental. Nevertheless, such a finding may still be benign and thereby "incidental" in relation to what was expected or searched for (i.e. metastases or malignant disease). In rare circumstances, the examination may reveal an unsuspected "second" malignancy, which then, by definition, is incidental in relation to the already known "first" malignancy.

The term incidental finding can also be discussed from other aspects. The meaning and use of the term incidental finding or incidentaloma depend on how much, and how specific, clinical information is given on the request form. This in turn may depend on the clinical situation and on the individual referring doctor formulating the request form. With a very specific clinical question, the likelihood of classifying other "nontargeted" radiological findings as incidental may be high, while the same radiological findings may be covered by a broader, more unspecific clinical question and thereby less likely to be called incidental. Incidental radiological findings also need to be related to previous radiological and other information. A finding that appears incidental in relation to the clinical question may already be known from previous studies and thereby not truly incidental, although it may be incidental to the reporting radiologist, if he or she does not have access to previous examinations. The term incidental finding or incidentaloma is therefore best applied to findings that are not previously shown on radiological examinations. The usually non-standardized text summarizing the patient history and clinical questions on radiological request forms and variations in interpretation by the radiologist of the clinical question, in addition to variations in diagnostic interpretation of the actual radiological images, means that comparisons of frequencies of incidental findings in different studies are, to be modest, uncertain.

One may also argue that if the frequency of a certain diagnosis in a defined population is known from previous studies, such as the frequency of abdominal aortic aneurysm (AAA) in 65-year-old men, the identification of such an aneurysm in a 65-year-old male patient is not entirely unexpected, even if not asked for by the referring doctor. On a population basis, such a finding is thereby not entirely incidental. However, the finding in the individual patient may still be incidental if not covered by the clinical question. The term incidental finding is therefore best applied on an individual patient basis.

Incidental findings that are masses or tumor-like are often called incidentalomas, for example if affecting the adrenal (adrenal incidentaloma). It is important to understand that the term incidentaloma is not a diagnosis but only a description of *how* a lesion was identified, i.e. incidentally. Not uncommonly, the term is incorrectly used by radiologists and clinicians to denote a benign finding. In fact, the term incidentaloma says nothing about the character or etiology of the lesion found. Thus, an incidentaloma may be benign or malignant – and it may be clinically unimportant or important.

2 How Common Are Incidental Findings on CT of the Abdomen?

2.1 Abdominal CT

The frequency of incidental findings in abdominal CT is strongly related to the age, sex, and clinical background of the studied population, and it also depends on the criteria used for definition of incidental findings.

In a recent retrospective study of 1,040 consecutive abdominal contrast-enhanced CT examinations, performed for a variety of reasons (mean age 66 years), "relevant incidental findings," i.e. findings leading to further imaging, clinical evaluation, or follow-up, were found in 19% of the examinations (Sconfienza et al. 2015). Such incidental findings were slightly more common in inpatients (23%) than in outpatients (15%), and there was an increase with patient age. The distribution among the involved organs was the kidneys (14%), gallbladder (14%), lung (12%), uterus (10%), adrenal (10%), and vessels (10%). The most common findings were gallstones (in 3% of the examinations), uterine lesions (2%), adrenal masses (2%), non-simple renal cysts (1%), lung nodules (1%), adnexal masses (1%), and kidney stones (1%). In total, 39 different types of relevant incidental findings were made on the 1040 contrast-enhanced abdominal CT examinations. It is notable that the frequency figures were based on a review of the radiology reports and not on a review of the CT images. Therefore, these figures should be considered minimum figures.

2.2 CT Colonography

In CT colonography, the clinical question is focused on the rectum and colon itself. However, a CT colonography examination covers the entire abdomen and pelvis, from the diaphragm to the symphysis pubis, and thereby allows full assessment of colonic as well as extracolonic organs and tissues. It may be argued that by using 3D virtual colonoscopy image reconstructions and 2D images zoomed-in at the colon with wide window-settings, it is theoretically possible to fully assess the colon and rectum without proper visualization of, and attention to, the extracolonic tissues. There is, however, a general agreement that evaluation of extracolonic organs and tissues should be an integral part of CT colonography. Thus, the ESGAR CT colonography Working Group states that "the extracolonic organs should be interrogated and abnormalities reported, noting the limitations if an unenhanced and/or low-dose technique was used" (Neri et al. 2013).

Extracolonic findings are very common on CT colonography, and the majority of these can be considered as incidental findings, although the terms are not entirely interchangeable. Extracolonic findings are commonly categorized as being of minor, moderate, or major importance. Findings of major importance are usually defined as those that potentially lead to further imaging, surgical procedures, or clinical follow-up. In a CT colonography study, mainly including screening subjects, at least one extracolonic finding was made in 55% of those aged 41–64 years and in 74% of those aged 65–92 years (Macari et al. 2011). More importantly, clinically significant findings leading to a recommendation for further radiological imaging were made in 4–6% of the same population. This suggests that the vast majority of incidental findings are of minor clinical importance but also that relevant findings are made in a smaller proportion of those screened. In two large CT colonography screening studies in asymptomatic individuals (over 10,000 and 2,000 participants, respectively), unsuspected extracolonic cancers were identified with similar frequency as (Veerappan et al. 2010), or even higher frequency than, in the colon itself (Pickhardt et al. 2010). In a more recent publication, 2.5% of an asymptomatic screening population had extracolonic findings of potentially major clinical importance, and in nearly 70% of these, significant pathology was proven at follow-up (Pooler et al. 2016a, b).The findings primarily involved the vascular system (26% of the cases, including aortic and other aneurysms), the urogenital system (18%), the liver (15%), the gastrointestinal system (10%), the lungs (9%), and the gynecological system (7%). Considering that screening for abdominal aortic aneurysms can be performed simultaneously, it has been suggested that CT colonography is a highly cost-effective screening method (Pickhardt et al. 2009). Nevertheless, the question about the potential and real impact of extracolonic findings on long-term morbidity and mortality, cost-effectiveness, and acceptance of CT colonography for screening remains a major issue, not least for decision-makers regarding general societal imbursement.

In symptomatic patients investigated with CT colonography, previously unknown extracolonic findings of major importance have been found in 7–13% of the cases (Hellstrom et al. 2004; Badiani et al. 2013) and in the symptomatic elderly in up to 24% (Tolan et al. 2007). In the large SIGGAR study on CT colonography in symptomatic patients, extracolonic findings were made in 59% and further investigated in 8.3% of the population (Halligan et al. 2015). Extracolonic findings are more common in older, as compared to younger, patients (Khan et al. 2007; Macari et al. 2011) and in females, due mainly to findings in the female reproductive organs (Khan et al. 2007).

It is obvious that extracolonic findings may constitute important medical information in both asymptomatic and symptomatic patients. Despite this, it has sometimes been suggested that extracolonic findings on CT colonography should be reported by the radiologist only if specifically asked for. However, the high frequency of significant extracolonic (incidental) findings implies that extracolonic findings should always be looked for and reported when of clinical significance.

Most studies on incidental findings classify the importance of the extracolonic findings as minor, moderate, or major, exemplified in a recent systematic review (Lumbreras et al. 2010). In order to standardize and facilitate reporting of extracolonic findings on CT colonography, classification within the CRAD CT colonography categorization system has been proposed (Zalis et al. 2005). Extracolonic findings are categorized as E0–E4:

- *E0*: "Limited examination. Compromised by artifact; evaluation of extra-colonic soft tissues is severely limited."
- *E1*: "Normal examination or anatomic variant. No extra-colonic abnormalities visible." Example: retroaortic left renal vein.
- *E2*: "Clinically unimportant finding. No work-up indicated." Examples: renal or hepatic cysts, gall stone without cholecystitis, or vertebral hemangioma.
- *E3*: "Likely unimportant finding, incompletely characterized. Subject to local practice and patient preference, work-up may be indicated." Example: minimally complex or homogeneously hyperattenuating kidney cyst.

- *E4*: "Potentially important finding. Communicate to referring physician as per accepted practice guidelines." Examples: solid renal mass, lymphadenopathy, aortic aneurysm, and nonuniformly calcified parenchymal lung nodule ≥1 cm.

3 How Extensively Should We Look for Incidental Findings on Abdominal CT?

The primary focus of abdominal CT is usually to reveal or exclude abnormal findings in the abdominal, retroperitoneal or pelvic organs, or soft tissues. This is normally done with soft tissue CT window settings, optimized for the liver, kidneys, and other soft tissues. However, organs and tissues outside the field of interest are also automatically included during scanning, e.g. the lung bases, the spine, the pelvic bones, and proximal parts of the femurs. Detection of abnormal findings in these locations requires that different CT window settings (window width, window level), optimized for the soft tissues, lung, and bone, respectively, are actively chosen. Also, full evaluation of the included parts of the lungs and bones may require evaluation in more than one image plane, such as axial and sagittal and/or coronal planes. In theory, full evaluation of an abdominal CT should thus include the abdomen in three planes with soft tissue and lung windows (for distribution of intra- and extraintestinal gas and abnormal gas collections), visible parts of the chest in three planes with CT windows for the lung and mediastinum, and visible parts of the spine and pelvic bones in three planes with bone window. Such a comprehensive analysis is rarely needed to answer the clinical question and is probably not routinely performed by most radiologists. In a busy clinical setting, the focus in abdominal CT is rather on the main clinical question, i.e. the intra-abdominal structures, using axial and coronal image planes with soft tissue windows, with image reconstructions in the sagittal plane used for problem-solving. Most radiologists probably also make an overview of the spine with bone window in the sagittal plane and of the pelvic bones in the axial or coronal plane to look for any unexpected clinically significant findings. The extent to which appropriate window settings are used in daily radiology practice is, however, largely unknown and probably depends on individual preferences, personal experience, and routines, as well as on the clinical situation, including patient age, comorbidity, clinical indication, and the radiologist's work situation (restrictions depending on emergency situations, workload, available reading time). On the other hand, ethical and medicolegal considerations and fear of malpractice, which have an impact on the radiologist's decision-making, may promote overly meticulous assessment routines that may become inefficient and expensive. Thus, it is uncertain to what extent radiologists in different clinical situations make full use of available image information in CT of the abdomen. This, of course, has an impact on the detection and reporting of incidental findings on abdominal CT.

4 Technical Factors Affecting the Detection and Characterization of Incidental Findings on Abdominal CT

One factor of importance for incidental findings is the image quality. In abdominal CT, it is today common to use low-radiation dose techniques, especially in younger patients. Using low x-ray tube current with fewer photons emitted creates more image noise, although this may to a large extent be compensated for by iterative reconstruction techniques that are used increasingly. Increased image noise may potentially make incidental findings less conspicuous and thereby less common but may also create artifacts that may be interpreted as potential pathology, findings that perhaps would have been dismissed as normal, if standard radiation dose had been used. In a study on CT pulmonary angiography (Kumamaru et al. 2014), a low kVp did not affect the detection of incidental lung findings, as compared to standard kVp. Other studies have reported the frequency of incidental findings using low mAs (Surov et al. 2014; Priola et al. 2013; Pickhardt and Hanson 2010) but without comparing incidental findings with standard radiation dose. Comparative studies on image quality of specific anatomical targets using low- and standard radiation doses have also been published (Bodelle et al. 2016). However, there is little information in the literature from comparative studies, using low- and standard radiation dose in the same patient.

Another technical factor of importance for abdominal incidental findings is the use of intravascular contrast media. Intravenous contrast media facilitates not only detection but also characterization of lesions on abdominal CT. Low-radiation dose and non-enhanced abdominal CT is typically used in patients with, e.g. flank pain in search for urinary stones and in acute abdomen when bowel obstruction or gastrointestinal perforation is searched for but also, e.g. in screening CT colonography. In CT colonography, it has been shown that extracolonic findings are more common in patients given intravenous contrast media than in those without (Yau et al. 2014). In symptomatic patients, CT colonography with routine use of both non-enhanced and contrast-enhanced image acquisition is recommended, thereby reducing the frequency of ambiguous interpretation of extracolonic organs and tissues, especially regarding cystic and solid lesions (Neri et al. 2013).

5 Kidneys

5.1 Solid Renal Tumors

Incidental findings in the kidneys are common and thus of special interest. An increasing proportion of renal cancers are detected incidentally on imaging examinations performed for unrelated reasons (The Swedish National Quality Registry for Kidney Cancer 2015). In 2015, 63% of newly diagnosed renal cancers in Sweden were detected incidentally, an increase from 43% in 2005. Most of these cancers are detected on CT examinations of the abdomen and sometimes on CT of the chest, while MRI of the abdomen and spine and abdominal ultrasonography contribute to a lesser extent. Data from The Swedish National Quality Registry for Kidney Cancer shows that incidentally detected renal cancers are smaller (mean 54 mm) than those presenting with symptoms (77 mm) and thereby of lower stage with potentially better prognosis. This is reflected in statistics on the mean size of all newly detected renal cancers over time, decreasing from mean 60 mm in 2005 to 50 mm in 2013 (The Swedish National Quality Registry for Kidney Cancer). The proportion of newly diagnosed renal cancers of stage 1a (<4 cm) increased from 22% in 2005 to 35% in 2014, most likely representing an effect of earlier diagnosis by incidental detection on radiological examinations.

Incidental detection of small renal cancers before they show local spread or metastasize may undoubtedly be lifesaving in some patients. Although not presently proven, the lower overall tumor stage at diagnosis should reasonably, in a longer perspective, be accompanied by improved survival for renal cancer patients as a group. Therefore, there seems to be good reasons for the radiologist to take the time and effort to thoroughly assess the kidneys in abdominal CT and other imaging examinations that may include the kidneys, irrespective of the clinical question.

On the other hand, many renal tumors detected incidentally are small or slow growing, being indolent in nature and perhaps of little clinical significance, especially in patients with significant comorbidity or a limited life expectancy. Such patients may die with, rather than from, renal cancer. Identification of an increasing number of small early cancers, together with the increased availability and use of relatively noninvasive interventions such as percutaneous tumor ablation techniques (radiofrequency, microwave, or cryoablation), increases the number of candidates for potential curative treatment. Incidental detection of renal tumors thereby creates a growing reservoir of potentially treatable patients (Welch and Black 2010). Not knowing which individual patients run a real risk of significant morbidity or mortality from their renal tumor may lead to overdiagnosis and overtreatment.

The term overdiagnosis is used when an increase in detection of a specific cancer is not accompanied by a corresponding decrease in clinical morbidity or mortality. A largely unchanged mortality rate, despite an increase in detection of renal cancers, may also be due to a parallel improvement in surgical and medical treatment and care, but overdiagnosis is probably a strong contributing factor, as suggested by Bae (2015). For clarity, "overdiagnosis" as a term is different from "false-positive" test results. Overdiagnosis means that the diagnosis of, e.g., cancer is correct, but the cancer is of no harm, while false-positive test result means diagnosis of cancer when there is no cancer.

Another complicating factor is that 10–15% of solid renal tumors are benign (Al Harbi et al. 2016) but difficult to differentiate from malignant tumor by imaging, even when using multiphase contrast-enhanced CT. Also when using biopsy, differentiation may sometimes be difficult. A remaining challenge for the future is therefore to find ways to better differentiate benign solid renal tumors from renal cancers and to differentiate those renal cancers that grow, metastasize, and thereby cause harm, from those that do not (Karlo et al. 2016). At present, incidentally detected renal masses of suspected solid nature on CT should be reported by the radiologist and further characterized by non-enhanced and contrast-enhanced CT in the corticomedullary and/or nephrographic phase as minimal requirements. Ideally, four-phase CT including also imaging in the excretory phase for visualization of the collecting system should be used, unless patient radiation is an issue, taking age and comorbidity into consideration. As tumor size and imaging characteristics have limited predictive capacity, percutaneous tumor biopsy has gained increased interest as a basis for decision-making, since it offers histologic parameters and molecular markers which may aid the individual therapeutic planning and prognostication (Bagrodia et al. 2012). In particular, image-guided biopsy should be performed when imaging findings are suggestive of lymphoma or metastasis. (Campbell et al. 2009).

The increasing proportion of incidentally detected renal cancers may evoke thoughts on general population screening for renal cancer. Using ultrasonography, large-scale screening studies have been employed in Japan. Tsuboi et al. (2000) screened over 60,000 persons in 1993–1997 with a wide age span (15–95 years). They found tumor-suspected renal lesions in 0.16% and confirmed cancers in 0.02% of the population. Mihara et al. (1999) examined nearly 200,000 persons with abdominal ultrasonography over a period of 13 years (1983–1996) with the majority in the age span of 30–60 years. Renal cell carcinoma was identified in 0.08%, and 38% of the tumors were 25 mm or smaller. Ninety-eight percent were operated, and the 5-year survival rate was 97.4%, much higher than for other abdominal cancers identified in the same screening population. They suggested a very good outcome for renal cancers detected at screening. However, a number of criteria need to be fulfilled to motivate general screening, and so far, screening for renal cancer has not been generally accepted as cost effective and medically relevant and is therefore not generally employed. As mentioned above, the risk of overdiagnosis (Bae 2015) is also an important factor when discussing general population screening for renal cancer. On the other hand, scrutinizing diagnostic information already available on clinical radiological examinations, such as abdominal CT, provides a form of opportunistic or collateral screening on behalf of the radiologist, with no extra radiation or cost. This is a different situation from general screening, and seems highly relevant, but the diagnostic information gained must be handled sensibly by the responsible clinicians, in symphony with the needs and preferences of the patient. Radiologists should also contribute to the better understanding of the biology of renal cancers by performing careful follow-up studies and developing methods for improved characterization of small, incidentally detected renal tumors.

Finally, radiologists need to care about incidental renal (and other) findings from ethical and medicolegal aspects. Neglected or missed "incidental" renal cancers may grow and metastasize over time. If the patient comes back a few years later with symptomatic metastatic renal cancer, it

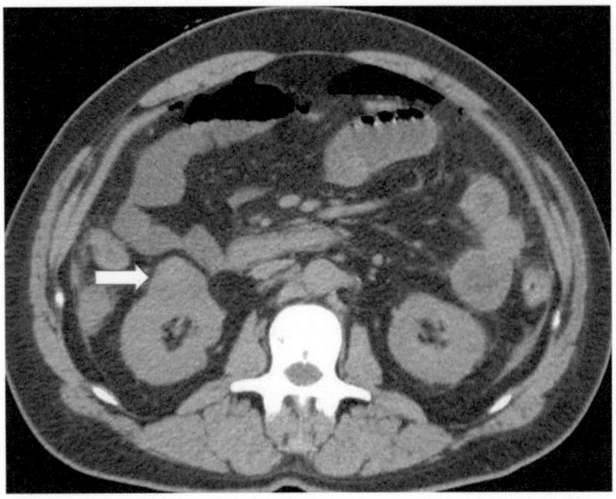

Fig. 1 A 46-year-old male with acute abdominal symptoms, unenhanced abdominal CT shows perforated diverticulitis with free abdominal gas (not shown). Incidentally, a right renal mass, isodense with renal parenchyma, was noted (*arrow*). Follow-up with contrast-enhanced CT showed clear cell renal carcinoma, histologically confirmed at surgery

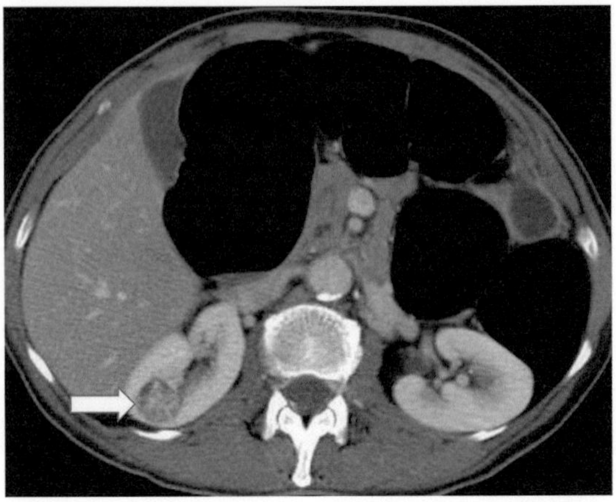

Fig. 2 A 61-year-old woman with bowel symptoms examined with CT colonography. On the supine, contrast-enhanced series (above), a 2 cm solid, diffusely contrast-enhancing tumor is noted in the right kidney (*arrow*). This lesion was not detectable on the prone, non-enhanced series, as it was isodense with normal parenchyma and not exophytic. Surgical removal showed clear cell renal carcinoma

is difficult for the radiologist to explain, and difficult for the patient to understand, that the kidneys were not the focus on the previous examination, when the potentially curable, small renal tumor was already apparent but not looked at or not reported. Clearly, such a scenario also evokes medicolegal issues.

On non-enhanced abdominal CT, solid renal tumors are easy to identify when large and exophytic, i.e. causing a bulge of the renal contour (Fig. 1). If endophytic, i.e. not reaching the normal renal outline, the tumor may be difficult to detect, unless contrast enhancement is used (Fig. 2). However, even a bulging tumor located in the upper or lower pole may be difficult to detect on axial images, as it may mimic a normal or somewhat prominent normal upper or lower renal pole, while it may be obvious on coronal or sagittal views. Similarly, tumors may be difficult to see on coronal views if located anteriorly or posteriorly. This emphasizes the importance of scrutinizing the kidneys in multiple views. If the tumor is large enough, density measurements (Hounsfield numbers) are reliable and may show values over 30–40 HU on native image series, indicating the solid, and not cystic, nature of the lesion, even without the proof of a contrast-enhanced image series. In any case, renal lesions suspected of being solid should be further characterized with CT without and with intravenous contrast medium, in order to determine the degree of contrast enhancement, tumor tissue heterogeneity, and tumor delineation and to rule out local overgrowth beyond Gerota's fascia or into adjacent organs, to rule out tumor thrombus into the renal vein and vena cava, and to assess lymph node involvement. An important aspect is also to assess the function and morphology of the contralateral kidney. Most renal tumors are well depicted in the nephrographic phase (Al Harbi et al. 2016). For preoperative assessment, especially when resection is planned, the arterial anatomy visualized at CT angiography in the corticomedullary phase is of interest. Ideally, a four-phase CT should therefore be performed: non-contrast phase, corticomedullary phase, nephrographic phase, and excretory phase. If radiation dose is a concern in younger patients, three-phase CT should be performed, including non-contrast phase, nephrographic phase, and excretory phase, i.e. CT urography as defined by ESUR (Van Der Molen et al. 2008). Additional radiation dose reduction may be obtained by split-bolus injection techniques, which limit the CT scanning to one pre-contrast scan and one

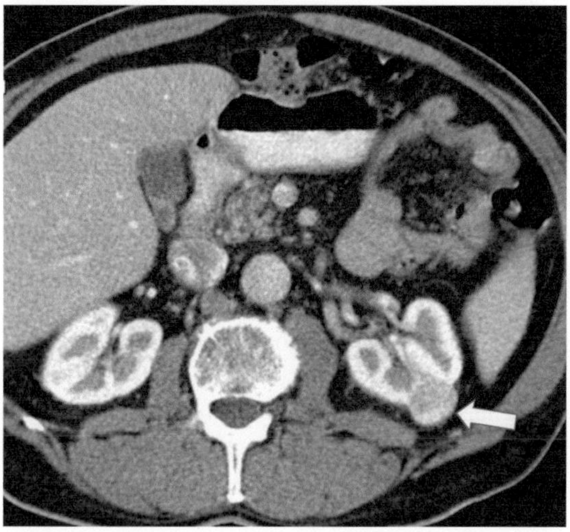

Fig. 3 Incidentally detected solid, renal mass in the posterior part of the left kidney (*arrow*). Subsequent surgical removal showed oncocytoma

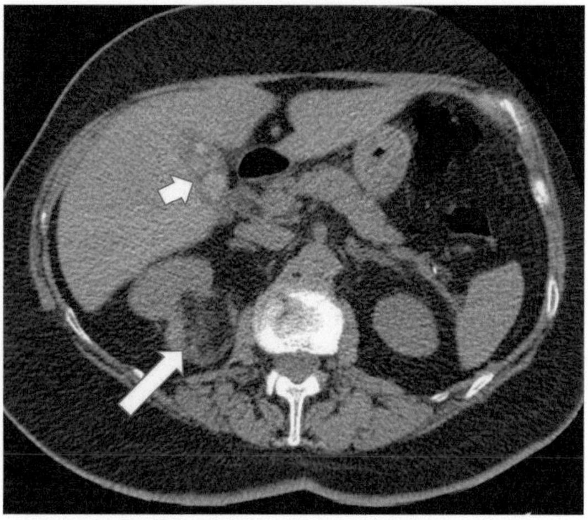

Fig. 4 Angiomyolipoma (AML) in the posterior part of the right kidney (*long arrow*), incidentally detected on acute non-enhanced abdominal CT in a 75-year-old woman with abdominal pain. The fatty components (mean − 45 HU) are characteristic for AML. The maximum diameter of the lesion was 7 cm, and due to the risk of spontaneous bleeding, the lesion was embolized. Note also faintly calcified stones in the normal-sized gallbladder (*short arrow*)

6–12 min post-contrast scan, providing a combined nephrographic and excretory phase (Chow et al. 2007).

5.2 Benign Renal Lesions

As mentioned above, in most cases, benign renal neoplasms cannot reliably be differentiated from malignant ones on non-contrast- or contrast-enhanced CT. Thus, oncocytomas, which are benign, may simulate renal cancer on CT (Fig. 3), and even at biopsy, it may sometimes be impossible to differentiate the two. Many of these tumors therefore go to surgery or percutaneous ablation without a definite diagnosis but with the chance of being malignant in 85–90% of the cases. All incidentally detected solid tumors in the kidneys should thus be considered potentially malignant and be fully investigated as such. One exception, however, is renal angiomyolipoma (AML), which is a benign tumor containing vascular, muscular, and fatty tissue components in varying proportions. In most cases, the fatty component is dominant or at least abundant enough to make it readily identifiable on non-contrast-enhanced CT (Fig. 4). Identification of macroscopic fatty components in regions of interest (density below −10 HU and preferably lower) is virtually diagnostic of AML (Jinzaki et al. 2014). Although these tumors are benign, they may occasionally show (benign) involvement of local lymph nodes. As most AMLs are asymptomatic, they are usually detected incidentally. Although these tumors are commonly clinically silent, with growth, there is a risk of bleeding, which may be acute and severe. Therefore, if an AML is 4 cm or larger, preventive embolization, ablation, or surgical removal is often considered. This means that incidentally detected AMLs smaller than 4 cm should be followed up in order to estimate their growth potential. Such follow-up is best performed with CT or MRI, which provide more reproducible size measurements than ultrasonography.

Occasionally, the fatty component of an AML is minimal and not readily identifiable on CT. Although fatty components may be identified by analysis on pixel level, such “fat-poor” AMLs may simulate renal cell carcinoma. Fat-poor angiomyolipomas may be hyperattenuating relative to renal parenchyma on non-enhanced CT with density measurements >45 HU, or, rarely isoattenuating and contrast enhancing, similar to some renal cell carcinomas. In questionable cases, MRI may be of help to demonstrate or rule out a fatty component (Jinzaki et al. 2014). Renal cancers do not exhibit fatty content, unless the tumor engulfs normal fatty tissue in the renal sinus, which has been described in rare cases.

If angiomyolipomas are detected at a young age, or if large, multiple, or bilateral, tuberous sclerosis should be suspected, as angiomyolipomas develop in over half of patients with tuberous sclerosis. Angiomyolipomas in patients with tuberous sclerosis seem to grow faster and may be more prone to bleeding and may therefore need treatment, including mTOR inhibitors, in a higher proportion than sporadic angiomyolipomas (Jinzaki et al. 2014).

5.3 Small Lesions

The risk of a solid renal mass lesion being malignant increases with the size of the lesion (Thompson et al. 2009). As pointed out above, solid renal masses tend to be small when detected incidentally. However, it is uncertain to what extent really small renal lesions (<1 cm) are reported by radiologists. Some subcentimeter lesions visually stand out as clearly low density compared to the surrounding enhancing parenchyma, suggesting a cystic character. However, objective measurements of density (HU numbers), to confirm cystic or solid nature of such small lesions, are problematic. This may be related to technical factors such as slice thickness, kilovoltage and amperage settings, contrast medium dose and timing, partial volume effects, and particularly pseudoenhancement due to beam hardening. Pseudoenhancement is more prone to occur with small (<1.5 cm) and centrally located lesions surrounded by contrast-enhancing renal parenchyma, while it is less apparent in larger lesions and in lesions with peripheral location (Tappouni et al. 2012; Patel et al. 2014). The risk of misinterpreting the nature of small renal lesions due to these factors should thus be considered. Commonly, 15 HU or even 10 HU increase in density after intravenous contrast injection, as compared to the native series, has been used to classify lesions as enhancing, thereby calling them solid. However, there is no consensus regarding the optimal cutoff, and lately even 15–20 HU enhancement has been considered indeterminate. In a recent study, the post-contrast-enhancement pattern in 137 verified solid renal tumors (85% malignant and 15% benign) measuring 1.0–3.9 cm (median 2.4 cm) was analyzed (Al Harbi et al. 2016). Using 15 HU post-contrast enhancement to define a mass as solid, 17% of the malignant lesions did not reach the threshold in the corticomedullary phase, 8% did not reach the threshold in the nephrographic phase, and 3% did not reach the threshold in both the corticomedullary and the nephrographic phases. Using 20 HU as the threshold, 21% of the malignant lesions did not reach the threshold in the corticomedullary phase, 12% did not reach the threshold in the nephrographic phase, and 9% did not reach the threshold in both phases. In particular, papillary cancers did not reach the 15 HU or 20 HU threshold in over half of the cases in the corticomedullary phase, while the corresponding figures in the nephrographic phase were 18% (15 HU threshold) and 32% (20 HU threshold). About a third of the chromophobe cancers did not reach the thresholds in any phase. Even the clear-cell cancers did not reach the 15 HU threshold in 11% (corticomedullary phase) and 7% (nephrographic phase), while the combination of corticomedullary and nephrographic phases reduced the proportion of clear-cell cancers not reaching the 15 HU and 20 HU thresholds to 5% and 6%, respectively. All of the benign lesions had post-contrast enhancement exceeding both thresholds in all phases (Al Harbi et al. 2016). It can be concluded that applying the 15 HU or 20 HU threshold on both the corticomedullary and nephrographic phases results in the best sensitivity for classifying a lesion as solid or not. Even so, benign and malignant renal tumors in most cases cannot be reliably separated on the basis of their enhancement pattern. Although most small renal cancers enhance above these thresholds with a wide margin, the fact that some do not enhance above 15 HU or 20 HU may pose a problem to differentiate e.g. a hyperdense cyst from a solid tumor. For indeterminate lesions, contrast-enhanced ultrasound or MRI should therefore be considered for problem-solving.

Lesion enhancement after contrast medium administration is a cornerstone in the differentiation between solid and cystic lesions, but other factors such as lesion demarcation, homogeneity, and occurrence of necrosis and calcifications must be taken into consideration. Reporting and decision-making must also take the clinical situation, especially the age of the patient and comorbidity, as well as the potential tumor growth potential, into consideration in order to avoid false-positive cases leading to unnecessary further examinations. If a subcentimeter lesion does not show any obvious malignant characteristics but is too small to characterize further by imaging, it is comforting that such small lesions are very unlikely to be malignant at the time (Berland et al. 2010). Even if a 1-cm renal tumor is malignant, it is very unlikely to have metastases at presentation (Thompson et al. 2009). Unless the patient is young and has a genetic risk or renal tumor is specifically searched for (which is not the case with an incidental finding), aggressive follow-up for further characterization of subcentimeter lesions is not generally recommended (Hindman 2015).

5.4 Cystic Renal Lesions

It is commonly stated that simple renal cysts occur in 50% of individuals over 50 years of age, based on autopsy findings. On abdominal CT, benign renal cysts are one of the commonest incidental findings (Carrim and Murchison 2003). There is a clear increase in the frequency and number of renal cysts with increasing age. Thus, cysts are rarely present under the age of 40 years (found in 8% of the patients), while it was found in 61% of patients aged over 80 years (Carrim and Murchison 2003). If multiple renal cysts occur in patients under 40 years of age, it may be indicative of autosomal dominant polycystic kidney disease (ADPKD) (see below). As simple renal cysts virtually always are symptom-free, they are nearly always incidental findings. Very rarely a large simple cyst may be suspected to cause pain or discomfort, and in such exceptional cases, a diagnostic percutaneous puncture and emptying of the cyst fluid may show if the cyst is the cause of the problem. After such drainage, the cyst usually refills in a short time, so if symptomatic and needing treatment, the cyst could be treated by surgical de-roofing.

The challenge for the radiologist when evaluating renal cyst-like lesions is to differentiate simple, benign cysts from atypical complex cysts and cystic tumors, which may require additional imaging or follow-up.

5.5 Simple Cysts

Benign simple cysts are characterized by a round or oval shape, low-density, homogeneous fluid content typically measuring <20 Hounsfield units (HU), and thin wall. After IV contrast injection, they should remain low in density, with less than 10–15 HU increase. However, one must consider that pseudoenhancement may occur, as discussed above. Most incidentally detected renal cysts can be easily dismissed on contrast-enhanced CT, based on the criteria above. A cyst which is well demarcated, thin walled, of low, homogeneous density, and without septa, solid parts, or calcifications should be called and reported as a benign cyst and does not require follow-up, regardless of the size of the cyst.

Renal cysts of benign appearance may also occur with a number of underlying specific disorders, which may be incidentally encountered on abdominal CT performed for various reasons. In patients on long-standing lithium therapy, renal dysfunction may develop, including a large number of small (1–2 mm), bilateral, cortical, and medullary "microcysts" in normally sized kidneys (Wood et al. 2015). Another cause of acquired cysts is end-stage renal disease and dialysis, which commonly are associated with the development of renal cysts (defined as at least three cysts in each kidney, usually in small, atrophic kidneys). This type of acquired cystic kidney disease is associated with occasional cyst bleeding and an increased risk of renal cancer development (Katabathina et al. 2010).

Occasionally, an unexpectedly large number of renal cysts in normal sized or enlarged kidneys are incidentally noted on abdominal CT. If this occurs in young or middle-aged patients, it may indicate autosomal dominant polycystic kidney disease (ADPKD). This is characterized by enlarged kidneys with multiple bilateral renal cysts, which develop and increase in number and size with age (Pei et al. 2015). The multitude of bilateral renal cysts may be accompanied by liver cysts, sometimes causing a considerable mass effect and occasionally pancreatic and other cysts (Kim et al. 2015). As the disorder is familial, most patients are aware of their potential disease at an early stage, but sometimes the diagnosis is first suspected at cross-sectional imaging in young or middle-aged adults, by incidental detection of multiple renal cysts. Normally, renal cysts are rarely detected in individuals under 30 years of age. APKD should be suspected if three or more cysts are found in one (or both) kidneys in patients under 40 years of age, two or more cysts in each kidney in patients 40–59 years, or four or more cysts in each kidney in patients aged 60 or more (Pei et al. 2009).

5.6 Complex Cysts

Cysts which do not fulfill the criteria for simple cysts are called complex cysts. These constitute a considerable part of incidentally detected cysts and cause considerable concern for radiologists and clinicians. Complex cysts are characterized by one or several of the following features: higher than expected density for a simple cyst (>20 HU), localized or global wall thickening, and internal septations, calcifications, or a solid component in a predominantly cystic lesion. Complex cysts may be entirely benign, but at the other end of the spectrum are cystic malignant tumors and cyst-like necrosis in malignant tumors. These latter cystic lesions may be easy to identify when they contain a clearly solid, contrast-enhancing component, and the concern is mainly about those that exhibit some of the above features, without convincing evidence of malignancy.

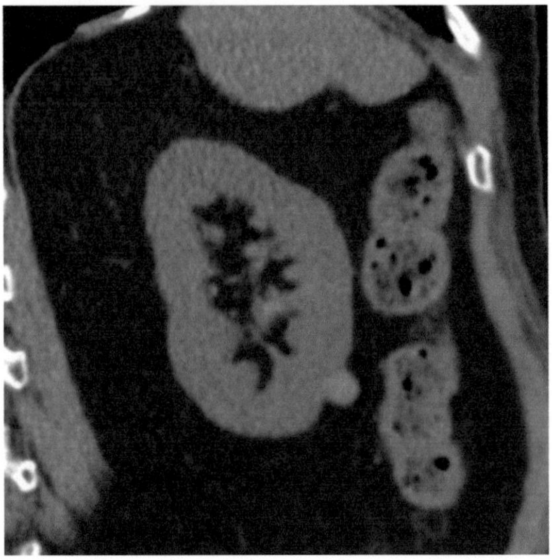

Fig. 5 Incidental detection of a 12 mm hyperdense exophytic renal lesion with homogeneous density of 67 HU on non-enhanced CT. After intravenous contrast injection, the density was unchanged. The finding is characteristic for cyst with high-protein content (hemorrhagic cyst)

One variant of complex cyst often detected incidentally is the protein-rich or hemorrhagic cyst (Fig. 5). These are cysts of high, homogeneous density above 20 HU on non-enhanced CT, without significant increase (<15 HU) in density after intravenous contrast administration and without any other features of complex cysts (i.e. absence of calcifications, septations, wall thickening, and solid components). As with any HU cutoff, there is overlap between normal and abnormal cyst density, variations depending on the choice of image slice and size and placement of the region of interest (ROI) as well as inherent variations between CT machines (Hammarstedt et al. 2013). As discussed above, HU cutoffs should be considered as rule of thumbs to be applied sensibly, taking all imaging characteristics into consideration.

Cysts may be rich in protein due to bleeding or infection, although the etiology cannot be proven in most cases. For example, in autosomal dominant polycystic kidney disease with a large number of cysts, the conversion of simple cysts to high-density cysts from one examination to another is not unusual. This is frequently interpreted as cyst bleeding, which usually is symptom-free, although it may occasionally be associated with pain. If a hyperdense renal lesion is incidentally detected on non-contrast-enhanced CT, differentiation between a hemorrhagic cyst and solid tumor should be affirmed by contrast-enhanced CT, MRI, or ultrasonography.

5.7 Bosniak Classification

Incidentally detected cysts which exhibit features of complexity are best classified by the Bosniak classification system. Originally presented in 1986 (Bosniak 1986), this system allows categorization of renal cysts according to the degree of complexity (Bosniak I–IV) and also provides recommendations on follow-up. Because of difficulties in separating Bosniak II and III, an additional category, Bosniak IIf (f for follow-up), was added (Israel and Bosniak 2003). The categorization is based on the cyst fluid density, post-contrast enhancement characteristics, degree of wall thickness, occurrence of internal septations and calcifications, and enhancing soft tissue nodules. A simple cyst is classified as Bosniak I if of water density, not contrast-enhancing, thin walled, and without septations, calcifications, or solid components (Fig. 6). Bosniak II cysts are characterized by "a few hairline-thin septa, fine calcification, or a short segment of slightly thickened calcification present in the wall or septa (Fig. 6). Uniformly, high-attenuation lesions (<3 cm) that are sharply marginated and do not enhance are included in this group." Bosniak II cysts are also considered to be benign. Bosniak IIf cysts exhibit somewhat more complexity: "These cysts may contain an increased number of hairline-thin septa. Minimal enhancement of a hairline-thin smooth septum or wall can be seen, and there may be minimal thickening of the septa or wall. The cyst may contain calcification that may be thick and nodular, but no contrast enhancement is present. There are no enhancing soft-tissue components. Totally intrarenal nonenhancing high-attenuation renal lesions that are 3 cm or larger are also included in this category. These lesions are generally well marginated." The recommendation for Bosniak IIf is to follow these lesions and to determine change in size or character.

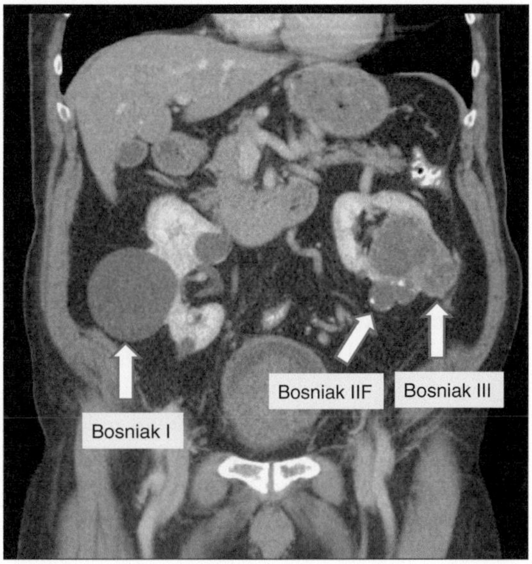

Fig. 6 Examples of Bosniak I, IIF, and III classification of cystic renal lesions. Note the solid, contrast-enhancing elements of the Bosniak III lesion. As additional incidental finding, a mass in the bladder, suggestive of enlarged prostate, is noted

Bosniak III cysts are defined as follows: "These lesions are indeterminate cystic masses that have thickened irregular walls or septa in which enhancement can be seen." Bosniak IV: "These lesions are clearly malignant cystic masses that not only have all the characteristics of category III lesions, but also contain enhancing soft-tissue components adjacent to but independent of the wall or septa" (Israel and Bosniak 2003) (Fig. 6).

It may be difficult to understand the details of the Bosniak classification by just reading the definitions. The classification system is better understood by looking at the clinical case illustrations presented in Bosniak's own original articles (Bosniak 1986, Israel and Bosniak 2003). Although not perfect in its prediction of malignant development, the Bosniak classification system offers a good help when complex cysts are incidentally encountered, including advice on follow-up. Decision on follow-up recommendations should be based on the Bosniak classification, but the patient comorbidity, age, and patient's own preferences must also be taken into consideration.

5.8 Renal Calcifications

Incidental renal calcifications are common, especially in the elderly. On unenhanced CT, even very small calcifications (1–2 mm) are easy to detect. When encountering a renal calcification, the following question should be asked: Does the calcification represent a urinary stone (located in a calyx, the renal pelvis, or ureter), a parenchymal calcification, or a vascular calcification? Vascular (arterial) calcifications are usually easy to identify by their location close to the renal hilum and in the course of the renal artery, and the finding may be supported by the coexistence of other vascular calcifications suggesting generalized atherosclerosis. In older patients with generalized vascular calcifications, renovascular calcifications are not commonly reported by the radiologist, as vascular calcifications can be considered as part of normal aging. However, in young patients, and in older patients with advanced calcifications, it might be worthwhile to report, as it may be related to treatable renal artery stenosis and renovascular hypertension (Glodny et al. 2012).

It may sometimes be difficult to differentiate a parenchymal calcification from a stone in the collecting system on non-enhanced CT and on CT obtained in the cortical or nephrographic phase, when there is not yet contrast medium filling of the collecting system, making it difficult to outline. This is rarely a problem in the excretory phase, when the collecting system is well depicted, although urinary stones may be hidden in the contrast-filled collecting system. Parenchymal calcifications are relatively rare and may be related to, e.g., nephrocalcinosis, tubular necrosis, tuberculosis, or other infections and sometimes to renal carcinoma. In case of tuberculosis, however, there are usually other typical manifestations such as corresponding parenchymal thinning and calyceal strictures and dilatation or tuberculosis manifestations in other organs. With renal carcinoma, calcifications rarely occur in small tumors, while larger calcified tumors usually are evident by their space-occupying characteristics.

Any calcifications suspected to be stones located in the collecting system should be reported, as they may potentially be displaced to the ureter causing obstruction. Even if small and not likely to cause pain or obstruction when located in a calyx, they may be of importance. Thus, they may increase in size with time, and the patient may benefit from early detection, follow-up, and perhaps treatment with extracorporeal shock wave lithotripsy (ESWL).

5.9 False-Positive Renal Masses

Focal compensatory hypertrophy associated with post-pyelonephritic parenchymal scar formation may sometimes simulate a renal mass lesion, although scar formation is more often associated with parenchymal atrophy, rather than giving an impression of mass lesion. As scar formation is a long-term effect of previous acute infection, scars may be encountered in symptom-free patients as incidental finding on CT. If in doubt, calyceal clubbing corresponding to the site of parenchymal scar formation should be looked for, to support post-pyelonephritic scarring, which is also characterized by multifocal, asymmetrical distribution in the kidney. This is different from persisting fetal lobulation, where smooth indentations of the renal outline are seen not opposite but between the pyramids. Another potential pitfall is hypertrophy of a column of Bertin, a normal variant occasionally interpreted as a renal tumor. A column of Bertin (columna renalis) represents normal cortical tissue extending deep into the kidney from the peripheral cortex, having exactly the same post-contrast attenuation as the rest of the renal cortex (Ramanathan et al. 2016).

5.10 Renal Size

The size of the kidneys should always be assessed, taking normal parenchymal thinning with age into consideration, and discrepancies in size of the two kidneys should be mentioned in the radiology report.

5.11 Normal Variants and Malformations

Among other clinically relevant incidental findings on abdominal CT, normal variants and malformations of potential clinical importance should be mentioned. Thus, congenital absence of a kidney or status post nephrectomy (single kidney) should be documented, as it may otherwise lead to confusion if the patient later undergoes, e.g. abdominal ultrasonography. Also, this information is of clinical value because of the risk of hyperfiltration and subsequent glomerulosclerosis that may occur after nephrectomy (Abdi et al. 2003). Likewise, duplication of the collecting system, ectopic and malrotated kidneys, and horseshoe kidney (Fig. 7) should be mentioned (Ramanathan et al. 2016). A horseshoe kidney is a renal fusion anomaly with functioning renal parenchyma or fibrotic tissue bridging the midline and the two renal units. Horseshoe kidneys usually have multiple renal arteries, sometimes originating from the distal aorta or iliac arteries, of importance in case of surgery or interventional procedures. Horseshoe kidneys occur in approximately 1/500 adults and are usually asymptomatic. However, they carry an increased risk for obstruction, infection, and stone formation, and it may be vulnerable in abdominal trauma. In some cases, horseshoe kidney can be linked to other malformations or a variety of genetic or other syndromes and to an increased risk of malignancy.

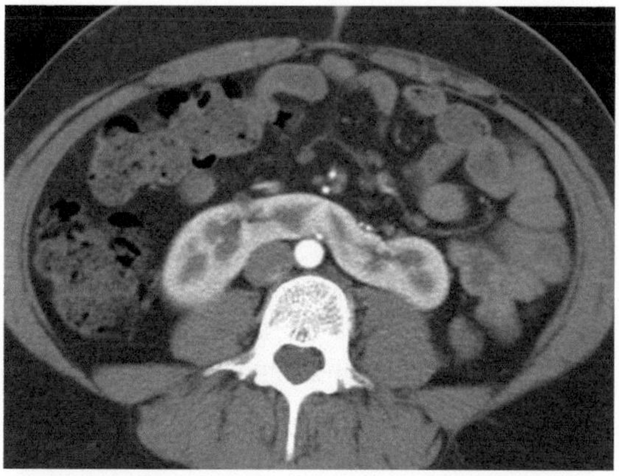

Fig. 7 Incidentally detected horseshoe kidney in a woman who had an arterial phase CT because of suspected aortic dissection. It was revealed that the patient had Turner's syndrome, which carries an increased risk of renal fusion anomaly (horseshoe kidney)

5.12 Hydronephrosis

Incidental detection of hydronephrosis and hydroureter, which may indicate urinary tract obstruction, should be mentioned. In such cases, it should be determined if it is uni- or bilateral, if it is associated with urteral dilatation, and if it is associated with generalized parenchymal thinning, which suggests more long-standing obstruction. Although hydronephrosis is usually related to urinary obstruction, this is not always the case, as dilatation may remain permanently after removal of an obstruction, if the obstruction has been long-standing and the system thereby lost some of its elasticity. Hydronephrosis on the basis of obstruction is associated with dilatation of the renal pelvis as well as calyces. It should be differentiated from a normal but large extrarenal renal pelvis without calyceal dilatation, which is not indicative of obstruction. If the CT is done with IV contrast administration, the function of the parenchyma and, with delayed scan in the excretory phase, the urinary outflow may be assessed. Another pitfall on non-enhanced and early post-contrast scanning is the existence of peripelvic cysts, which also may simulate hydronephrosis. However, in the excretory phase, differentiation between hydronephrosis and a cluster of peripelvic cysts is usually straightforward (Fig. 8). Less commonly, a parapelvic cyst, i.e. an ordinary cyst originating from the renal parenchyma and extending into the renal sinus region, may be mistaken for hydronephrosis.

6 Urinary Bladder and Upper Urinary Tract Tumors

The urinary bladder has traditionally been the domain for the urologists, cystoscopy being the primary method for tumor detection. However, improved quality of CT allows detection of bladder tumors in many instances (Raman and Fishman 2014). The vast majority of patients

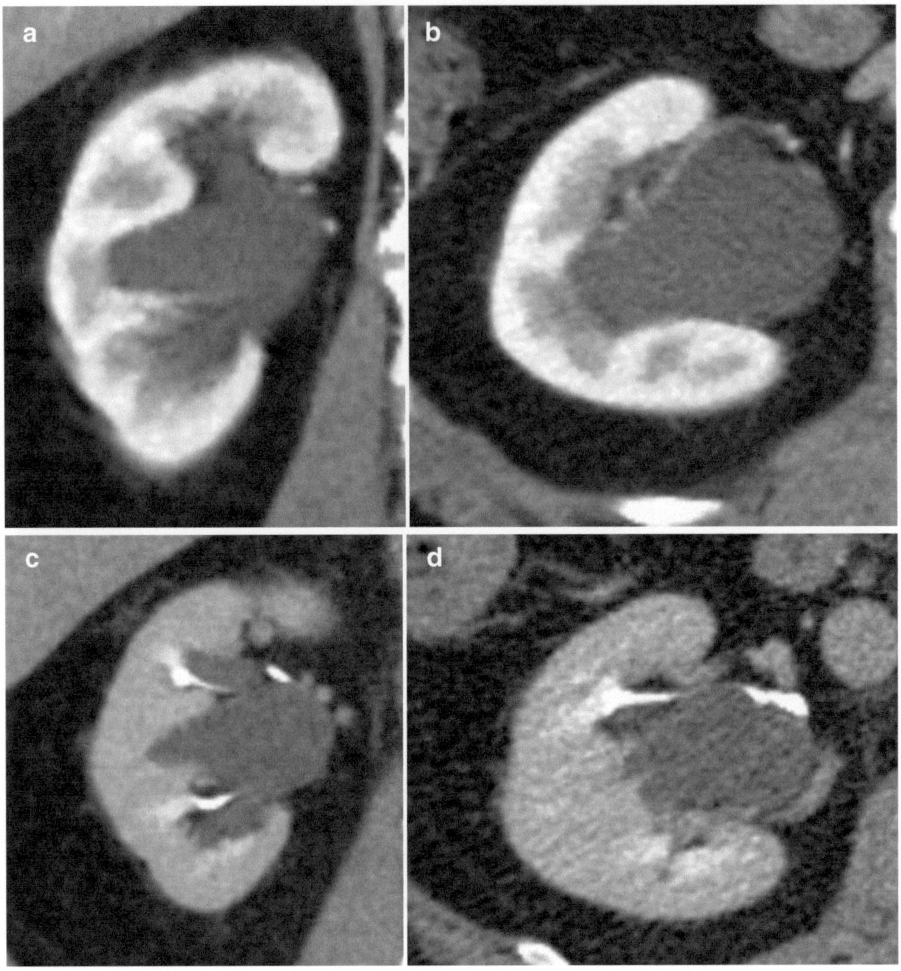

Fig. 8 Incidental finding suggestive of hydronephrosis on contrast-enhanced abdominal CT in the corticomedullary phase, before iodine contrast material arrives in the collecting system (*upper row*: coronal (**a**) and axial (**b**) planes, respectively). Images obtained a few minutes later (in the excretory phase) clearly show that the collecting system has normal width (*lower row*: coronal (**c**) and axial (**d**), respectively) and that the hypodense fluid-containing structures represent peripelvic cysts. Peripelvic cysts are not uncommon and are claimed to develop from lymphangiectasia, in contrast to parapelvic cysts which represent ordinary cysts protruding into the sinus region

with bladder or upper urinary tract cancer present with hematuria, and the workup includes cystoscopy and CT urography. The frequency of incidentally detected bladder and upper urinary tract cancers is largely unknown but appears to be low.

Unless grossly space occupying, bladder tumors are best visualized in the corticomedullary phase, as compared to the nephrographic and excretory phases (Helenius et al. 2016), due to their high attenuation in the arterial phase. As early detection of bladder cancer may improve prognosis, the bladder should routinely be scrutinized for incidental tumor detection, especially in middle-aged and older individuals, having in mind the better chance of tumor detection on contrast-enhanced CT series. Nevertheless, many bladder tumors can be depicted also on non-enhanced CT (Fig. 9).

Tumors of the calyces, renal pelvis, and ureters are much less common than urothelial bladder tumors, representing about one tenth of the total number of urothelial tumors. Thus, they are relatively rare tumors, not commonly detected as incidental findings. Typical findings

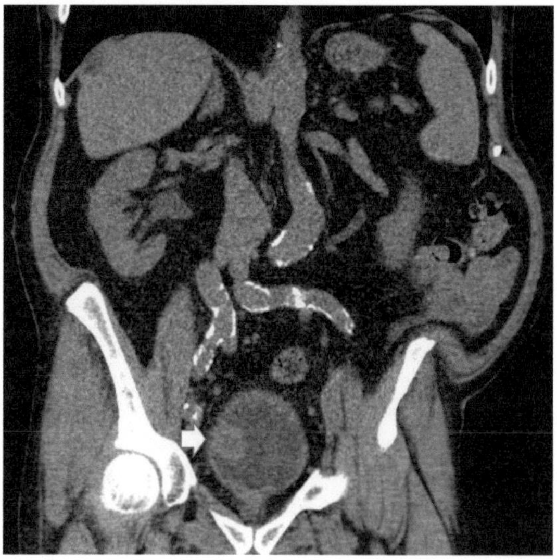

Fig. 9 Two centimeter rounded bladder wall tumor (*arrow*), hyperdense relative to the urine and protruding into the bladder lumen, on non-enhanced CT

at careful assessment of the collecting system and ureters are wall-thickening and contrast-filling defects on images obtained in the excretory phase, with or without dilatation depending on the degree of outflow obstruction (Xu et al. 2010). The nephrographic phase has been shown to demonstrate upper urinary tract tumors in a higher frequency compared to the excretory phase (Metser et al. 2012), but the combination of the two provides a better diagnostic accuracy. However, as for bladder cancer, the best possibility for incidental detection of upper urinary tract tumors appears to be in the corticomedullary or arterial phase.

7 Adrenals

Adrenal masses are among the most common incidental findings on CT of the abdomen. Hammarstedt et al. found a frequency of 4.5% in a reevaluation of 3,801 unselected clinical abdominal CT examinations, from a cohort of over 30,000 CT examinations (Hammarstedt et al. 2010). The same study showed a considerable variation in the frequency of reported lesions between hospitals (range 1.8–7.1%), suggesting considerable under-reporting in clinical practice, although differences in patient population profiles and other factors also may be a factor. The frequency of adrenal incidentalomas increases with age. Figures from autopsy studies suggest figures in the range of 7–8% (Abecassis et al. 1985) or even higher in the elderly, depending on diagnostic criteria used and the age and character of the studied populations. The vast majority of adrenal incidentalomas are non-hyperfunctioning adenomas, but the task of the radiologist is to determine, with reasonable certainty, if the lesion is a benign adenoma, cyst or other benign lesions, or malignant primary or metastatic tumor.

When an unexpected adrenal lesion is identified on CT, three questions should be raised: First, does the patient have a known malignancy? Second, does the lesion have benign, indeterminate, or malignant CT characteristics? Third, is the lesion hyperfunctioning or not?

The first question – does the patient have a known malignancy – is very relevant as the risk of an incidentally detected adrenal mass being malignant is very low if the patient has no known malignancy. Thus, Song et al. (2008) found no case of malignant adrenal lesion in 1,049 adrenal incidentalomas in patients without malignant disease. In a patient with known malignancy, on the other hand, an adrenal mass may represent a metastasis or an unrelated benign lesion. In patients with a previous history of extra-adrenal malignancy, incidentally detected adrenal lesions were found to be benign in 74% of the cases. In patients with concurrent extra-adrenal malignancy without metastases, the adrenal lesion was benign in 53%, and in patients with extra-adrenal malignancy with metastases, the adrenal lesion was benign in 25% of the cases (Hammarstedt et al. 2012). Thus, an adrenal lesion in a patient with a malignancy should not automatically be taken for a metastasis, especially in a situation where it is the only suspected metastatic site, as the existence of a metastasis may change treatment dramatically.

The second question – does the lesion have benign, indeterminate, or malignant CT characteristics – can ideally be answered already at the time of detection, if the CT examination includes

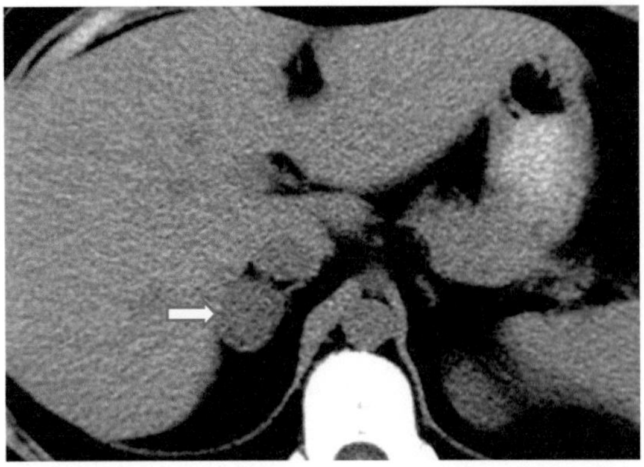

Fig. 10 Non-enhanced abdominal CT showed an incidental right-sided, oval-shaped, well-demarcated, homogeneous adrenal mass (*arrow*), with low density (5–7 HU). This suggests high lipid content characteristic of adrenal adenoma. In the absence of extra-adrenal malignancy, the risk that it is a malignant lesion is very small

a non-contrast-enhanced series. This is based on the size, morphology, and attenuation measurements of the lesion. It has been shown that adrenal lesions which are homogeneous, well defined with regular outlines, and have a density of 10 HU or less on native images (without contrast medium administration) can confidently be classified as benign (Fig. 10). This density value has also been accepted as a reasonable cutoff in the recently published guidelines from the European Society of Endocrinology (Fassnacht et al. 2016), based on a systematic review and meta-analysis of the literature (Dinnes et al. 2016). Some lesions with ≤10 HU are benign cysts or myelolipomas (Fig. 11), with low density due to their fluid or fatty content, respectively. Myelolipomas are mixed tumors from fatty and myelopoietic cells and are characterized by areas of macroscopic fat, easily identifiable on CT (mean density − 70 HU). They are not hormone producing and therefore usually asymptomatic, unless very big (Lattin et al. 2014). The majority of benign adrenal lesions are, however, adenomas. Most adenomas are rich in intracytoplasmic lipid, which explains the low-density values (≤10 HU). A minority of adenomas are lipid poor, with density measurements >10 HU, partly overlapping with malignant lesions which are also lipid poor.

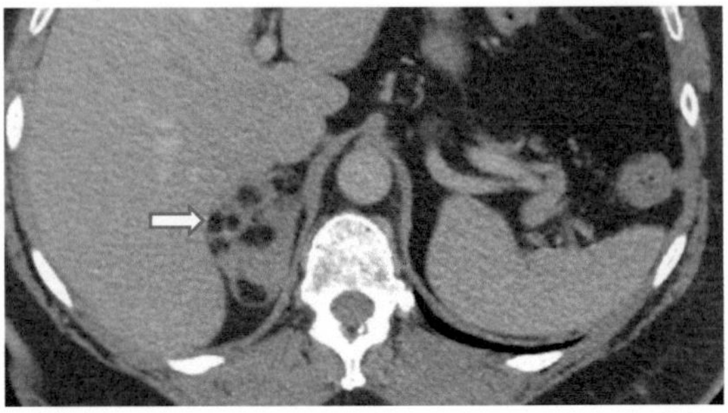

Fig. 11 Incidental finding of right adrenal mass with multiple well-defined components of macroscopic fat. The finding is typical for benign adrenal myelolipoma

However, malignant lesions often have other characteristics, such as irregular outlines, necrosis, and uneven parenchymal contrast enhancement. Contrast medium washout calculation on CT has been suggested to separate benign from malignant adrenal lesions, when native density measurements are indeterminate, i.e. >10 HU. Absolute washout measurements require that CT scans are obtained before intravenous contrast administration, during the portal phase, and after 10 or 15 min, while relative washout can be calculated on early- and delayed-phase contrast-enhanced images.

Using 60–75 s delay for early contrast enhancement scan and 15 min for delayed scan, a washout of 60% or more is a characteristic for benign (adenoma). However, according to a recent meta-analysis, the scientific evidence is not sufficient to motivate washout calculations for regular use for differentiating malignant from benign incidentalomas (Dinnes et al. 2016; Fassnacht et al. 2016).

The third question – is the lesion hyperfunctioning or not – cannot be answered based on its imaging appearance. Each patient with a newly discovered adrenal incidentaloma should be checked for hormonal overproduction of cortisol, aldosterone, or adrenalin/noradrenalin, by deepened clinical history, physical examination, and hormonal laboratory test (Lattin et al. 2014). This is the responsibility of the referring clinician, but the radiologist can point out the need of hormonal testing in his/her report.

7.1 Shape and Size of Adrenals

Identifying adrenal masses may be difficult as the shape and size of the adrenals differ between individuals and between the right and left side within the patient. Vincent et al. (1994) presented CT-based normal values for the size of the adrenal limbs and adrenal body on the right and left side, which may be of some help. The maximum width of the adrenal body was 6.1 mm and 7.9 mm on the right and left side, respectively; the maximum width of the right and left medial limbs were 2.8 mm and 3.3 mm, respectively; and the width of the lateral limb was 2.8 mm and 3.0 mm, respectively. More useful, though, is to look for any localized mass that alters the outline of the adrenal.

The ESE-ENSAT guidelines (Fassnacht et al. 2016) concern only incidentalomas measuring 1 cm or more in size, and workup or follow-up is recommended only if the lesion is 1 cm or more, unless clinical signs and symptoms suggest hormonal overproduction. It is acknowledged that this cutoff is arbitrary, based on the difficulties to confidently identify, measure, and characterize subcentimeter lesions and considering the variations in size and shape of the adrenal. Nevertheless, it should be recognized that even subcentimeter nodules may be hormonally active.

7.2 Management of Adrenal Incidentalomas

Until recently, workup and follow-up of adrenal incidentalomas have been quite extensive, including repeated CT examinations for up to 2 years with and without contrast medium administration to ensure a benign course. With increasing knowledge that adrenal incidentalomas in patients without malignancy very rarely are, or become, malignant, these investigational programs have now been shortened substantially for many patients. For those with indeterminate imaging findings and those with evidence of hormone excess, multidisciplinary expert team meetings are recommended in new guidelines (Fassnacht et al. 2016).

Patients without known extra-adrenal malignancy: non-enhanced CT is recommended for classifying an adrenal lesion as benign or indeterminate. A benign-appearing, well-defined, homogeneous lesion measuring <4 cm and with density ≤10 HU should be considered benign and needs no follow-up. However, evaluation for hormonal excess should be performed. If a similar lesion is 4 cm or larger, it is still likely to be benign, but due to lack of scientific evidence, follow-up with unenhanced CT after 6–12 months for size assessment is recommended. Size (largest diameter) increase of 20% and at least 5 mm is considered suspicious for malignancy and possible indication for surgery.

A patient without known extra-adrenal malignancy and an incidental adrenal mass with indeterminate density characteristics (>10 HU on non-enhanced CT) but otherwise benign appearance, should have non-enhanced CT in 6-12 months for growth assessment. If, on the other hand, the imaging findings do not support a benign etiology (heterogeneous, ill-defined or large lesion), if growth occurs, or if there is hormone overproduction, the patient may be a candidate for surgery. The decision should ideally be taken in a multidisciplinary team, taking clinical circumstances and patient preferences into account (Fassnacht et al 2016). With MRI, the differentiation between benign and malignant lesions is best done using chemical shift technique. Due to its rich lipid content, benign adenomas usually demonstrate a reduction in signal intensity on out-of-phase images, while the signal intensity of lipid-poor adenomas and malignant lesions remains unchanged on in-phase and out-of-phase images. Unlike CT which provides absolute measurements of density, MRI can provide only relative measures of signal intensity. Visual assessment of the MRI signal drop appears to be as useful as these measurements. However, the evidence base for chemical shift evaluation is weak, and CT is recommended as first choice, except in young patients and pregnant women.

7.3 Patients with a History of Extra-Adrenal Malignancy

If the adrenal lesion fulfills the criteria for benign etiology on non-contrast CT, it should be considered benign and requires no follow-up. If the lesion is indeterminate on non-enhanced CT, biopsy, PET-CT, or surgical resection can be considered to rule out metastasis. Regarding biopsy, it must be preceded by hormonal analysis to rule out pheochromocytoma, as the biopsy may release catecholamines causing severe symptoms.

7.4 Young Patients with Adrenal Incidentaloma

In patients under 40 years of age, the likelihood that an adrenal lesion is malignant is higher than in older patients. Therefore, immediate assessment and management rather than 6–12 months follow-up are recommended (Fassnacht et al. 2016).

8 Liver

Simple cysts, hemangiomas, and focal nodular hyperplasia are the most common hepatic lesions detected incidentally. Solid, malignant liver tumors are uncommon as incidental findings in patients without extrahepatic malignancy. In a large CT colonography screening study for colorectal cancer in nearly 8,000 asymptomatic individuals with a mean age of 57 years, unexpected extracolonic findings were analyzed on the unenhanced CT examinations (Pooler et al. 2016a, b). Individuals with extracolonic findings classified on CT colonography as C-RADS category E3 or E4 (Zalis et al. 2005), i.e. likely unimportant but incompletely characterized extracolonic findings (E3) or potentially important extracolonic findings (E4), were followed for 2–10 years. It is notable that all E3 (Pooler et al. 2016a) and E4 (Pooler et al. 2016b) liver masses in patients without known malignancy or cirrhosis were found to be benign liver cysts or cavernous hemangiomas on follow-up. It is thus comforting that incidentally detected isolated liver lesions on CT examinations very rarely seem to represent malignancy, providing that the patient has no known malignant disease or known underlying liver disease. Nevertheless, any solid-appearing liver lesion detected incidentally should be fully characterized by multiphase CT (if not obtained at detection), MRI, or contrast-enhanced ultrasonography. Solid-appearing liver lesions should be clearly highlighted in the radiology report, as underlying malignancy may be unknown to the radiologist. Also, even if benign, adenomas, focal nodular hyperplasia, and other solid liver lesions may be of clinical importance, causing symptoms and requiring intervention in some patients.

8.1 Cystic Lesions

Simple liver cysts are benign lesions without malignant potential and need no follow-up when identified incidentally on abdominal CT examinations. In autopsy studies, liver cysts have been demonstrated in up to half of patients without malignant disease. Benign liver cysts are characterized on CT as other benign, simple cysts, i.e. they are rounded or oval shaped with a thin wall and homogeneous, low density, water-like content (<20 HU) which does not enhance after intravascular contrast medium administration. Cysts that are difficult to characterize on non-enhanced CT are usually easy to confirm on contrast-enhanced CT, unless subcentimeter in size. In doubtful cases, contrast-enhanced ultrasonography, and in particular MRI, may be used for problem-solving. If multiple liver cysts are identified, the kidneys and pancreas should be scrutinized for additional cysts as part of autosomal dominant polycystic kidney disease, which occasionally occurs as an incidental finding in young- or middle-aged patients, although most of such cases are known from family history (Kim et al. 2015).

Any unclear cystic lesion that does not fulfill the CT criteria for a simple cyst, i.e. those that are multilocular or have a thick or irregular wall, septations, solid components, or suspicious contrast enhancement, should be suspected for malignancy and further characterized with ultrasonography or MRI. Such cystic lesions may represent a wide range of etiologies, including biliary cystadenoma or cystadenocarcinoma, cystic degeneration of hepatocellular cancer, and metastasis from ovarian carcinoma and a range of benign disorders, such as biloma, abscess, or echinococcal cysts (Qian et al. 2013). Most of these conditions are, however, unlikely to be incidental findings as they are commonly associated with symptoms. One exception is echinococcal (hydatid) disease, which may be encountered incidentally, as symptoms may develop slowly. Although not encountered commonly as an incidental finding, increasing international migration from endemic areas makes it an important differential diagnosis also in non-endemic countries. Echinococcal disease is caused by the larval stage of the *Echinococcus granulosus* or multilocularis tapeworm, by ingestion of eggs of the parasite transmitted from animals to humans. Echinococcus disease is endemic in large parts of the world. The ingested eggs release oncospheres which penetrate the gastrointestinal tract to the portal system and invade the liver parenchyma, causing characteristic cystic lesions. These may become symptomatic when large enough to compress the biliary tree or portal vessels, causing jaundice or portal hypertension, or by rupture into surrounding tissues or spaces (Alghofaily et al. 2016). Although the liver is the most common location for echinococcal disease, echinococcal cysts may be seen in virtually any organ. The typical appearance is that of liver cysts containing so-called daughter cysts, i.e. cysts within a mother cyst, sometimes with wall enhancement. The cyst walls, and detached floating membranes, may give the impression of septations. Commonly, characteristic calcifications of the cyst walls occur (Marrone et al. 2012).

8.2 Hemangioma

Hemangiomas are the most common non-cystic focal liver lesions, occurring in about 20% in autopsy series. As these lesions are mostly asymptomatic, it is a common incidental liver finding. The reported frequency of hemangiomas may be higher on MRI (7%) than on CT, where the prevalence on abdominal CT was 2.4% in a recent retrospective analysis of 70,000 abdominal CT examinations (85% incidental) (Mocchegiani et al. 2016). These are minimum figures, considering the retrospective design of the study. On non-enhanced CT, the most common type of hemangioma, the cavernous hemangioma, has attenuation similar to that of other vascular structures and may therefore be difficult to characterize. After intravenous contrast medium injection, hemangiomas appear well defined, with nodular, peripheral-enhanced vascular structures becoming apparent, surrounding the low-attenuating center, followed by gradual centripetal contrast medium fill-in, which typically will be noted over several minutes until more or less complete fill-in will occur (Fig. 12). In most cases, hemangiomas can be confidently diagnosed on contrast-enhanced CT. Normally, hemangiomas are asymptomatic and require no further follow-up (Marrero et al. 2014). However, if large (>4 cm), there is a risk, albeit small, of spontaneous rupture that may motivate follow-

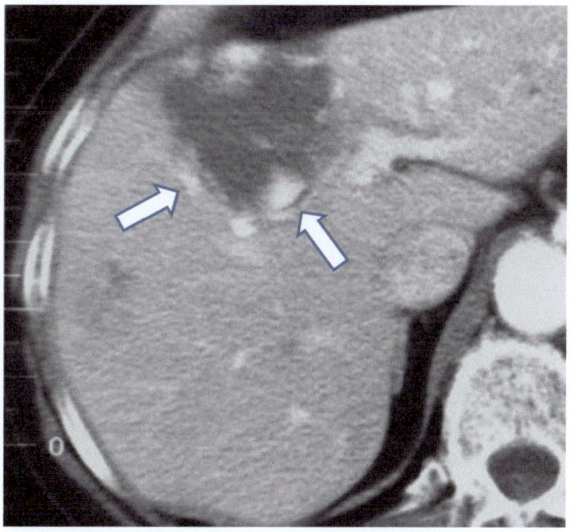

Fig. 12 Incidental detection of a low density liver lesion with nodular peripheral contrast enhancement (*arrows*) on early phase contrast-enhanced CT. The finding is highly suggestive of hemangioma, which can be confirmed by progressive centripetal contrast fill-in on a later phase imaging

up and possible intervention (Mocchegiani et al. 2016). Considering that rupture occurred mainly in large lesions with a peripheral location, the size and location of the hemangioma should be clearly stated in the radiology report. If an hemangioma is incidentally suspected on non-enhanced CT, the lesion, like other lesions that do not fulfill the criteria for simple cysts, should be further characterized by contrast-enhanced CT or MRI, if necessary including delayed imaging to confirm a hemangioma. Heavily T2-weighetd MRI is particularly effective to differentiate hemangioma from a malignant lesion (McFarland et al. 1994). As an alternative, contrast-enhanced ultrasound may be used, providing that a trained examiner is available (D'Onofrio et al. 2015).

8.3 Non-cystic Benign Liver Lesions

After hemangioma, focal nodular hyperplasia (FNH) is the second most common benign liver tumor. Although it occurs also in males, it is much more common in women, in whom it commonly presents in the third or fourth decade of life. In 85% of the cases, the lesion is less than 5 cm in size at detection. It is usually asymptomatic, and therefore most lesions are detected incidentally on cross-sectional imaging, including abdominal CT. However, with increasing size, it may cause pain, discomfort, or a palpable mass. Rarely, several FNH lesions may coexist. The appearance on CT is that of a slightly lobulated soft tissue mass, which is iso- or hypoattenuating as compared to the surrounding parenchyma on non-enhanced CT. In the arterial post-contrast phase, the lesion is typically homogeneously hyperattenuating as compared to the liver parenchyma, with a central "scar" of less enhancement. In the portal phase and later, the FNH is more or less isoattenuating with the parenchyma (Fig. 13), while the central scar often shows gradual enhancement on later phases (Hussain et al. 2004). In rare cases, the central scar remains hypoattenuating after intravenous contrast administration, making distinction from fibrolamellar hepatocellular carcinoma with central necrosis difficult. In some cases (16–40%), the central scar is small or not clearly recognizable on CT, making the diagnosis less specific (Mortele et al. 2000). In such cases, MRI may be helpful to establish the diagnosis (Hussain et al. 2004).

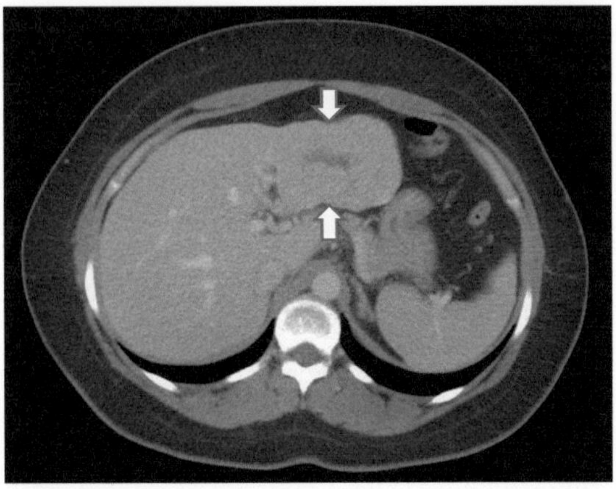

Fig. 13 A 32-year-old, previously healthy female with acute lower abdominal pain admitted for acute abdominal CT, which showed acute appendicitis. As incidental finding, a 7 × 6 cm solid, slightly lobulated lesion of the left lobe of the liver was found. The lesion appeared isoattenuating with the liver in the portal phase (*arrows*) and showed a central scar suggestive of, but not proving, focal nodular hyperplasia (FNH). It could not be confidently classified on single-phase CT, but FNH was confirmed by subsequent liver MRI

Hepatic adenomas are less common than cysts, hemangiomas, and FNH. As with FNH, they are more common in women of childbearing age, but a stronger association with oral contraception medication has been shown for adenomas, in addition to a strong association with steroid (mis-)use. There is also a long-term increased risk of malignancy, not seen with FNH. A hepatic adenoma may cause symptoms, such as pain, discomfort, or other symptoms related to a mass effect, but symptoms may also be more acute, related to rupture and bleeding. With increased use of abdominal CT, an increasing proportion of hepatic adenomas are identified as incidental findings on CT. Their detection and differentiation from FNH (and hepatocellular carcinoma) are important, as hepatic adenomas may be candidates for more intense follow-up or surgical removal, which is not usually the case for FNH.

Apart from occasional bleeding, some adenomas develop necrosis, recognizable on imaging examinations. In 5–10% of cases, calcifications may be seen on CT. Hepatic adenomas usually occur as single lesions, mostly in the right lobe of the liver but may be multiple. They are usually well circumscribed, non-lobulated, and isoattenuating with the liver parenchyma before contrast enhancement. Due to varying elements of intra-tumoral fat and post-hemorrhage tissue reactions, they may appear irregularly hypo- or hyperdense. In case of liver steatosis, they may occur as hyperdense in comparison with the liver. After intravenous contrast administration, small adenomas tend to be hyperattenuating on imaging in the arterial phase and isoattenuating in the portal phase (Grazioli et al. 2001). Unlike FNH, there is no central scar in adenomas, unless mimicked by central necrosis. Overlapping CT imaging features between hepatocellular carcinoma, FNH, and adenoma makes characterization at incidental detection on CT difficult. In the clinical situation, this is not trivial, and, therefore, a combination of multiphase CT and MRI is often necessary to obtain a final diagnosis (Grazioli et al. 2005).

8.4 Approach to an Incidental Liver Mass Detected on CT

Many liver lesions detected incidentally on abdominal CT are small and of uncertain clinical importance. An isolated 8 mm liver lesion of unclear etiology in an 85-year-old patient without known malignancy is probably of very minor clinical importance, while a similar finding in a 30-year-old male body builder using anabolic steroids may be of potential clinical importance, requiring follow-up. Both lesion size and patient background factors, as well as comorbidity and life expectancy, clearly have to be taken into consideration when evaluating incidentally detected liver lesions. The American College of Radiologists (ACR) Incidental Findings Committee has published guidelines regarding the management of incidental liver masses (Berland et al. 2010). They suggest that patients with incidental liver lesions be categorized according to risk status, into those with low, average, or high risk: *Low risk individuals* are defined as "young patients (≤40 years old), with no known malignancy, hepatic dysfunction, hepatic malignant risk factors or symptoms attributable to the liver." *Average risk individuals* are defined as those ">40 years old, with no known malignancy, hepatic dysfunction, abnormal liver function tests or hepatic malignant risk factors or symptoms attributable to the liver". *High risk individuals* are defined as those "with known primary malignancy with a propensity to metastasize to the liver, cirrhosis, and/or other hepatic risk factors. Hepatic risk factors include hepatitis, chronic active hepatitis, sclerosing cholangitis, primary biliary cirrhosis, hemochromatosis, hemosiderosis, oral contraceptive use, anabolic steroid use" (Berland et al. 2010).

Although multidetector CT with thin slices may sometimes reveal focal liver lesions measuring only 2–3 mm in size, characterization of lesions measuring 0.5 cm or even 1 cm in size may be difficult and uncertain. The ACR suggests that incidental liver *lesions < 0.5 cm* in low- or average-risk patients (as defined above) should be considered as benign, requiring no follow-up. In high-risk patients, follow-up in 6 months by CT or MRI is recommended, for example, in case of cirrhosis. *Lesions measuring 0.5–1.5 cm* with benign features, i.e. typical hemangioma or homogeneous, sharply marginated, low-attenuation lesions (up to about 20 HU), with no contrast enhancement, should be considered as benign, requiring no follow-up in any of the risk groups. Apart from hemangiomas, cysts and hamartomas are included in this group. *Lesions 0.5–1.5 cm* with low attenuation but suspicious imaging features, such as ill-defined margins, enhancement >20 HU, or heterogenous appearance, should have follow-up (6 months or closer) in all risk groups. *Lesions 0.5–1.5 cm* with "flash filling" ("robustly enhancing"), such as typical hemangioma or FNH in patients with low or average risk, need no further follow-up. If "flash filling" or robustly enhancing lesion occurs in high-risk patient, evaluation with MRI or follow-up in 6 months should be considered. For high-risk patients, comprehensive guidelines for the identification of hepatocellular carcinoma have been published by EASL-EORTC (2012). For *lesions > 1.5 cm* with low attenuation and benign appearance, no further follow-up is needed. *For lesions > 1.5 cm* with low attenuation but suspicious imaging features (as above), low-risk patients should have follow-up in 6 months, average-risk patients should have prompt evaluation, preferably with MRI, and for high-risk patients, biopsy should be considered. For *lesions > 1.5 cm* with "flash filling" (robustly enhancing) and benign imaging features, hemangioma, FNH, or other benign etiologies should be confirmed, if not confidently diagnosed with CT. If the CT shows robust enhancement but no benign diagnostic features, multiphasic MRI and possibly biopsy should be performed to confirm or rule out hepatocellular carcinoma and metastatic liver disease.

A structured approach to incidentally detected liver lesion on CT examinations as described above (Berland et al. 2010) is certainly valuable and helpful but not always possible to follow. Shortage of staff or machines, long waiting lists, cost containment, and priorities versus other patient groups come into play in daily clinical work and in scheduling patients for evaluation and follow-up. In the era of patient-centered care, also the preferences of the patient need to be taken into account. Structured guidelines should therefore be seen as guidelines for obtaining reasonably safe and adequate patient care.

8.5 Steatosis

Steatosis of the liver parenchyma is a very common finding on abdominal CT, if actively looked for. Using a threshold of 40 HU, Boyce et al. (2010) found steatosis in 6.2% of 3,357 asymptomatic individuals undergoing screening CT colonography at a mean age of 57 years (Boyce et al. 2010). Steatosis may vary in degree over time, as measured on abdominal CT (Hahn et al. 2015). When marked, steatosis may be apparent for to the naked eye when the hepatic vasculature has a higher density than the surrounding liver parenchyma on non-enhanced CT (Fig. 14). Considering the potential relationship between liver steatosis and the metabolic syndrome and other metabolic and hormonal disorders, it seems reasonable to regularly scrutinize the liver for steatosis on abdominal CT and to report it to the referring physician, although there is no immediate therapeutic action or patient benefit coupled to such a finding, at present.

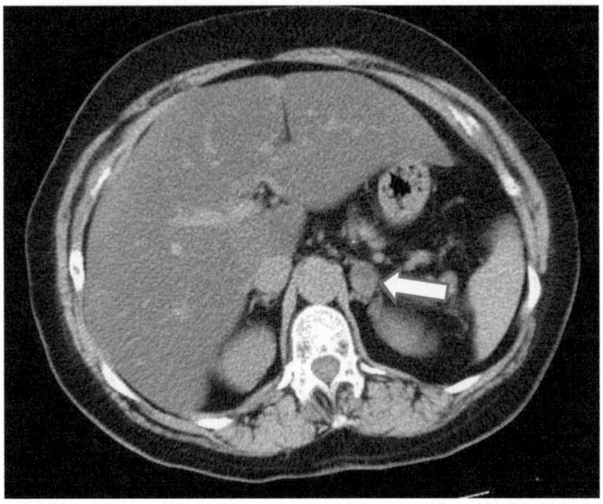

Fig. 14 A 69-year-old female with acute abdominal pain. Non-enhanced CT of the abdomen was performed, showing no bowel obstruction or other acute disorders. Incidentally, a 2.3 cm left adrenal lesion was found (*arrow*), with low but slightly irregular density (5–18 Hounsfield units). Seventeen months follow-up showed no change and no hormonal overproduction. As a second incidental finding, marked liver steatosis was noted (density values <10 Hounsfield units). Note that the normal non-contrast-enhanced hepatic vessels appear hyperdense in comparison with the low-density liver parenchyma

9 Gallbladder and Biliary Tree

Asymptomatic gallstones are one of the most common incidental findings on abdominal CT. In the study of Sconfienza et al. (2015) of about 1,000 abdominal CT examinations, gallstones were the most frequent incidental finding. In most cases, this is a trivial finding, but it should be mentioned in the radiology report for clinical correlation. CT is very sensitive to calcium deposits, meaning that most calcified gallstones are identified, but many gallstones are only faintly or not at all calcified and are easily missed on CT, while they are apparent on ultrasonography. When gallstones are encountered, the gallbladder wall should be scrutinized to reveal inflammatory or chronic general wall thickening. Similarly, widening of the extra- and intrahepatic biliary tree should be search for. A common bile duct >7 mm in a patient with the gallbladder present and >10 mm after cholecystectomy can be considered as dilated and indicative of obstruction (Sebastian et al. 2013).

Gallbladder wall calcification (porcelain gallbladder) has been claimed to be associated with gallbladder cancer, but the association appears weak, and the ACR Incidental Findings Committee does not generally recommend follow-up for calcified gallbladder wall without an associated soft tissue mass (Sebastian et al. 2013).

Uniform gallbladder wall thickening over 3 mm without a mass lesion can be associated with previous inflammation (chronic cholecystitis) but, importantly, also with, e.g., congestive heart failure and hypoproteinemia.

Although seen more commonly on ultrasonography, gallbladder polyps and cancer may occasionally be detected incidentally on CT (Mellnick et al. 2015). Soft tissue filling defects with contrast enhancement are suggestive of polyps. If <10 mm in size, these are likely benign, but follow-up with ultrasonography for growth is recommended if 5–10 mm, while removal should be considered if >10 mm (Sebastian et al. 2013). Irregular focal gallbladder wall thickening with contrast enhancement can be indicative of gallbladder cancer, which is the most common biliary tract cancer. It is frequently incidental, but only in the meaning that it is unsuspected until detected at laparoscopic or open gallstone surgery in a symptomatic patient (Cavallaro et al. 2014).

10 Spleen

Most incidental findings of the spleen are benign and of no clinical consequence. Malignant splenic abnormalities are often accompanied by other findings indicative of malignancy. There is considerable overlap in the CT appearance of benign and malignant abnormalities. A comprehensive overview of incidental splenic lesions and their management have been presented by the ACR Incidental Findings Committee (Heller et al. 2013).

11 Lymph Nodes

Incidental detection of single, clustered, or generalized lymph node enlargement is an important finding, which may indicate lymphoma or other malignancies. If not generalized, however, it is difficult to determine the clinical importance of the finding, considering the normal variation in size and the overlap in appearance of inflammatory, reactive, and malignant nodes. Lymph nodes in the abdomen and pelvis tend to have different sizes in different compartments, and there is a variation normally in the number of visible nodes on CT. Short-axis node diameter provides stronger correlation to malignancy than long axis and is recommended for assessment. Short axis of 1 cm or more can be considered as abnormal in the retroperitoneum (Heller et al. 2013), although nodes in, e.g. the retrocrural space, normally are smaller. In patients with malignancy, enlarged nodes on CT are likely to be malignant but may also be reactive and benign. Conversely, normal node size does not exclude malignant involvement. An increased number of normal-sized nodes may be indicative of a pathological process. It has been suggested that a cluster of three or more nodes in a single node station or a cluster of two or more nodes in two nodal stations is suspicious. If encountered in the absence of clinical explanation, a 3-month follow-up for growth may then be motivated (Heller et al. 2013).

Isolated enlargement of mesenteric lymph nodes is sometimes detected incidentally, combined with an infiltrated, encapsulated fatty mesenteric tissue and a perivascular fatty rim. These findings are indicative of sclerosing mesenteritis (panniculitis) (Sabate et al. 1999), which may be asymptomatic or present with vague abdominal symptoms.

12 Pancreas

12.1 Solid Tumors

Solid tumors of the pancreas usually represent ductal adenocarcinoma or neuroendocrine neoplasms. Incidental detection of solid pancreatic adenocarcinoma is uncommon and probably contributes only marginally to the overall survival for this patient group at large. Neuroendocrine tumors may be functional, i.e. hormone producing, named after the hormones produced, e.g. insulinomas and gastrinomas. Incidentally detected neuroendocrine neoplasms are likely to be nonfunctional and symptom-free. In a retrospective review of cases referred for assessment of solid pancreatic masses, 24 (7%) of 321 cases were detected incidentally (Goodman et al. 2012). Of these, 14 were adenocarcinomas and ten were neuroendocrine tumors, initially identified on CT performed for various unrelated reasons and with varying examination protocols. Only two of the tumors were located in the head of the pancreas, the rest being located in the body, tail, or uncinate process. Of the 14 adenocarcinomas, eight were hypodense and six were isodense with the pancreatic parenchyma, while seven of the ten neuroendocrine tumors were hyperdense. In total, 16 of the 24 tumors exhibited an obvious mass. The remaining eight cases were identified by indirect signs, such as subtle deformity of the pancreatic contour, a dilated main pancreatic duct (>3 mm) (interrupted duct sign) due to obstruction by the tumor (Goodman et al. 2012), or an effacement of the normal intrapancreatic fat. It seems likely that such subtle signs may be overlooked in many clinical circumstances. Eleven of the 24 patients had metastases already at the time of incidental detection, and the overall survival in those with adenocarcinoma was only 22 months, reflecting the dismal prognosis in pancreatic adenocarcinoma, despite presymptomatic detection. Incidental detection of a hyperdense contrast-enhancing pancreatic mass suggests neuroendocrine etiology (Fig. 15) with a slightly better prognosis (mean survival 42 months, range 16–82 months).

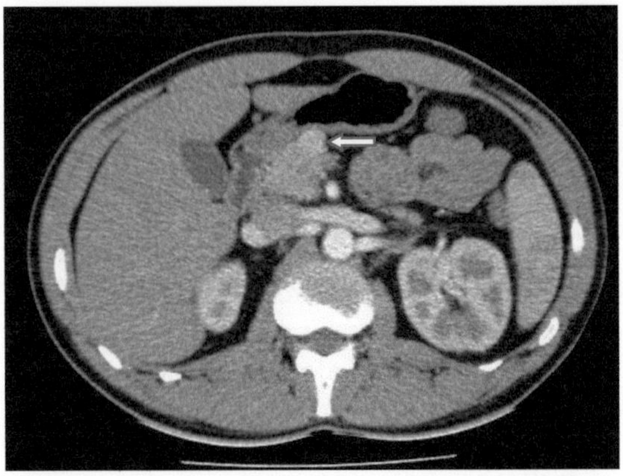

Fig. 15 A 44-year-old male with incidentally detected 1.7 cm hyperattenuating solid lesion in the anterior part of the pancreas (*arrow*), visualized on arterial phase CT. After further characterization with MRI and somatostatin-receptor scintigraphy, the lesion was surgically removed. Histological analysis showed benign neuroendocrine tumor

12.2 Cystic Lesions

As compared to solid pancreatic tumors, cystic pancreatic lesions are more common as incidental findings on CT and much more likely to be benign. Over the last decades, there has been a marked increase of incidentally detected cystic pancreatic lesions, due to the increased use and improved resolution and overall image quality of multidetector CT and due to increased awareness of their existence. In an analysis of consecutive cystic pancreatic lesions subjected to surgery over a 33-year time period, there was an increase of incidental detection from 22% in 1978–1989 to 50% in 2005–2011 (Valsangkar et al. 2012). Laffan et al. (2008) retrospectively reexamined 2,832 contrast-enhanced abdominal outpatient CT examinations, excluding those with symptoms or history of pancreatic disorders. In that population with a mean age of 58 years, they found cystic pancreatic lesions in 73 cases (2.6%). No pancreatic cysts were found in those under 40 years of age, while the frequency in the age group 80–89 years was 8.7%. The incidental detection rate in ordinary clinical situations may be lower as the purpose of the study (Laffan et al. 2008) was to specifically look for pancreatic lesions, not considering other perhaps more clinically urgent conditions, which in a clinical situation may have drawn attention away from the pancreas. It should also be noted that only contrast- enhanced CT examinations were evaluated. In non-contrast-enhanced CT examinations, the incidental detection rate may be lower, due to less conspicuity of the lesions in the absence of intravenous contrast injection. On the other hand, the real frequency of cystic pancreatic lesions may be considerably higher than that found on CT, as MRI has shown a frequency of 13.5% (Lee et al 2010), and autopsy studies revealed cystic pancreatic lesions in up to 24% of the studied population (Kimura et al. 1995).

In a recent, large, retrospective analysis of predominantly men (88%), including all cyst etiologies, patients with pancreatic cysts had nineteen times higher risk of developing pancreatic cancer over 8 years observation, compared to those without a diagnosis of pancreatic cysts (Munigala et al. 2016).

When the radiologist encounters an incidental cystic pancreatic lesion, the first question to be asked is if it could represent a pseudocyst associated with previous acute pancreatitis or chronic pancreatitis. This may be apparent from available earlier radiological examinations or from medical files and may also be indicated by CT findings such as parenchymal calcifications, necrotic areas, dilatation of the main duct and side branches, parenchymal atrophy, and extrapancreatic location of the pseudocyst. In other cases, the differentiation between a pseudocyst and a mucinous cystic neoplasm may be difficult and of concern, as the clinical handling and prognosis are different.

If a pseudocyst and cyst-like necrosis in a solid pancreatic cancer can be ruled out, the cyst is likely to represent a serous cystadenoma (SCA), mucinous cystic neoplasm (MCN), or intraductal papillary mucinous neoplasm (IPMN) (Fig. 16). Comprehensive guidelines on the management of MCN and IPMN have recently been published (Tanaka et al. 2012). Serous cystadenomas are benign tumors with female preponderance, occurring in elderly women (median age 68 years), therefore sometimes called "grandmother tumor" (Zaheer et al. 2013). On CT, they may occur as

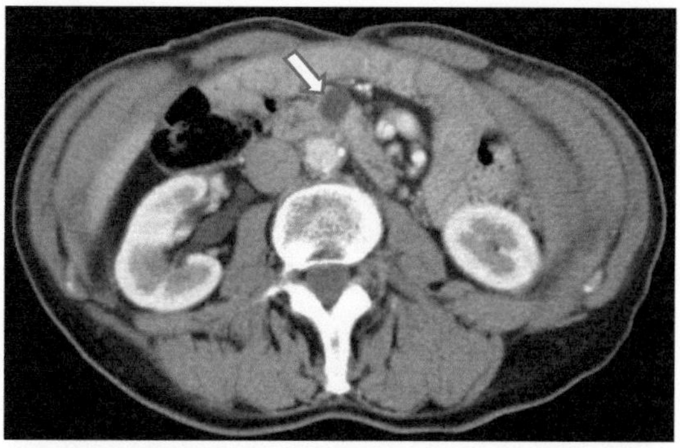

Fig. 16 Incidentally detected 1.5 cm cystic mass in the body of pancreas (*arrow*) on contrast-enhanced CT in a 75-year-old male. Further characterization with MRI was suggestive of side-branch intraductal papillary mucinous neoplasm (IPMN). Surgical removal confirmed IPMN with high-grade dysplasia

a mass consisting of small, multiple cysts with multiple septations and sometimes a characteristic central scar with or without calcification.

Further investigation of incidentally detected cystic pancreatic lesions includes a multiphase CT, including native, arterial, as well as venous phase imaging. MRI has a similar, or better, accuracy in differentiating benign from malignant cystic pancreatic lesions, and together with MRCP allows visualization of the pancreatic duct, and in case of branch duct IPMN, the connection to the main pancreatic duct (Tanaka et al. 2012). Although not performed as first-line investigation, PET-CT has the highest accuracy in this respect (Kauhanen et al. 2015). If uncertainty remains, endoscopic ultrasonography with fine needle aspiration is a recommended option (Muthusamy et al. 2016).

13 Gastrointestinal Tract

Incidental findings of the gastrointestinal tract on abdominal CT occur occasionally but constitute a difficult area depending on the wide normal variation of the bowel wall appearance. In a series of 2,014 individuals undergoing CT colonography screening, an unsuspected tumorous lesion of the extracolonic gastrointestinal tract was found in ten asymptomatic individuals (0.5%) (Pickhardt et al. 2007). The lesions measured 1.0–3.4 cm.

Three of them were located in the stomach (one lipoma, one polyp, one leiomyoma), two in the jejunum (one lipoma, one hamartoma), three in the ileum (one lipoma, one hamartoma, one leiomyoma), and two in the appendix (two mucinous adenomas).

13.1 Stomach

Mass lesions in the stomach are notoriously difficult to detect and characterize, as a non-distended stomach has a thick wall, difficult to differentiate from true wall thickening. Likewise, a normal thick-folded stomach wall is easily misinterpreted as tumorous or infiltrated. This means that radiologists should be very careful in evaluating the stomach wall thickness, unless the stomach is well distended, or a clear abnormality is indicated by, e.g. focal thickening and distinctly abnormal contrast enhancement.

13.2 Small Bowel

Obstruction, perforation, and acute inflammatory intestinal disorders rarely present as incidental findings. Chronic inflammatory or postinflammatory bowel wall thickening may occur as an incidental finding in asymptomatic patients examined for unrelated reasons, while tumors of the small bowel are rare, both as symptomatic and incidental findings (see above). Asymptomatic duodenal or other diverticula may be occasional findings. Incidental Meckel's diverticula are frequently missed on CT of asymptomatic patient, but their identification is facilitated if bowel loops are separated by abundant intraperitoneal fat (Kawamoto et al. 2015).

13.3 Large Bowel

Colon cancer is the second or third most common cancer in both men and women in the western world. It is well known that early diagnosis is beneficial and associated with better outcome, as shown in screening studies using fecal occult blood tests followed by colonoscopy and removal of precancerous polyps (Hardcastle et al. 1986; Mandel et al. 1993; Kronborg et al. 1996). Opportunistic screening by scrutinizing the colon in abdominal CT examinations performed for unrelated reasons, in order to find such cancer tumors or precancerous polyps, may therefore seem like a good idea. Although colon cancer and large adenomas sometimes are incidentally identified on standard abdominal CT, small- and medium-sized colonic polyps cannot be expected to be identified without preceding bowel cleansing and rectal gas distension of the bowel. Localized, tumor-like colon wall thickening or "stricture" is frequently reported by radiologists as an incidental, tumor-suspected finding on abdominal CT. Such findings may represent asymptomatic colon cancer or adenoma and may, when detected and reported, contribute to early treatment by endoscopic or surgical removal and thereby better prognosis. Not seldom, however, the endoscopist finds no lesion, suggesting that the incidental CT finding was false positive. This reflects the difficulty in differentiating the normal colonic wall "thickening" that occurs with bowel wall relaxation, from wall thickening caused by a colonic mass lesion, in a non-distended colon. Radiologists should be aware of this normal variability in appearance of the colon walls, frequently depicted on CT colonography, where a poorly distended segment in one body position may show tumor-like symmetrical or asymmetrical wall thickening, while it appears completely normal when well distended in the other body position (Fig. 17). In order to avoid misinterpretation, one has to critically assess the degree of bowel distension and the symmetry and extent of wall thickening. Bowel content may also lead to false-positive findings. Unlike most polyps, fecal material frequently shows angular shape and often contains gas components, and density measurements show lower HU values than organic tissue.

Despite the risk of false-positive findings and overdiagnosis of colonic tumors, the colon should be scrutinized in every abdominal CT in middle-aged and elderly patients, considering the potential benefits of detecting an early cancer or precancerous adenoma.

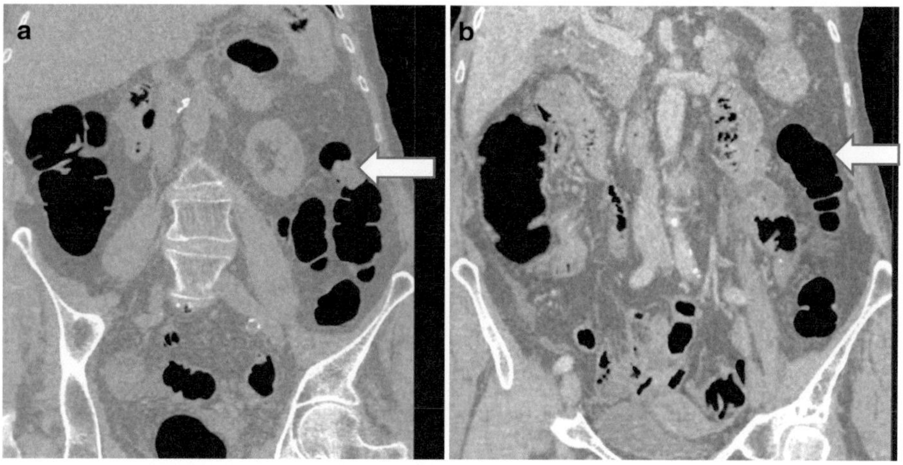

Fig. 17 (**a**, **b**) Patient admitted because of large bowel symptoms. CT colonography shows focal mass-like structure in the descending colon in prone position (**a**, *arrow*), while the same colon segment appears normal on images obtained shortly thereafter in the supine position (**b**, *arrow*). The finding represents a focal contraction of the colon, sometimes seen on abdominal CT, and represents a potential source of false-positive colonic finding on abdominal CT

13.4 Appendix

Occasionally, a mucocele of the appendix may be incidentally detected on abdominal CT, as approximately 25% of these are asymptomatic. Mucoceles occur primarily in patients over 50 years of age, with some female preponderance. Mucocele is an important incidental finding for two reasons. First, with growth it may rupture, causing dissemination of mucinous material in the abdominal cavity, resulting in pseudomyxoma peritonei. Second, a mucocele may be malignant, and the patient can benefit from early surgical removal. A mucocele is a fluid-filled tubular pelvic lesion anatomically in contact with the cecum (Fig. 18). It may simulate other pelvic cystic masses (Moyle et al. 2010). The absence of a normal-appearing appendix may be a clue to the diagnosis on CT. Depending on the degree of lumen obstruction, the mucocele gradually distends, so it can be of variable size at detection. There may be irregular wall thickening and occasionally calcifications. Mucoceles are usually benign, originating from either a nonneoplastic occlusion of the appendiceal lumen or from an obstruction due to mucinous cystadenoma or adenocarcinoma of the appendix. Thus, a mucocele may be malignant. Importantly, if a mucocele is suspected, no biopsy or percutaneous drainage should be attempted, as this may cause spillage of the content into the peritoneal cavity.

14 Vascular Structures

The most important incidental vascular finding on abdominal CT is abdominal aortic aneurysm (AAA). It is defined as an abdominal aortic diameter of 3 cm or more or an increase of 1.5 times the normal diameter. The ACR Committee on Incidental Findings recommend follow-up every 5 years for patients with ectatic aortas measuring 2.5–2.9 cm, every 3 years for aortas measuring 3.0–3.4 cm, every 2 years for 3.5–3.9 cm, every year for 4.0–4.4 cm, every 6 months for 4.5–4.9 cm, and every 3–6 months for larger aneurysms (Khosa et al. 2013). AAA is more frequent in men than in women, and there is an increased incidence with age. Due to the risk of rupture, many countries have introduced ultrasound screening for AAA in men, in order to identify those in need of follow-up or preventive surgery. However, measurements of aortic diameters on non-enhanced or enhanced CT are also easily obtained (Fig. 19) and provide an opportunity for collateral or opportunistic AAA screening,

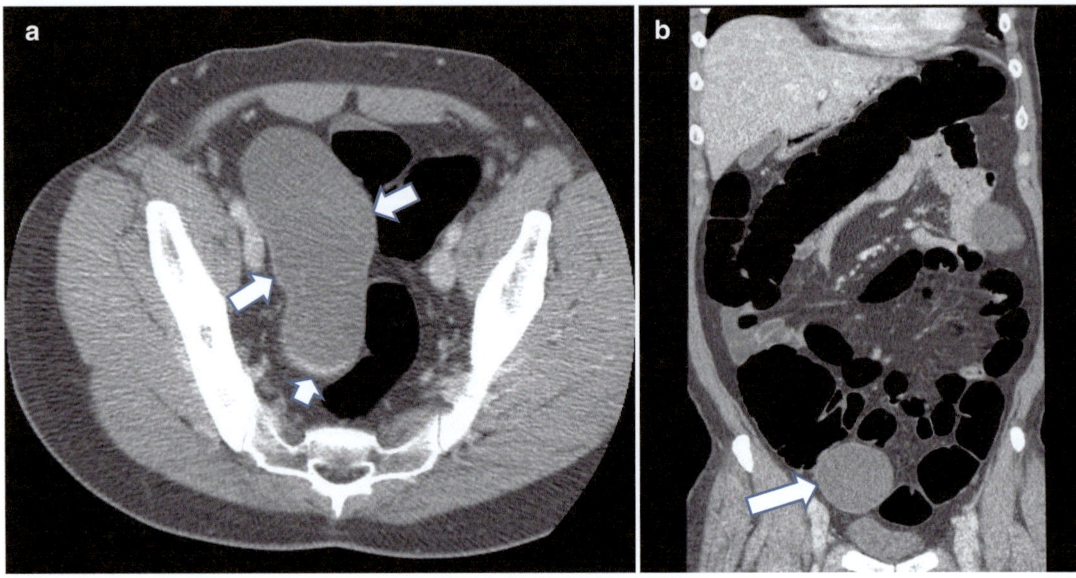

Fig. 18 A 55-year-old symptom-free male screened with CT colonography, which revealed no intra-colonic tumor but a large extracolonic tubular, low-density (20–30 HU) lesion (**a**, **b**) *long arrows*), in anatomical connection with the cecum. Thin calcifications were noted in part of the wall of the lesion (a, *short arrow*). No normal-appearing appendix could be identified. Appendiceal mucocele was suggested and confirmed at surgery. The lesion ruptured when surgically removed. Histological analysis confirmed a benign appendiceal mucocele

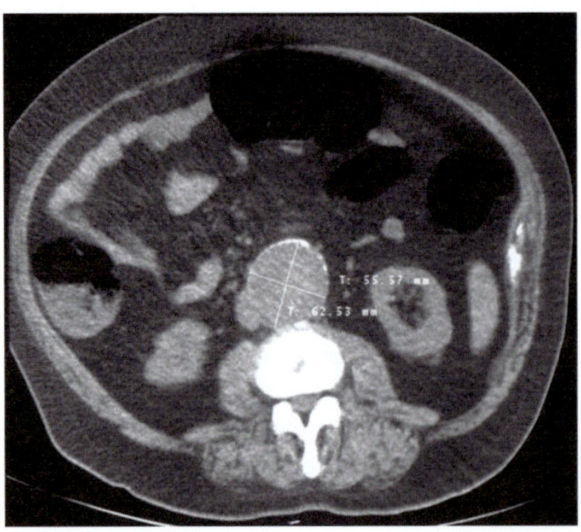

Fig. 19 A 6.2 cm abdominal aortic aneurysm incidentally detected on CT colonography. With this size of aneurysm, the patient is a candidate for elective endovascular aortic repair (EVAR)

which may be beneficial considering the long-term risk of aneurysm rupture and death. Iliac artery aneurysms are also common incidental findings, defined as a diameter of 2.5 cm or more (Khosa et al. 2013). Iliac artery aneurysms, like aneurysms in the splenic and renal arteries, are usually part of generalized atherosclerosis and sometimes coexist.

Incidental detection of calcifications in the aorta and abdominal arteries can be considered normal features of aging. However, if occurring in young patients, especially if there is suspicion of bowel ischemia (mesenteric arteries) or drug-resistant hypertension (renal artery stenosis), it may be beneficial information that should be conveyed to the referring physician.

15 Adnexal and Uterine Lesions (Not Including Incidental Lesions in Children or Pregnant Women)

In some settings, gynecological imaging is mostly handled by gynecologists, with transvaginal ultrasonography as their main imaging tool. This tends to make radiologists less involved in the imaging and workup of the gynecological organs. When there is a need for complementary imaging, MRI is usually the first choice, although CT has an important role in the workup of symptomatic patients with, for example, pain or infection and in preoperative assessment. Nevertheless, incidental findings in the female reproductive organs on CT of the abdomen and pelvis are common and need to be tackled by the radiologist. In fact, incidental gynecological findings were made in 9.5% of 749 women undergoing CT colonography, and 20% of these underwent further radiological or surgical workup – all with a benign outcome (Stitt et al. 2009). This suggests that radiological reports to some extent may convey "false alarms." In a recent study of contrast-enhanced abdominal CT (mean age 67 years), gynecological findings comprised 7% of the clinically significant (C-RADS E4 findings) incidental findings (Sconfienza et al. 2015). The impact of incidental gynecological findings on abdominal CT is also indicated by the fact that women accounted for 79% of follow-up costs for extracolonic findings in a CT colonography study, mostly attributed to suspected gynecological findings (Xiong et al. 2006).

Clearly, incidental gynecological findings on abdominal CT should not be ignored but must be handled sensibly by the radiologist, as most of the findings are benign. In a retrospective study of postmenopausal women undergoing hysterectomy for various reasons, the prevalence and histology of coexisting adnexal mass lesions were investigated (Annaiah et al. 2012). They found ovarian pathology in 31% of 200 adnexa. Over half of these were unilocular cysts, 15% were multilocular cysts, 18% were solid tumors, and 11% were uni- or multilocular cysts with solid nodules. Malignant lesions were found in 5% and borderline tumors in 4%. However, all tumors below 2 cm in size were benign, and all unilocular cysts below 5 cm were benign. Further support for a benign course of unilocular ovarian cysts was provided in a large screening study of 15,000 women aged 50 years or more, followed periodically with transvaginal ultrasound (Modesitt et al. 2003). Unilocular ovarian cysts were found in 18% of the population. The mean size of the lesions at the time of detection was 2.7 cm, and 69% had a diameter below 3 cm. Sixty-nine percent of the cysts resolved spontaneously during a mean of 6.5 years follow-up, most of them within 3 months. Over time, 16.5% of the cystic lesions developed septations and 5.8% developed a solid area, but none of the women with an isolated unilocular ovarian cyst developed malignancy during the study period. The authors concluded that a clearly unilocular ovarian cyst at ultrasonography carries an extremely low risk to develop cancer (Modesitt et al. 2003). Although findings at ultrasonography are not always identical to those at CT, it has been recommended (Patel et al. 2013) that similar guidelines should be applied for CT as for ultrasonography, with only slight modifications (Levine et al. 2010).

Factors which add to the complexity in interpretation of adnexal lesions is the normal variation in appearance of the reproductive organs in the different menstrual phases and their different appearances in pre-and postmenstrual women, as well as potential effects of, e.g., contraceptive medication and hormone replacement therapy. A particular problem in clinical practice is that the date of the last menstrual period is often unknown for the individual radiologist. After menopause, the postmenopausal period is divided into an early phase (within 5 years after menopause) and a late phase (later than 5 years after menopause). In a White Paper from The American College of Radiology (ACR), it is suggested that when the menstrual status is not known, women up to 50 years of age could be considered premenopausal and those over 50 years postmenopausal (Patel et al. 2013), although in reality, there is a considerable overlap.

15.1 Adnexal cysts and teratomas

The most common adnexal lesion likely to present as an incidental finding on CT is a cyst or cyst-like lesion. In a woman of premenopausal age, an incidentally detected cystic adnexal lesion often represents a dominant physiologic ovarian follicle, which normally develops during the follicular phase of the menstrual period. These follicles are sometimes counted as cysts, and they fulfill the criteria for simple, benign adnexal cysts, i.e. unilocular cysts of round or oval shape, with uniform fluid attenuation and regular or imperceptible wall and without solid areas or mural nodules (Patel et al. 2013). In other cases, the cystic lesion may represent a corpus luteum cyst, which is seen normally during the second half of the menstrual cycle (and during the first trimester of pregnancy). The typical CT appearance of a corpus luteum cyst is that of a 1–3 cm cystic lesion with homogeneous non-enhancing cyst content and a thick wall, which is clearly enhancing after intravenous contrast administration, sometimes called the "hyperenhancing rim sign" (Bonde et al. 2016). On Doppler ultrasonography, this vascularized wall has been termed a "wall of fire," due to its rich blood supply. This enhancing wall is, however, not unique for a corpus luteum cyst, as similar findings may be made in, e.g., ectopic pregnancy (Lin et al. 2008) and in abscesses which, however, are unlikely to occur as incidental findings. Occasionally, the corpus luteum cyst may bleed, causing fluid layering and rupture. Bleeding into the cyst may make the cyst content irregular with increased internal density, making it more difficult to differentiate on CT from other lesions, such as endometrioma or ovarian neoplasms (Bonde et al. 2016). In contrast, endometrioma can be clearly differentiated using MRI. Adnexal cystic lesions may also be located outside the ovary, para-ovarian cysts, and sometimes peritoneal cysts or tortuous tubular structures, such as a dilated fallopian tube (sactosalpinx) may mimic an adnexal cyst on CT. The ACR (Patel et al. 2013) suggests that incidentally detected benign-appearing adnexal cysts 5 cm or smaller in premenopausal women need no follow-up, while those larger than 5 cm should have follow-up with ultrasonography at 6–12 weeks. In postmenopausal women, a similar benign-appearing cyst needs no follow-up if 3 cm or smaller, while larger cysts should have prompt follow-up with ultrasonography (Patel et al. 2013). However, based on results from combined autopsy and ultrasound studies, benign cysts are very frequent and merely a normal finding in postmenopausal women (Valentin et al. 2003), and it is therefore suggested that unilocular, benign-appearing cysts <5 cm need no follow-up in postmenopausal women, due to the small risk of malignancy (Timmerman et al. 2005).

The ACR Incidental Findings Committee on Adnexal Findings also defines a category with "probably benign cyst," i.e. cysts that fulfill the CT criteria for a benign cyst, except for one of the following observations: angulated margins, not round or oval in shape, or if the cyst is poorly imaged. In premenopausal women, such cysts should have ultrasound follow-up if 3 cm or larger, and if 5 cm or larger, prompt ultrasound examination. In postmenopausal women, such a finding should initiate prompt ultrasound examination if the cyst is 3 cm or more. For women in the late postmenopausal phase, the ACR guidelines suggest that even 1 cm cysts with such characteristics should be subjected to prompt ultrasonography, but patient age, comorbidity, and patient preferences have to be taken into account in the decision-making.

Incidental cystic adnexal lesions which do not fulfill the criteria for benign or probably benign cysts on CT (except dermoid cysts, see below) should be promptly referred to ultrasonography for further characterization, treatment, or follow-up. These are lesions with a large size (see above) and/or other characteristics that disqualify them as benign cysts on CT examination, such as solid components, papillary vegetations, necrosis, thick septations, or wall thickening (Fig. 20). It should be noted, however, that thick septations and wall thickening also are features of tubo-ovarian abscesses, endometriomas, and some benign tumors and therefore not specific for malignancy. Nevertheless, any non-cystic solid incidental adnexal lesion should be sent for prompt ultrasound examination or MRI if indicated. The ovary itself may appear on contrast-enhanced CT as hypodense as related to the surrounding tissues and the myometrium. This should not be mistaken for a cystic mass.

Among other incidental findings on CT, dermoid cysts or teratomas should be mentioned. These are mixed tumors, with elements from ectoderm, mesoderm, and endoderm, in varying proportions. Mature cystic teratomas (dermoid cysts) may occur in young women, can be

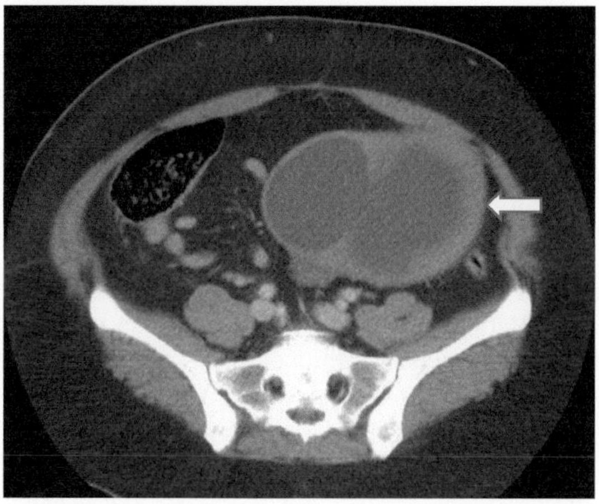

Fig. 20 Cystic mass incidentally detected in a woman examined with abdominal CT for an unrelated reason. The lesion was septated and thick walled (*arrow*). Mucinous cystadenoma was histologically confirmed

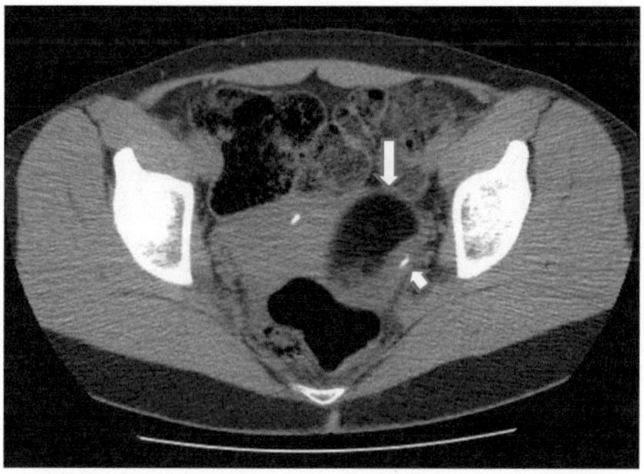

Fig. 21 Dermoid cyst with components of fat (*long arrow*), soft tissue, and bone or teeth (*short arrow*) incidentally detected on abdominal CT in a 44-year-old woman. The patient was operated and histology confirmed a benign dermoid cyst (teratoma)

bilateral (10%), and are slow growing. They are filled with liquid sebaceous material and contain elements from e.g. hair, skin, teeth, bone, and fat, which are present in most cases and tend to protrude locally from the wall (Rokitansky nodule), projecting into the cyst. The key to CT diagnosis is the occurrence of fatty content and elements of bone or teeth in a mixed pelvic mass, easily recognized on CT (Outwater et al. 2001) (Fig. 21). In a pelvis with a lot of fatty tissue, the fatty component of a teratoma may be difficult to distinguish at first glance, but the characteristic calcifications located outside the uterus and vascular tree should raise the suspicion of a dermoid. Cystic teratomas are usually benign tumors, but about 1% are, or develop into, malignant variants. In particular, immature ovarian teratomas, which are more common in younger women, may have a malignant course, showing more solid tissue components and less fatty elements. Benign ovarian dermoids are usually symptom-free but may sometimes be the cause of painful rupture or torsion. Dermoids should always be reported by the radiologist, in order to allow the referring doctor and the patient to discuss and decide if the lesion should be removed.

15.2 Uterus

The most common incidental finding in the uterus is leiomyomas (fibroids), benign tumors of the uterine myometrium. Using ultrasonography, fibroids have been found in 21% of women aged 30–60 years (Marino et al. 2004), and even higher frequencies have been suggested from autopsy materials. Although it cannot be expected that CT will identify all fibroids seen on ultrasonography, they still are the most common incidental CT findings in the uterus. Typical finding on CT is a bulky or enlarged uterus with bumpy outline or a mass in continuity with the uterus. Although they may cause menorrhagia, pain, discomfort, or impaired fertility, many cause no symptoms and are detected incidentally. They are hormone dependent, develop after menarche, are most common after 30 years of age, and usually undergo reduction in size after menopause. On CT, they are commonly isoattenuating with the surrounding myometrium and usually appear slightly hypoattenuating after intravenous contrast administration. Occasionally, they may undergo degeneration and can attain a cystic appearance. In postmenopausal women, patchy, sometimes dense calcifications are commonly seen. Uterine leiomyosarcoma may have a similar appearance, and the two cannot confidently be differentiated on CT (Gaetke-Udager et al. 2016). However, uterine leiomyosarcomas are exceedingly rare as incidental findings. Incidental detection of an enlarged uterus may also indicate uterine adenomyosis, a disease with ectopic deposits of endometrial tissue within the uterine myometrium, which may cause diffuse gynecological symptoms including menorrhagia and pain. Adenomyosis may be associated with a globally enlarged uterus with thickened myometrium and focal or diffuse distribution of multiple subcentimeter myometrial cysts, sometimes detectable on CT (Woodfield et al. 2009). If suspected on CT examination, the diagnosis should be confirmed by MRI or transvaginal ultrasonography, which provides more specific findings of adenomyosis (Yitta et al. 2011).

Mass lesions of the uterine cervix are difficult to detect on CT, unless large or clearly necrotic. The uterine cervix may normally appear hypoattenuating, depending on the degree of enhancement of the myometrium, and should not be mistaken for a cervical mass. If a cervical mass is suspected, patency and secondary widening of the endocervical canal and uterine cavity should be looked for, to support the finding.

A common incidental finding in the uterine cervix is a nabothian cyst, i.e. benign, mucinous retention cysts usually 2–10 mm in size. Nabothian cysts are better depicted on MRI, and small nabothian cysts may not be discernible on CT, but otherwise they appear as low density lesions in the cervix. They may be single or multiple and are thin walled with a low-density, nonenhancing, water-like content. They are usually asymptomatic. Only rarely may they reach several centimeters in size, possibly causing symptoms. They are caused by blockage of normal glands in the cervix, sometimes related to an infectious process in the cervix. When confidently identified on CT, there is no need for further imaging or treatment, as they are benign, usually asymptomatic and may disappear (and recur) spontaneously.

Of potential clinical importance is the incidental detection on CT of a thickened endometrium, as it may indicate an endometrial neoplasm. Endometrial thickness is easily assessed with transvaginal ultrasound, while on CT it may be difficult to define the endometrium thickness, unless grossly increased, and to differentiate the endometrium from fluid in the uterine cavity. Likewise, the endometrium may have different appearance related to the imaging plane and to the anatomical variations in the shape of the uterus (ante- and retroflexion). These difficulties are reflected in a study where endometrial thickness was qualitatively assessed by two readers on CT, using transvaginal ultrasonography as reference standard. The sensitivity of CT in identifying endometrial thickening in pre- and postmenopausal women was only 53% (specificity 93.5%), and CT overcalled endometrial thickness in one third of cases (Grossman et al. 2008). The authors emphasized the value of sagittal reconstructions in addition to standard axial and coronal reformats when assessing endometrial thickness, especially when the endometrium appears triangular and thickened on axial views. Using sagittal views and measuring the hypoattenuating inner-to-inner diameter on contrast-enhanced CT, Kang et al. (2014) found a high accuracy in determining the endometrial thickness, using the established criteria for ultrasonography (16 mm for premenopausal and 5 mm for postmenopausal women). It can be concluded that the endometrium should be scrutinized on CT performed for unrelated reasons in pre- and postmenopausal women, but the limitations mentioned above must be taken into account, while cases of clearly thickened endometrium should be further evaluated by endovaginal ultrasonography, taking effects of e.g. hormonal replacement into account.

16 Prostate

The prostate gland is usually not in focus in abdominal-pelvic CT. Most radiologists probably report incidentally detected prostatic enlargement, at least if gross or causing hydronephrosis. Prostate calcifications are common and become more frequent with age, but many prostate gland calcifications go undetected or unreported and are usually considered clinically nonsignificant. Using ultrasound, 7% of over 1,000 adults aged 21–50 years had prostate calcifications (Geramoutsos et al. 2004). Two types of calcifications were identified. The more common type was characterized by multiple small calcifications and had no relationship with symptoms. Coarse, larger calcifications were associated with prostatitis, pain, or other lower urinary tract symptoms, although the vast majority of patients with such calcifications were asymptomatic.

Of greater clinical interest is the incidental detection of prostate cancer. It is usually claimed that prostate cancer cannot be reliably identified using CT, especially in view of PSA (prostate-specific antigen) testing, multiparametric MRI, and ultrasound-guided biopsy becoming more and more available. Considering that early detection and treatment of aggressive prostate cancer may improve survival and that many men with undetected prostate cancer are going through abdominal CT for various unrelated reasons, it is important to know if the prostate really can be ignored when reading CT. The role of CT for incidental detection of prostate cancer has been highlighted in two recent articles. Glazer et al. (2015) have suggested that an enhancing localized mass in the peripheral zone (especially if 1 cm or larger) is suspicious for highly relevant clinical cancer (Gleason 3 + 4 or higher grade) when detected on a venous phase contrast-enhanced CT. Other enhancing lesions had little diagnostic value. The findings are supported by another study, which compared CT findings with multiparametric MRI of the prostate (Jia et al. 2016). It must be pointed out, however, that CT has a poor overall ability to identify prostate cancer. But when focal contrast enhancement occurs in the peripheral zone, there is a high likelihood that it may correspond to a clinically significant prostate cancer. With this in mind, it seems that the prostate gland cannot any longer be ignored when routinely assessing the pelvic region on a CT examination.

17 Skeletal Lesions

Degenerative changes of the spine, such as disc height reduction and osteophytes, as well as osteoarthritis of the hips, can be detected in a large proportion of elderly persons on abdominal CT, providing that the skeleton is assessed in an appropriate image plane and with appropriate window settings (Fig. 22). As most of subtle or moderate degenerative spinal changes in the elderly can be considered as normal aging, they are not regularly reported by all radiologists. However, at least in younger patients and if the abnormalities are extensive in the elderly, the findings could be of clinical importance and should be reported.

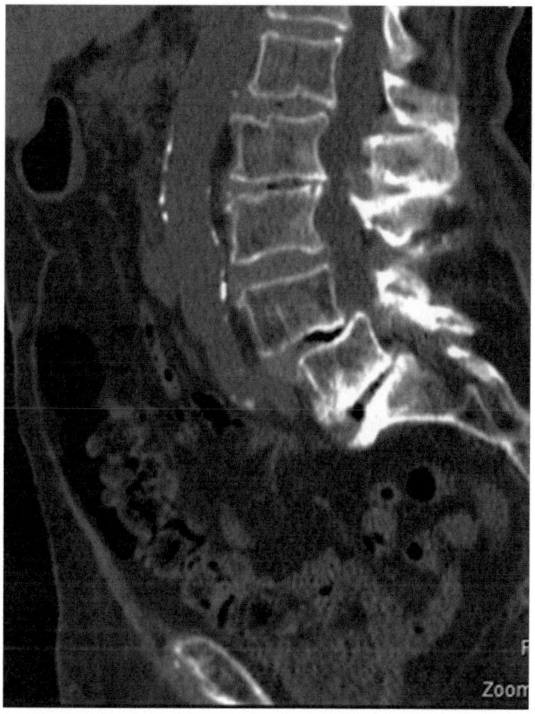

Fig. 22 Abdominal CT for acute abdominal pain, but not back pain, in an elderly woman revealed degenerative changes in the lumbar spine, including severe disc degeneration with vacuum phenomenon in several discs and spondylolisthesis with L4 slipped anteriorly on L5

18 To What Extent Are Incidental Findings Reported?

In clinical work, retrospective reviews of abdominal CT examinations can often reveal incidental findings that have not been mentioned in the radiology report. Published frequency figures on incidental findings can therefore be assumed to represent minimum figures of the real frequency of abnormalities. For example, in an analysis of incidental lung nodules on abdominal CT, it was shown that of 95 patients with lung nodules, only eight had this mentioned in the radiology report (Rinaldi et al. 2010). In a prospective multicenter study of adrenal incidentaloma frequency, the frequency of reported cases from the study centers was 0.9%, while a dedicated and systematic reevaluation of cases showed a frequency of 4.5% (Hammarstedt et al. 2010). Forty-seven percent of the incidentalomas found at reevaluation had not been reported to the study center and were also not mentioned in the original radiology report. This suggests that abnormalities that are not related to the main clinical question are commonly missed or ignored.

19 Why Do Radiologists Report or Not Report Incidental Findings?

Apart from real variations in frequencies of abnormal findings in different study populations, variations may be due to varying propensity to report such findings. Reasons for radiologists to report or not report incidental findings may be many. First of all, organs or tissues displayed at abdominal CT may not be fully scrutinized if they are not in clinical focus. Parts of the anatomy included in the CT scan may not be looked at, or not looked at with proper CT window settings, thereby making abnormalities less obvious. Another reason may be "satisfaction of search," i.e. feeling satisfied when having identified some relevant pathology, and not focusing enough on the rest (Berbaum et al. 1990). Even if properly displayed at the CT examination, and looked at, the incidental finding may erroneously be interpreted as normal by the radiologist (false-negative finding). Finally, the incidental finding may be correctly identified but not considered important enough to be reported, depending on the clinical question, the size, and nature of the finding and factors such as patient age and comorbidity. This is a common scenario, considering that modern CT (and MRI and ultrasound) has a high spatial and contrast resolution that allows the detection of many lesions in the size range 2–10 mm, especially in the solid organs such as the liver and kidneys. In this size range, CT density measurements (CT numbers, Hounsfield units) are unreliable, and even contrast medium enhancement is difficult to evaluate. Therefore, characterization of small lesions (<10 mm) is difficult, and this may be a reason not to report such findings. However, this does not explain non-reporting of larger lesions.

In the decision process, to report or not report, not only the size and character of the lesion but also the potential present and future clinical importance of the finding, as well as patient comorbidity and age, are crucial factors. Reporting of all detected small findings in all organs and tissues would be impractical and leads to confusion and uncertainty among referring clinicians on how to handle the findings, and it may potentially lead to unnecessary follow-up studies with associated risks of complications and increased costs, with no certain benefit. Thus, the radiologist has an important role to judge which findings should be conveyed to the clinician and which findings should be ignored, a task which is not always easy and has ethical implications. Reporting of "too many" small or insignificant findings leads to difficulties for the referring physician to decide which information is relevant and what should be conveyed to the patient. On the other hand, not detecting and reporting an incidental finding that may represent, e.g., early cancer may be catastrophic. Thus, if the lesion grows and is detected only a few years later, when it may have metastasized, and the patient (and doctor) is aware of a previous CT examination which retrospectively shows the lesion, important medicolegal and ethical questions may be raised.

20 Do the Patients Want to Know About Incidental Findings?

It is often claimed that reporting incidental findings to the patient may cause unnecessary patient worry, as it may lead to repeated follow-up studies and even interventions, often with no real benefit. It may also cause significant costs and sometimes even risk to the patient, from ionizing radiation at radiological examinations, surgery, to other interventions that may follow an incidental finding. An important question is then what the patients think about it – do patients want to know about incidental findings?

Ghanouni et al. (2012) interviewed asymptomatic middle-aged persons about about their preferences in a screening situation with either CT colonography or colonoscopy, after the accuracy, side effects, and possibility to detect abnormalities outside the colon were described for both methods. Overall preference was similar for the two methods, but the ability to visualize extracolonic organs (incidental findings) was considered an advantage of CT colonography.

Plumb et al. (2014) made a discrete choice experiment of perceived benefits versus harms with CT colonography in a hypothetical colorectal screening situation. They tried to "determine the maximum rate of false-positive diagnoses that patients and health care professionals were willing to accept in exchange for detection of an extracolonic malignancy." They examined the opinions of 50 healthcare professionals and 52 patients admitted for reasons unrelated to colon symptoms. They had to make a choice between CT colonography which looks inside and outside the colon (unrestricted CT colonography), and CT colonography that looks inside, but not outside, the colon (restricted CT colonography). It was explained that the unrestricted test had a 1/600 chance of detecting a curable extracolonic cancer, but that it also had a risk of inducing unnecessary additional imaging tests or interventions, such as biopsies, endoscopies and surgery. Surprisingly, both patients and healthcare professionals stated that they would tolerate a very high rate of false-positive extracolonic diagnoses in order to find the 1/600 curable extracolonic cancer. The anticipated problem with false positive extracolonic findings at screening CTC, as seen from a patient perspective, may therefore be exaggerated. On the other hand, the study was based on a hypothetical screening scenario, which may not reflect opinions in a real life situation. Also, it did not take into account the downstream cost of such screening scenario, which may influence the overall net benefits.

Muth et al. (2013) examined the patient experience of being part of a 2-year follow-up program with repeated abdominal CT examinations, after a benign-appearing and non-hyperfunctioning adrenal lesion had been incidentally detected on a CT examination. Of the 110 patients, 85% reported some degree of worry at diagnosis but only a few remained worried during follow-up, and the overall impression was that such a follow-up program was well tolerated by the patients. It must be emphasized, though, that the patient experience of incidental findings and subsequent follow-up is heavily dependent on the amount and quality of information given from the healthcare provider. If patient information is insufficient, it can be assumed that the patient experience may be very different.

21 Who Should Decide Which Information to Convey to the Referring Physician and to the Patient?

This also raises the question who should decide what information to be conveyed to the patient. The radiologist acts as a first filter, presenting in the radiology report those findings that he or she finds relevant to report. This means that certain information, considered unimportant by the radiologist, may be left out of the report. The next filter is the referring physician, who receives the radiology report. This physician may choose to convey all or only part of the information in the radiology report to the patient, depending on personal preferences and patient situation. The third filter is the patient himself or herself. The patient may want to be informed about all findings, including reading the report, or may be satisfied with what the clinician presents as being relevant and of interest. In this chain, the radiologist is the key person, as the information that he or she conveys forms the basis for the actions of the referring physician.

Importantly, the wording of the radiology report appears to have a great impact on how an incidental finding is understood and acted upon by the referring physician and by the patient. For example, the way a radiologist describes a clearly benign cyst ("cyst," "benign cyst," "most likely a cyst" etcetera) has an impact on the degree of concern among the referring physicians and to an even larger extent among the patients, as shown in a recent questionnaire study on perceived concern over the message in the radiology report (Rosenkrantz 2017).

The radiologist must therefore not only be accurate in detecting abnormalities but also be knowledgeable about the relative importance and impact of various findings in the short- and long-time perspective. Finally, the radiologist has to put the information into proper wording in the report, not to cause unnecessary workup or patient worry, while at the same time clearly indicating if such follow-up is needed. In order do this successfully, the radiologist, in turn, needs adequate and concise clinical information on the radiology request form about the patients' medical history, other than just the indication for the current radiological examination. Knowledge about, for example, malignant or other diseases, previous surgery, and radiation therapy in patients referred for unrelated symptoms may greatly facilitate the understanding of "incidental" findings – findings that many times should not be considered incidental, but expected – providing that the clinical information was given.

22 Potential Impact of e-Medicine

A factor of potential future importance for this issue is Internet Web-based access to medical files for patients, as presently being introduced at a larger scale in several countries. This may include patients' own access to their medical records, including radiology reports, at home or anywhere by digital media. The benefits and harms of this "open access" for patients are largely unknown, but reading radiology reports and images on one's own, including descriptions of incidental findings not related to the patients main complaint, may certainly create questions and perhaps patient confusion and worry. Knowing that patients may read the reports may also have an impact on what is reported and how radiologists and physicians formulate their descriptions of findings. Further studies are needed to fully understand the benefits and problems with this development.

Conclusion

It can be concluded that detection and reporting of incidental findings on CT of the abdomen may occasionally be lifesaving, but the majority of such incidental findings are clinically irrelevant. The following advice can be given to radiologists when analyzing abdominal CT examinations:

- Make it a routine to do systematic search for incidental findings on abdominal CT, using appropriate window settings and multiple image planes.
- When identifying an incidental finding, look for prior imaging examinations. If there is, determine if there is any interval change in size or character of the lesion.
- Consider potential severity of the finding, short and long term.
- Put the finding in context of the individual patient, taking patient age, clinical history, comorbidity, and life expectancy into account.
- Moderate the radiology report according to the above.

It is the delicate task of the radiologist to balance potential benefits and risks when reporting incidental findings and recommending certain actions. On one hand, it may lead to early diagnosis and treatment, improving health and prognosis. On the other hand, this must be balanced against the risk of providing no added diagnostic or therapeutic value, creating unnecessary workup, patient worry and anxiety, and increased costs and diverting resources from more important healthcare work.

Acknowledgement The author is grateful for constructive review of parts of the manuscript provided by radiology colleagues Mats Andersson, Kjell Geterud, Henrik Leonhardt, and Fredrik Thorén Thorén, all at the Department of Radiology, Sahlgrenska University Hospital, Gothenburg, Sweden.

References

Abdi R et al (2003) Correlation between glomerular size and long-term renal function in patients with substantial loss of renal mass. J Urol 170(1):42–44

Abecassis M et al (1985) Serendipitous adrenal masses: prevalence, significance, and management. Am J Surg 149(6):783–788

Al Harbi F et al (2016) Enhancement threshold of small (< 4 cm) solid renal masses on CT. AJR Am J Roentgenol 206(3):554–558

Alghofaily KA et al (2017) Hepatic hydatid disease complications: review of imaging findings and clinical implications. Abdom Radiol (NY) 42(1): 199–210

Annaiah TK et al (2012) Histology and prevalence of ovarian tumours in postmenopausal women: is follow-up required in all cases? J Obstet Gynaecol 32(3):267–270

Badiani S et al (2013) Extracolonic findings (ECF) on CT colonography (CTC) in patients presenting with colorectal symptoms. Acta Radiol 54(8):851–862

Bae JM (2015) Epidemiological evidences on overdiagnosis of prostate and kidney cancers in Korean. Epidemiol Health 37:e2015015

Bagrodia A et al (2012) Risk prediction in the management of small renal masses. Curr Opin Urol 22(5):347–352

Berbaum KS et al (1990) Satisfaction of search in diagnostic radiology. Invest Radiol 25(2):133–140

Berland LL et al (2010) Managing incidental findings on abdominal CT: white paper of the ACR incidental findings committee. J Am Coll Radiol 7(10):754–773

Bodelle B et al (2016) Benefits of sinogram-affirmed iterative reconstruction in 0.4 mSv ultra-low-dose CT of the upper abdomen following transarterial chemoembolisation: comparison to low-dose and standard-dose CT and filtered back projection technique. Clin Radiol 71(1):e11–e15

Bonde AA et al (2016) Radiological appearances of corpus luteum cysts and their imaging mimics. Abdom Radiol (NY) 41(11):2270–2282

Bosniak MA (1986) The current radiological approach to renal cysts. Radiology 158(1):1–10

Boyce CJ et al (2010) Hepatic steatosis (fatty liver disease) in asymptomatic adults identified by unenhanced low-dose CT. AJR Am J Roentgenol 194(3):623–628

Campbell SC et al (2009) Guideline for management of the clinical T1 renal mass. J Urol 182(4):1271–1279

Carrim ZI, Murchison JT (2003) The prevalence of simple renal and hepatic cysts detected by spiral computed tomography. Clin Radiol 58(8):626–629

Cavallaro A et al (2014) Managing the incidentally detected gallbladder cancer: algorithms and controversies. Int J Surg 12(Suppl 2):S108–S119

Chow LC et al (2007) Split-bolus MDCT urography with synchronous nephrographic and excretory phase enhancement. AJR Am J Roentgenol 189(2):314–322

D'Onofrio M et al (2015) Contrast-enhanced ultrasound of focal liver lesions. AJR Am J Roentgenol 205(1):W56–W66

Dinnes J et al (2016) Management of Endocrine Disease: imaging for the diagnosis of malignancy in incidentally discovered adrenal masses: a systematic review and meta-analysis. Eur J Endocrinol 175(2): R51–R64

EASL-EORTC (2012) EASL-EORTC clinical practice guidelines: management of hepatocellular carcinoma. J Hepatol 56(4):908–943

Fassnacht M et al (2016) Management of adrenal incidentalomas: European Society of Endocrinology Clinical Practice Guideline in collaboration with the European Network for the Study of Adrenal Tumors. Eur J Endocrinol 175(2):G1–g34

Gaetke-Udager K et al (2016) Diagnostic accuracy of ultrasound, contrast-enhanced CT, and conventional MRI for differentiating leiomyoma from leiomyosarcoma. Acad Radiol 23(10):1290–1297

Geramoutsos I et al (2004) Clinical correlation of prostatic lithiasis with chronic pelvic pain syndromes in young adults. Eur Urol 45(3):333–337; discussion 337–338

Ghanouni A et al (2012) Public perceptions and preferences for CT colonography or colonoscopy in colorectal cancer screening. Patient Educ Couns 89(1):116–121

Glazer DI et al (2015) Mass-like peripheral zone enhancement on CT is predictive of higher-grade (Gleason 4 + 3 and higher) prostate cancer. Abdom Imaging 40(3):560–570

Glodny B et al (2012) Prediction of the presence of renal artery stenosis by calcium scoring of the abdominal aorta. Eur J Radiol 81(7):1393–1399

Goodman M et al (2012) Incidentally discovered solid pancreatic masses: imaging and clinical observations. Abdom Imaging 37(1):91–97

Grazioli L et al (2001) Hepatic adenomas: imaging and pathologic findings. Radiographics 21(4):877–892; discussion 892–874

Grazioli L et al (2005) Accurate differentiation of focal nodular hyperplasia from hepatic adenoma at gadobenate dimeglumine-enhanced MR imaging: prospective study. Radiology 236(1):166–177

Grossman J et al (2008) Efficacy of contrast-enhanced CT in assessing the endometrium. AJR Am J Roentgenol 191(3):664–669

Hahn L et al (2015) Longitudinal changes in liver fat content in asymptomatic adults: hepatic attenuation on unenhanced CT as an imaging biomarker for steatosis. AJR Am J Roentgenol 205(6):1167–1172

Halligan S et al (2015) Identification of Extracolonic Pathologies by Computed Tomographic Colonography in Colorectal Cancer Symptomatic Patients. Gastroenterology 149(1):89–101.e105

Hammarstedt L et al (2010) Adrenal lesion frequency: a prospective, cross-sectional CT study in a defined region, including systematic re-evaluation. Acta Radiol 51(10):1149–1156

Hammarstedt L et al (2012) Adrenal lesions in patients with extra-adrenal malignancy – benign or malignant? Acta Oncol 51(2):215–221

Hammarstedt L et al (2013) Adrenal lesions: variability in attenuation over time, between scanners, and between observers. Acta Radiol 54(7):817–826

Hardcastle JD et al (1986) Fecal occult blood screening for colorectal cancer in the general population. Results of a controlled trial. Cancer 58(2):397–403

Helenius M et al (2016) Comparison of post contrast CT urography phases in bladder cancer detection. Eur Radiol 26(2):585–591

Heller MT et al (2013) Managing incidental findings on abdominal and pelvic CT and MRI, part 3: white paper of the ACR Incidental Findings Committee II on splenic and nodal findings. J Am Coll Radiol 10:833–839

Hellstrom M et al (2004) Extracolonic and incidental findings on CT colonography (virtual colonoscopy). AJR Am J Roentgenol 182(3):631–638

Hindman NM (2015) Approach to very small (<1.5 cm) cystic renal lesions: ignore, observe, or treat? AJR Am J Roentgenol 204(6):1182–1189

Hussain SM et al (2004) Focal nodular hyperplasia: findings at state-of-the-art MR imaging, US, CT, and pathologic analysis. Radiographics 24(1):3–17; discussion 18–19

Israel GM, Bosniak MA (2003) Follow-up CT of moderately complex cystic lesions of the kidney (Bosniak category IIF). AJR Am J Roentgenol 181(3):627–633

Jia JB et al (2016) Prostate cancer on computed tomography: a direct comparison with multi-parametric magnetic resonance imaging and tissue pathology. Eur J Radiol 85(1):261–267

Jinzaki M et al (2014) Renal angiomyolipoma: a radiological classification and update on recent developments in diagnosis and management. Abdom Imaging 39(3):588–604

Kang SK et al (2014) Performance of multidetector CT in the evaluation of the endometrium: measurement of endometrial thickness and detection of disease. Clin Radiol 69(11):1123–1128

Karlo CA et al (2016) Renal cell carcinoma: a nomogram for the CT imaging-inclusive prediction of indolent, non-clear cell renal cortical tumours. Eur J Cancer 59:57–64

Katabathina VS et al (2010) Adult renal cystic disease: a genetic, biological, and developmental primer. Radiographics 30(6):1509–1523

Kauhanen S et al (2015) Accuracy of 18F-FDG PET/CT, multidetector CT, and MR imaging in the diagnosis of pancreatic cysts: a prospective single-center study. J Nucl Med 56(8):1163–1168

Kawamoto S et al (2015) CT detection of symptomatic and asymptomatic Meckel diverticulum. AJR Am J Roentgenol 205(2):281–291

Khan KY et al (2007) Frequency and impact of extracolonic findings detected at computed tomographic colonography in a symptomatic population. Br J Surg 94(3):355–361

Khosa F et al (2013) Managing incidental findings on abdominal and pelvic CT and MRI, Part 2: white paper of the ACR Incidental Findings Committee II on vascular findings. J Am Coll Radiol 10(10):789–794

Kim H et al (2015) Clinical correlates of mass effect in autosomal dominant polycystic kidney disease. PLoS One 10(12):e0144526

Kimura W et al (1995) Analysis of small cystic lesions of the pancreas. Int J Pancreatol 18(3):197–206

Kronborg O et al (1996) Randomised study of screening for colorectal cancer with faecal-occult-blood test. Lancet 348(9040):1467–1471

Kumamaru KK et al (2014) Incidental findings detection using low tube potential for CT pulmonary angiography. Int J Cardiovasc Imaging 30(8):1579–1588

Laffan TA et al (2008) Prevalence of unsuspected pancreatic cysts on MDCT. AJR Am J Roentgenol 191(3):802–807

Lattin GE Jr et al (2014) From the radiologic pathology archives: adrenal tumors and tumor-like conditions in the adult: radiologic-pathologic correlation. Radiographics 34(3):805–829

Lee KS, Sekhar A, Rofsky NM, Pedrosa I (2010) Prevalence of incidental pancreatic cysts in the adult population on MR imaging. Am J Gastroenterol 105(9):2079–2084

Levine D et al (2010) Management of asymptomatic ovarian and other adnexal cysts imaged at US Society of Radiologists in Ultrasound consensus conference statement. Ultrasound Q 26(3):121–131

Lin EP et al (2008) Diagnostic clues to ectopic pregnancy. Radiographics 28(6):1661–1671

Lumbreras B et al (2010) Incidental findings in imaging diagnostic tests: a systematic review. Br J Radiol 83(988):276–289

Macari M et al (2011) CT colonography in senior versus nonsenior patients: extracolonic findings, recommendations for additional imaging, and polyp prevalence. Radiology 259(3):767–774

Mandel JS et al (1993) Reducing mortality from colorectal cancer by screening for fecal occult blood. Minnesota Colon Cancer Control Study. N Engl J Med 328(19):1365–1371

Marino JL et al (2004) Uterine leiomyoma and menstrual cycle characteristics in a population-based cohort study. Hum Reprod 19(10):2350–2355

Marrero JA et al (2014) ACG clinical guideline: the diagnosis and management of focal liver lesions. Am J Gastroenterol 109(9):1328–1347; quiz 1348

Marrone G et al (2012) Multidisciplinary imaging of liver hydatidosis. World J Gastroenterol 18(13):1438–1447

McFarland EG et al (1994) Hepatic hemangiomas and malignant tumors: improved differentiation with heavily T2-weighted conventional spin-echo MR imaging. Radiology 193(1):43–47

Mellnick VM et al (2015) Polypoid lesions of the gallbladder: disease spectrum with pathologic correlation. Radiographics 35(2):387–399

Metser U et al (2012) Detection of urothelial tumors: comparison of urothelial phase with excretory phase CT urography – a prospective study. Radiology 264(1):110–118

Mihara S et al (1999) Early detection of renal cell carcinoma by ultrasonographic screening – based on the

results of 13 years screening in Japan. Ultrasound Med Biol 25(7):1033–1039
Mocchegiani F et al (2016) Prevalence and clinical outcome of hepatic haemangioma with specific reference to the risk of rupture: a large retrospective cross-sectional study. Dig Liver Dis 48(3):309–314
Modesitt SC et al (2003) Risk of malignancy in unilocular ovarian cystic tumors less than 10 centimeters in diameter. Obstet Gynecol 102(3):594–599
Mortele KJ et al (2000) CT and MR imaging findings in focal nodular hyperplasia of the liver: radiologic-pathologic correlation. AJR Am J Roentgenol 175(3):687–692
Moyle PL et al (2010) Nonovarian cystic lesions of the pelvis. Radiographics 30(4):921–938
Munigala S et al (2016) Risk of pancreatic cancer in patients with pancreatic cyst. Gastrointest Endosc 84(1):81–86
Muth A et al (2013) Patient-reported impacts of a conservative management programme for the clinically inapparent adrenal mass. Endocrine 44(1):228–236
Muthusamy VR et al (2016) The role of endoscopy in the diagnosis and treatment of cystic pancreatic neoplasms. Gastrointest Endosc 84(1):1–9
Neri E et al (2013) The second ESGAR consensus statement on CT colonography. Eur Radiol 23(3):720–729
Outwater EK et al (2001) Ovarian teratomas: tumor types and imaging characteristics. Radiographics 21(2):475–490
Patel MD et al (2013) Managing incidental findings on abdominal and pelvic CT and MRI, part 1: white paper of the ACR Incidental Findings Committee II on adnexal findings. J Am Coll Radiol 10(9):675–681
Patel J et al (2014) In vivo predictors of renal cyst pseudoenhancement at 120 kVp. AJR Am J Roentgenol 202(2):336–342
Pei Y et al (2009) Unified criteria for ultrasonographic diagnosis of ADPKD. J Am Soc Nephrol 20(1):205–212
Pei Y et al (2015) Imaging-based diagnosis of autosomal dominant polycystic kidney disease. J Am Soc Nephrol 26(3):746–753
Pickhardt PJ, Hanson ME (2010) Incidental adnexal masses detected at low-dose unenhanced CT in asymptomatic women age 50 and older: implications for clinical management and ovarian cancer screening. Radiology 257(1):144–150
Pickhardt PJ et al (2007) Extracolonic tumors of the gastrointestinal tract detected incidentally at screening CT colonography. Dis Colon Rectum 50(1):56–63
Pickhardt PJ et al (2009) CT colonography to screen for colorectal cancer and aortic aneurysm in the Medicare population: cost-effectiveness analysis. AJR Am J Roentgenol 192(5):1332–1340
Pickhardt PJ et al (2010) Colorectal and extracolonic cancers detected at screening CT colonography in 10,286 asymptomatic adults. Radiology 255(1):83–88
Plumb AA et al (2014) Detection of extracolonic pathologic findings with CT colonography: a discrete choice experiment of perceived benefits versus harms. Radiology 273(1):144–152
Pooler BD et al (2016a) Indeterminate but likely unimportant extracolonic findings at screening CT colonography (C-RADS Category E3): incidence and outcomes data from a clinical screening program. AJR Am J Roentgenol 207(5):996–1001
Pooler BD et al (2016b) Potentially important extracolonic findings at screening CT colonography: incidence and outcomes data from a clinical screening program. AJR Am J Roentgenol 206(2):313–318
Priola AM et al (2013) Clinical implications and added costs of incidental findings in an early detection study of lung cancer by using low-dose spiral computed tomography. Clin Lung Cancer 14(2):139–148
Qian LJ et al (2013) Spectrum of multilocular cystic hepatic lesions: CT and MR imaging findings with pathologic correlation. Radiographics 33(5):1419–1433
Raman SP, Fishman EK (2014) Bladder malignancies on CT: the underrated role of CT in diagnosis. AJR Am J Roentgenol 203(2):347–354
Ramanathan S et al (2016) Multi-modality imaging review of congenital abnormalities of kidney and upper urinary tract. World J Radiol 8(2):132–141
Rinaldi MF et al (2010) Incidental lung nodules on CT examinations of the abdomen: prevalence and reporting rates in the PACS era. Eur J Radiol 74(3):e84–e88
Rosenkrantz AB (2017) Differences in perceptions among radiologists, referring physicians, and patients regarding language for incidental findings reporting. AJR Am J Roentgenol 208:140–143
Sabate JM et al (1999) Sclerosing mesenteritis: imaging findings in 17 patients. AJR Am J Roentgenol 172(3):625–629
Sconfienza LM et al (2015) Relevant incidental findings at abdominal multi-detector contrast-enhanced computed tomography: a collateral screening? World J Radiol 7(10):350–356
Sebastian S et al (2013) Managing incidental findings on abdominal and pelvic CT and MRI, Part 4: white paper of the ACR Incidental Findings Committee II on gallbladder and biliary findings. J Am Coll Radiol 10(12):953–956
Song JH et al (2008) The incidental adrenal mass on CT: prevalence of adrenal disease in 1,049 consecutive adrenal masses in patients with no known malignancy. AJR Am J Roentgenol 190(5):1163–1168
Stitt IA et al (2009) Incidental gynecological findings on computed tomographic colonography: prevalence and outcomes. Gynecol Oncol 115(1):138–141
Surov A et al (2014) Non-osseous incidental findings in low-dose whole-body CT in patients with multiple myeloma. Br J Radiol 87(1041):20140185
Swedish National Quality Registry for Renal Cancer (2015) http://www.cancercentrum.se/samverkan/cancerdiagnoser/urinvagar/njurcancer/kvalitetsregister/
Tanaka M et al (2012) International consensus guidelines 2012 for the management of IPMN and MCN of the pancreas. Pancreatology 12(3):183–197

Tappouni R et al (2012) Pseudoenhancement of renal cysts: influence of lesion size, lesion location, slice thickness, and number of MDCT detectors. AJR Am J Roentgenol 198(1):133–137

Thompson RH et al (2009) Metastatic renal cell carcinoma risk according to tumor size. J Urol 182(1):41–45

Timmerman D et al (2005) Logistic regression model to distinguish between the benign and malignant adnexal mass before surgery: a multicenter study by the International Ovarian Tumor Analysis Group. J Clin Oncol 23(34):8794–8801

Tolan DJ et al (2007) Replacing barium enema with CT colonography in patients older than 70 years: the importance of detecting extracolonic abnormalities. AJR Am J Roentgenol 189(5):1104–1111

Tsuboi N et al (2000) Renal masses detected by general health checkup. Int J Urol 7(11):404–408

Valentin L et al (2003) Frequency and type of adnexal lesions in autopsy material from postmenopausal women: ultrasound study with histological correlation. Ultrasound Obstet Gynecol 22(3):284–289

Valsangkar NP et al (2012) 851 resected cystic tumors of the pancreas: a 33-year experience at the Massachusetts General Hospital. Surgery 152(3 Suppl 1):S4–12

Van Der Molen AJ et al (2008) CT urography: definition, indications and techniques. A guideline for clinical practice. Eur Radiol 18(1):4–17

Veerappan GR et al (2010) Extracolonic findings on CT colonography increases yield of colorectal cancer screening. AJR Am J Roentgenol 195(3):677–686

Vincent JM et al (1994) The size of normal adrenal glands on computed tomography. Clin Radiol 49(7):453–455

Welch HG, Black WC (2010) Overdiagnosis in cancer. J Natl Cancer Inst 102(9):605–613

Wood CG 3rd et al (2015) CT and MR imaging for evaluation of cystic renal lesions and diseases. Radiographics 35(1):125–141

Woodfield CA et al (2009) CT features of adenomyosis. Eur J Radiol 72(3):464–469

Xiong T et al (2006) Resources and costs associated with incidental extracolonic findings from CT colonography: a study in a symptomatic population. Br J Radiol 79(948):948–961

Xu AD et al (2010) Significance of upper urinary tract urothelial thickening and filling defect seen on MDCT urography in patients with a history of urothelial neoplasms. AJR Am J Roentgenol 195(4):959–965

Yau TY et al (2014) Is intravenous contrast necessary for detection of clinically significant extracolonic findings in patients undergoing CT colonography? Br J Radiol 87(1036):20130667

Yitta S et al (2011) Normal or abnormal? Demystifying uterine and cervical contrast enhancement at multidetector CT. Radiographics 31(3):647–661

Zaheer A et al (2013) Incidentally detected cystic lesions of the pancreas on CT: review of literature and management suggestions. Abdom Imaging 38(2):331–341

Zalis ME et al (2005) CT colonography reporting and data system: a consensus proposal. Radiology 236(1):3–9

Incidental Findings in ^{18}F-FDG PET/CT and PET/MR

Benedikt M. Schaarschmidt
and Christian Buchbender

Contents

1	**Introduction**	169
2	**Incidental Tracer Uptake in ^{18}F-FDG PET/CT**	170
2.1	Head and Neck	170
2.2	Thorax	173
2.3	Abdomen	176
2.4	Small Pelvis	177
2.5	Bone	179
2.6	Inflammatory Lesions and Immunological Responses	179
2.7	Miscellaneous	180
3	**Non-^{18}F-FDG Avid Incidental Findings in PET/CT**	186
3.1	Lung Nodules	186
3.2	Liver Lesions	186
3.3	Adrenal Lesions	187
4	**Incidental Findings in PET/MR: Differences in Comparison to PET/CT**	188
4.1	Introduction	188
4.2	PET/MR Protocols: Basic Principles	189
4.3	Advantages of ^{18}F-FDG PET/MR in Comparison to PET/CT	189
4.4	Disadvantages of ^{18}F-FDG PET/MR in Comparison to PET/ CT	191
References		192

B.M. Schaarschmidt (✉) • C. Buchbender
Medical Faculty, Department of Diagnostic and Interventional Radiology, University Dusseldorf, Dusseldorf D-40225, Germany
e-mail: benedikt.schaarschmidt@med.uni-duesseldorf.de

Abstract

By combining functional and morphological imaging in one single modality, hybrid imaging scanners such as PET/CT and PET/MR have become essential modalities in in whole-body imaging of inflammatory and oncological diseases. As the number of incidental findings is increased due to the simultaneous acquisition of morphological and functional information, it is of utmost important to correctly identify and interpret these findings. Therefore, this chapter provides an overview of the most common incidental findings in ^{18}F-FDG PET/CT and PET/MR. Incidental ^{18}F-FDG uptake is covered in the first part of the chapter, followed by a brief outline of frequent findings in morphological CT that demand special attention in hybrid imaging. At the end of the chapter, potential advantages and pitfalls of ^{18}F-FDG PET/MR imaging in the detection and characterization of incidental findings are discussed.

1 Introduction

New hybrid imaging scanners have become essential modalities in state-of-the-art oncological imaging by uniting morphological and functional imaging in one single examination. Especially the combination of computed tomography (CT) and positron emission tomography (PET) in an integrated PET/CT scanner is a success (Bockisch et al. 2004). First, attenuation correction of PET

Med Radiol Diagn Imaging (2016)
DOI 10.1007/174_2016_36, © Springer International Publishing Switzerland
Published Online: 07 May 2016

data can be performed more quickly by using CT data acquired in the same scanner than with a separate attenuation scan on a stand-alone PET scanner. Secondly, CT images can be accurately fused with the PET dataset facilitating lesion localization and providing additional morphological information at the same time. Especially in lymphoma and lung cancer, the benefits of this technology have led to the introduction of PET/CT in the latest guidelines and imaging recommendations (Antoch et al. 2003a; Leyn et al. 2007; Cheson et al. 2014). The great success of PET/CT laid the foundation for the development of integrated positron emission tomography/magnetic resonance (PET/MR) scanners (Antoch and Bockisch 2009; Pichler et al. 2010). Apart from the superior soft tissue contrast of MRI in comparison to CT, which might be advantageous in several tumor entities such as gynecological malignancies and tumors of the head and neck, the combination of functional magnetic resonance imaging (MRI) with functional data derived from PET offers unprecedented possibilities in tumor characterization and therapy response evaluation (Buchbender et al. 2012a, b).

For hybrid imaging, however, the choice of an adequate tracer is crucial. Although multiple tracers are in development that are specific for certain metabolic pathways or bind on specific receptors, most hybrid imaging examinations are still performed using ^{18}F-FDG. As a substitute for glucose, intracellular uptake of this unspecific tracer is achieved by active transporters and passive glucose transport proteins. After reaching the cytoplasm, hexokinase phosphorylates ^{18}F-FDG to ^{18}F-FDG-6-phosphate which cannot be further processed by glucose-6-phosphate isomerase leading to accumulation of the radioactive tracer (Avril 2004). To accurately quantify tracer accumulation, the so-called standardized uptake value (SUV) is used, which is calculated by dividing regional tracer activity through the injected activity per body weight (Thie 2004).

Except for some areas such as the brain or inflammatory lesions, glucose uptake is increased in neoplastic cells due to increased glucose consumption compared to the surrounding tissue, a mechanism first described by Warburg in 1956 and therefore called "Warburg effect" (Warburg 1956; Boellaard et al. 2015). Still, tracer uptake can be observed in nonneoplastic lesions or tissue with an increased glucose consumption. Hence, two types of incidental findings can be regularly observed in hybrid imaging examinations:

- Increased tracer uptake in PET imaging with or without a morphological correlate (incidental tracer uptake)
- Incidental lesion in morphological imaging that show no increased tracer uptake in PET imaging

As most hybrid imaging examinations are performed for distant metastasis evaluation, it is of utmost importance to correctly identify incidental tracer uptake. Additionally, the reporting physician has to be aware in which cases the lack of increased metabolic activity in incidentally detected morphological findings can exclude neoplastic lesions or not. Therefore, incidental tracer uptake will be discussed in the first part of this chapter. In the second part of this chapter, the benefits and the limitations of the additional PET data for the interpretation of frequently found morphological incidental findings will be reviewed. In the last part, potential specific benefits for the interpretation of incidental findings of PET/MR as a new modality will be explored.

Although incidental tracer uptake can also be observed in specific tracers (such as ^{64}Ga-PSMA in the salivary glands), presently, the most widely used tracer today is ^{18}F-FDG, which is, thanks to the establishment of distribution networks, even available in remote departments. Therefore, this chapter will focus on ^{18}F-FDG.

2 Incidental Tracer Uptake in ^{18}F-FDG PET/CT

2.1 Head and Neck

Incidental tracer uptake in the head and neck is frequent. While the salivary glands usually only show a mild tracer uptake, even highly increased metabolic activity in Waldeyer's ring, the eye muscles or the larynx can be normal. The key to a swift and correct assessment of tracer uptake in the head and neck is symmetry. While symmetrical tracer uptake can nearly always be considered

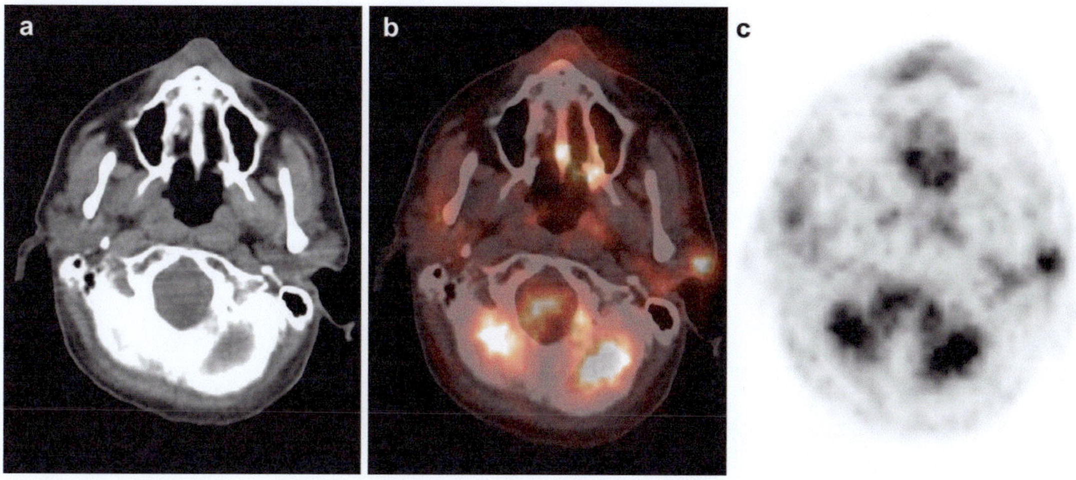

Fig. 1 A 44-year-old male patient undergoing PET/CT suffering from fever of unknown origin. Contrast-enhanced CT (**a**), fused PET/CT (**b**), and PET images (**c**) are displayed. Increased tracer uptake in the left parotid gland was observed. Warthin's tumor was confirmed by histopathology

as benign, asymmetrical tracer uptake demands further investigation.

2.1.1 Salivary Glands and Waldeyer's Ring

^{18}F-FDG is physiologically absorbed by the salivary glands and excreted into the saliva (Stahl et al. 2002). Henceforth, a mild, symmetrical tracer uptake can be frequently observed, but also increased tracer uptake is not uncommon in patients with inflammatory diseases of the salivary glands such as infections, obstructive sialadenitis, and inflammatory changes after radiation therapy. Focal tracer uptake in the salivary glands is observed in 2.1 % of all ^{18}F-FDG PET/CT examinations and is a diagnostic dilemma.

The majority of parotid tumors are benign, while benign as well as malignant lesions are equally distributed in the submandibular gland. Still, tracer uptake does not predict malignancy, and up to 66.7 % of all lesions with an increased tracer uptake are benign (Skolnik et al. 1977; Okamura et al. 1998; Seo et al. 2015). Especially the two most common benign tumors of the parotid gland, pleomorphic adenoma and Warthin's tumor, show a strong ^{18}F-FDG accumulation and are therefore frequently discovered in PET/CT, while a markedly reduced tracer uptake can be noted in malignant tumors such as adenocystic carcinoma or necrotic squamous cell carcinoma (Horiuchi et al. 1998, 2008; Purohit et al. 2014, see Fig. 1). As a definite differentiation of benign from malignant lesions is difficult in PET and CT, further diagnostic workup by MRI and ultrasound can be recommendable.

Waldeyer's ring constitutes of lymphoid tissue located in the naso- and oropharynx including the lingual, the palatinal, and the nasopharyngeal tonsils. Due to the increased tracer uptake of lymphatic cells, tracer uptake can be frequently observed. Still, non-Hodgkin lymphoma and squamous cell carcinomas are frequently found in this location. Although physiological tracer accumulation can be highly variable and range from mild to intense, it is usually symmetrical (Nakamoto et al. 2005; Wong et al. 2007). Therefore, asymmetrical tracer uptake should trigger further investigation, for example, by endoscopy or local inspection (Wong et al. 2007, see Fig. 2).

2.1.2 Thyroid

^{18}F-FDG uptake in the thyroid can be highly heterogeneous. Most frequently, a mild to moderate tracer uptake can be observed. In patients with thyroiditis and goiter, however, the overall tracer uptake can be markedly increased (Börner et al. 1998; Yasuda et al. 1998). Special attention has to be paid to focal tracer uptake: In whole-body hybrid imaging examinations, it can be observed with an incidence of up to 4 % in patients without suspected thyroid malignancy. Despite the fact

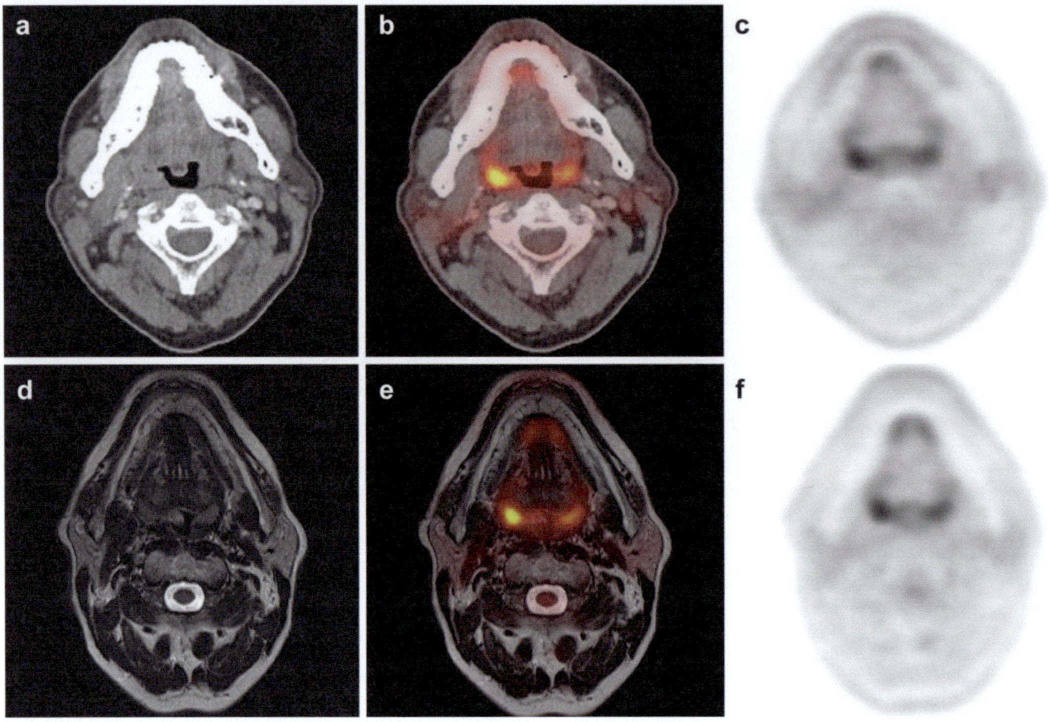

Fig. 2 64 year old male patient suffering from cancer with unknown primary. Morphological, fused and PET images are displayed for PET/CT (**a–c**) and PET/MR (**d–f**). Asymmetrical tracer uptake was noted in the tonsils by PET (right tonsil: SUVmax 10.0; left tonsil: SUVmax 6.2, **c** and **f**). The shape of the tonsils was symmetrical and no tumor was detected by contrast enhanced CT (**a**) or MRI (**d**). Histopathological sampling during endoscopic evaluation detected a squamous cell carcinoma in the right tonsil

that thyroid adenoma and carcinoma show an increased tracer uptake, malignant cells are detected in up to 36.7 % of all investigated ^{18}F-FDG avid nodules (Choi et al. 2006; Boeckmann et al. 2012; Soelberg et al. 2012).

In histopathological analysis, the most frequently observed malignancy is thyroid carcinoma, as thyroid carcinoma cells are known to overexpress the glucose transport protein GLUT1 and therefore exhibit an increased tracer uptake (Haber et al. 1997). Another, albeit frequently forgotten, reason for focal tracer uptake is metastatic disease of the thyroid gland. Thyroid metastases are typically clinically occult, although they are found in up to 9.5 % of patients dying from a nonthyroid tumor in autopsy studies and can be macroscopically detected in 42 % of these cases. Especially malignant melanoma, breast cancer, renal cancer, head and neck cancer, and colorectal cancer are known to metastasize to the thyroid (Abrams et al. 1950; Shimaoka et al. 1962, see Fig. 3).

The risk of malignancy is higher in lesions with an increased metabolic activity than in lesions only detected on morphological imaging and demand more thorough investigation. Although some authors proposed cutoff values for the maximum standardized uptake value (SUVmax) to differentiate benign from malignant lesions, more recent publications indicate no significant differences between benign and malignant lesions in SUVmax, even if higher values, in general, might be indicative of a malignant lesion (Choi et al. 2006; Boeckmann et al. 2012). As contrast-enhanced CT does not allow a definite diagnosis of a thyroid nodule, an additional ultrasound examination of the thyroid with fine needle aspiration is recommended by the latest ACR white paper if a focal tracer uptake is detected by ^{18}F-FDG PET and the life expectancy of the patient is not significantly reduced (Hoang et al. 2015).

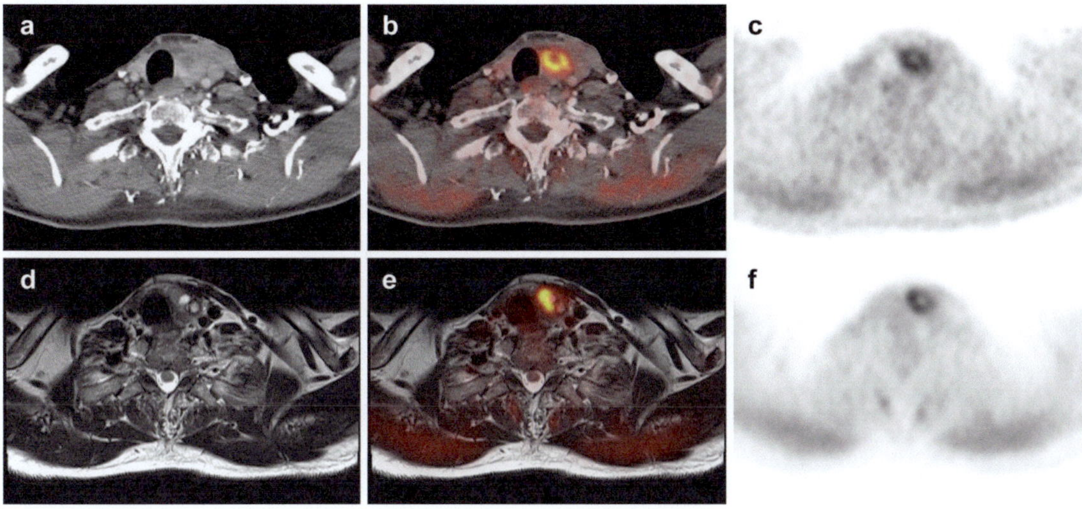

Fig. 3 55 year old male patient who underwent hybrid imaging for staging of recurrent tongue cancer. Morphological, fused and PET images are displayed for PET/CT (**a–c**) and PET/MR (**d–f**). The nodule in the left thyroid lobe shows an inhomogeneous appearance and a blurred delineation to the surrounding tissue in CT (**a**) and MRI (**d**) as well as a focal FDG-uptake (**c** and **f**). The nodule was considered as possibly malignant in both modalities due to the intense tracer accumulation, but neither the morphological information from CT nor from MRI provided additional information. After resection, a thyroid metastasis of a squamous cell carcinoma was histopathologically confirmed

2.1.3 Larynx

Laryngeal uptake is frequently observed in patients that speak after tracer injection. Symmetrical uptake, for example in the vocal cords, does not pose any diagnostic uncertainty. Palsy of the recurrent laryngeal nerve, caused by prior trauma, thyroid surgery, or local tumor invasion, leads to an increased metabolic activity in the contralateral vocal cord. This asymmetrical tracer uptake can mimic early stage laryngeal cancer or even lymph node metastases in inaccurately fused PET/CT datasets. Here, tracer uptake can be avoided by preventing patients from speaking after tracer injection (Kostakoglu et al. 1996; Purohit et al. 2014).

2.2 Thorax

2.2.1 Lung

Due to the low cellular density of lung parenchyma, overall glucose metabolism in the lungs is low. In combination with CT, tracer uptake due to inflammatory changes can be differentiated from malignant lung lesions in most cases.

In 0.15 % of all PET/CT examinations, intense focal tracer uptake in the lung can be observed that is not related to a pulmonary mass but rather a pulmonary vessel. As these findings are not detectable on follow-up scans, most authors believe that these lesions represent pulmonal microembolism: During radioactive tracer injection via an intravenous line, a small thrombus at the intravenous end of the intravenous line is loaded with a high concentration of ^{18}F-FDG during tracer injection, dissoluted and finally stopped in the pulmonary capillaries (Hany et al. 2003; Chondrogiannis et al. 2015). Even if this finding does not demand any further investigation, the CT and the PET datasets have to be checked for misregistration to exclude malignancy.

2.2.2 Thymus

The thymus is located in the upper ventral mediastinum and harbors an important role in lymphocyte development. While it can be clearly visualized in pediatric patients, the volume of the organ reduces over time and is rarely visible in the adult population. In accordance with organ volume, the ^{18}F-FDG uptake decreases over time (Brink et al. 2001; Nakahara et al. 2001). In patients after chemotherapy or radioactive iodine ablation, however, an enlargement of the thymus and an increased tracer uptake, the so-called

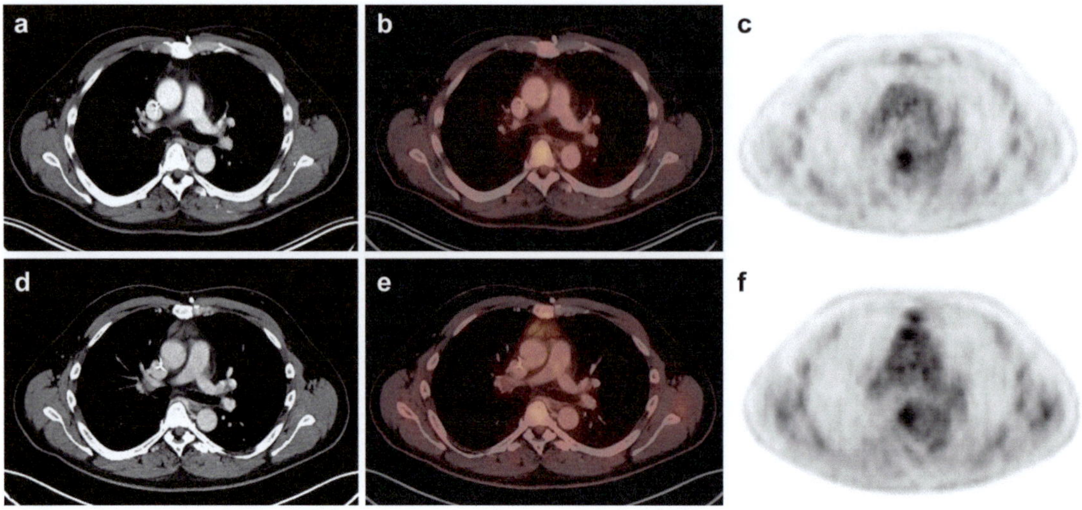

Fig. 4 48 year old male patient suffering from metastatic rectal cancer undergoing PET/CT for whole-body tumor staging. Morphological CT, fused PET/CT and PET images are displayed before (**a–c**) and after chemotherapy (**d–f**). After treatment, a new mass in the anterior mediastinum with a faint tracer uptake can be observed, indicating thymus rebound

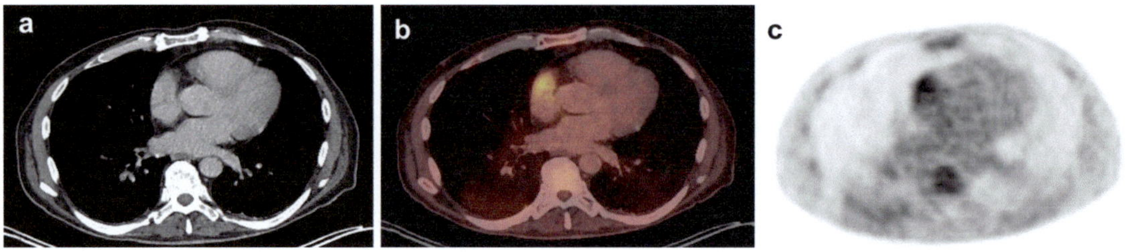

Fig. 5 66 year old male patient undergoing PET/CT for tumor detection with known atrial fibrillation. Contrast enhanced CT (**a**), fused PET/CT (**b**) and PET images (**c**) are displayed. A strong tracer uptake was noted in the left and the right atrium (displayed here) without morphological correlate indicating functional tracer uptake

thymus rebound, can be sometimes observed and should not be mistaken for metastases or lymphoma (Cohen et al. 1980; Jeon et al. 2014, see Fig. 4).

2.2.3 Heart

In the regular, nonfasting state, the heart mainly metabolizes carbohydrates, while fasting leads to an increased consumption of fatty acids. As the myocardial layer of the left ventricle is thicker than in the other cavities of the heart, the strongest metabolic activity can be observed here in nonfasting patients. Therefore, the preparation of the patient is highly dependent on the clinical indication. To improve the detection of small tracer avid lesions in oncological patients, it is mandatory that patients fast for at least 4 h prior to ^{18}F-FDG injection. Longer fasting times might be necessary when a lesion is closely related to the myocardium due to the high variability of cardiac glucose consumption (Boellaard et al. 2015).

This high variability can lead to multiple appearances of the heart in ^{18}F-FDG PET, ranging from absent to a diffusely increased ^{18}F-FDG uptake pattern. Furthermore, focal tracer uptake in the papillary muscles as well as regional tracer uptake, most notably in the lateroposterior and in the anterobasal region, is frequent. In patients with coronary artery disease, however, this regional uptake can be altered due to increased glucose consumption of hibernating myocardium (Mäki et al. 1996; Maurer et al. 2011).

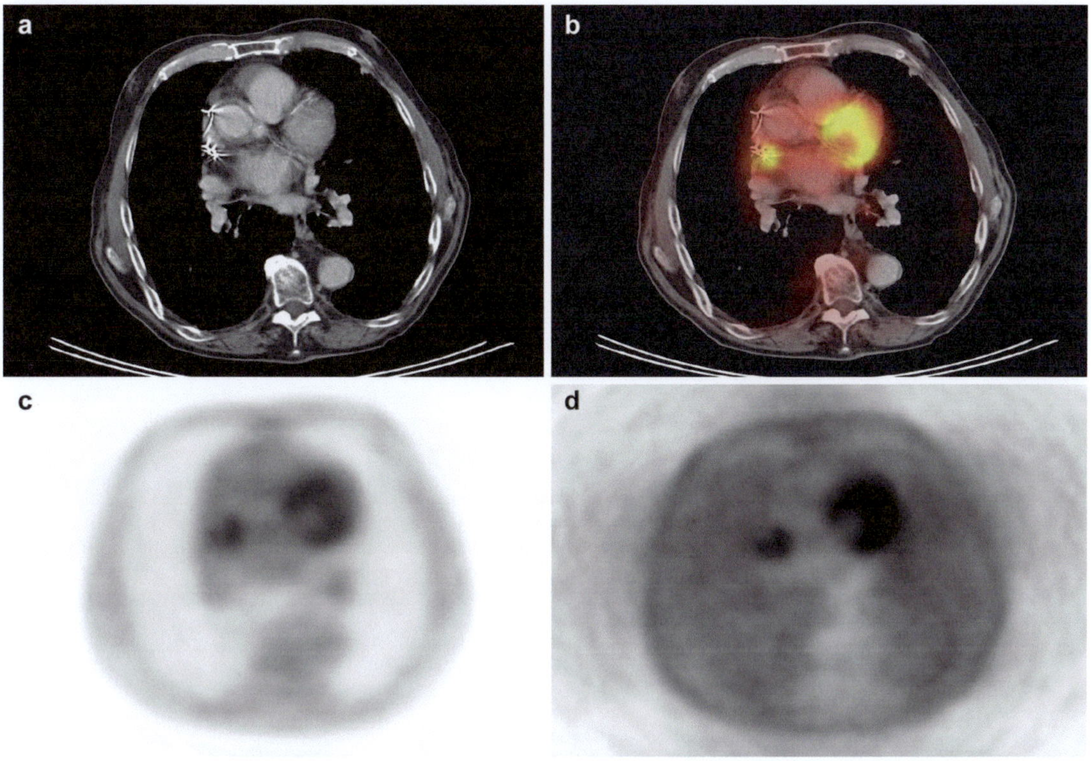

Fig. 6 74 year old male patient suffering from metastatic squamous cell carcinoma undergoing PET/CT for whole-body tumor staging. Morphological CT (**a**), fused PET/CT (**b**) as well as attenuation corrected (**c**) and non attenuation corrected (**d**) PET images are displayed. Increased interatrial fat is observed in morphological CT (**a** and **b**) with an increased tracer accumulation that can be observed in the attenuation corrected (**c**) and non attenuation corrected PET images (**d**), proving that the increased tracer uptake in the attenuation corrected PET images is not an artifact but indicates a lipomatous hypertrophy of the interatrial septum (LHIAS)

In patients with atrial fibrillation, an increased uptake in the atrial wall can be observed that can be mistaken for mediastinal lymph nodes without careful analysis of the fused PET/CT images (Dong et al. 2014, see Fig. 5).

Rare cases of diffuse tracer uptake are inflammatory diseases such as pericarditis, myocarditis, and epicarditis as well as sarcoidosis, but its relevance in oncological PET imaging has to be evaluated further (James et al. 2011).

Albeit extraordinarily rare, benign as well as malignant cardiac masses can lead to an increased focal tracer accumulation, although a high SUVmax is a strong predictor of malignancy (Nensa et al. 2015). A far more frequent explanation for focal tracer accumulation than a malignant process is lipomatous hypertrophy of the interatrial septum, which is found in up to 2.2 % in CT imaging (Heyer et al. 2003). Albeit not a focal tumor, the increased fatty deposition in the intraatrial septum can show a markedly increase glucose uptake in ^{18}F-FDG PET (Fan et al. 2005; Kuester et al. 2005, see Fig. 6).

2.2.4 Esophagus and Gastroesophageal Junction

Tracer uptake in the esophagus can be frequently observed, most notably in the gastroesophageal junction. Apart from increased smooth muscle activity, the prevalence of esophagitis seems to be the most common cause (Wu et al. 2014). Due to its focal appearance, it can be easily mistaken for a carcinoma of the esophageal junction. Without a morphological correlate, increased tracer uptake at this location is not a predictor of malignancy (see Fig. 7). The combination of a high SUVmax with a soft tissue mass or focal esophageal wall thickening, however, has to be considered a strong predictor of malignancy (Heusner et al. 2009; Stagg et al. 2014).

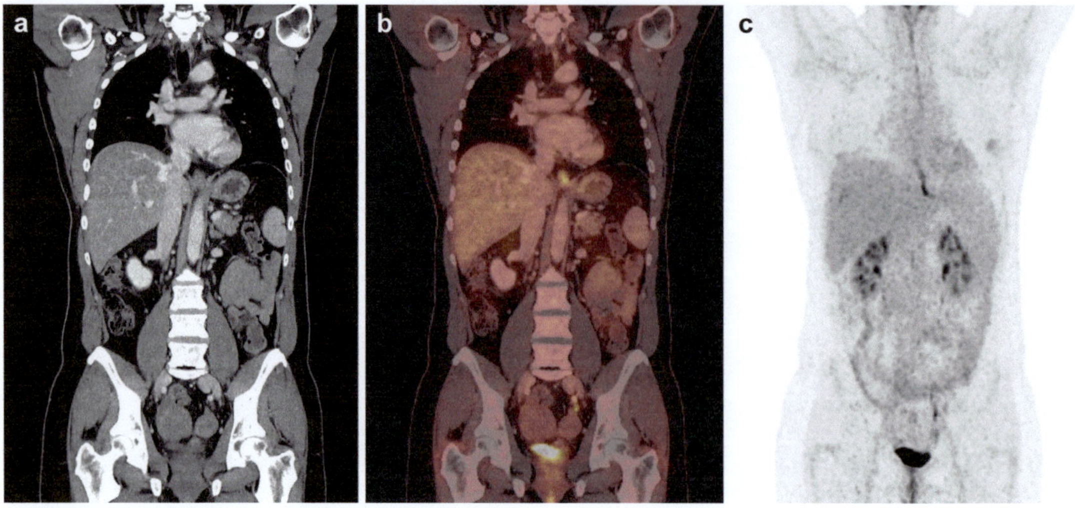

Fig. 7 45 year old female patient undergoing PET/CT suffering from an adenomatous cancer with unknown primary after six cycles of chemotherapy. Contrast enhanced CT (**a**), fused PET/CT (**b**) and PET images (**c**) are displayed. Increased functional uptake of the gastroesophageal junction can be observed. A mild reflux esophagitis was discovered during endoscopy

2.3 Abdomen

2.3.1 Stomach and Bowel

Gastrointestinal uptake in the stomach and the bowel is frequently observed in a multitude of different shapes and can be caused by many different reasons. Patchy, segmental, or diffuse tracer enhancement without a morphological correlate originates from ^{18}F-FDG uptake of smooth muscle cells or the mucosa as well as intestinal microorganisms. Especially lymphoid tissue in the cecum can also exhibit a markedly increased tracer uptake (Rosenbaum et al. 2006). Furthermore, inflammatory lesions, for example, in patients with inflammatory bowel disease or patients with gastritis, can show a markedly increased tracer uptake. Special caution is necessary in patients with type 2 diabetes that are treated with metformin, an oral biguanide. Metformin increases glucose consumption in the gastrointestinal tract and leads to a markedly increased, segmental and continuous tracer uptake in the colon and, to a lesser extent, in the small intestine (Bailey 1995; Gontier et al. 2007, see Fig. 8). Although this effect can be reduced by stopping metformin intake 2–3 days prior ^{18}F-FDG PET examinations, no definite recommendations are available concerning ^{18}F-FDG administration and metformin intake (Özülker et al. 2010; Oh et al. 2010; Boellaard et al. 2015).

Focal tracer uptake in the colon, however, is observed in 1–3 % and associated with a high risk of a malignant or premalignant lesion and demands further colonoscopic evaluation (Kamel et al. 2004; Israel et al. 2005). Still, it has to be kept in mind that although focal tracer uptake in PET/CT has a specificity of 80.2 % for the detection of a colonic pathology, the sensitivity is only 14.8 %. Therefore, the presence of colonic pathologies does not have to coincide with focal tracer uptake (Shim et al. 2012; Keyzer et al. 2015).

2.3.2 Urinary Tract

In the kidneys, a strong tracer uptake of ^{18}F-FDG can be regularly observed as sugars are excreted due to glomerular filtration. In contrast to glucose, however, the radioactive-labeled tracer is not reabsorbed in the tubuli, leading to a markedly increased tracer accumulation in the urinary tract (Rosenbaum et al. 2006). Sometimes, the radioactive urine causes nodal enhancement along the ureter imitating tracer avid lymph nodes on the PET images. In combination with the morphological CT images, the tracer accumulation can be normally clearly attributed to the ureter. Still, the intense tracer accumulation in the bladder caused by the radioactive urine might obscure adjacent lymph nodes.

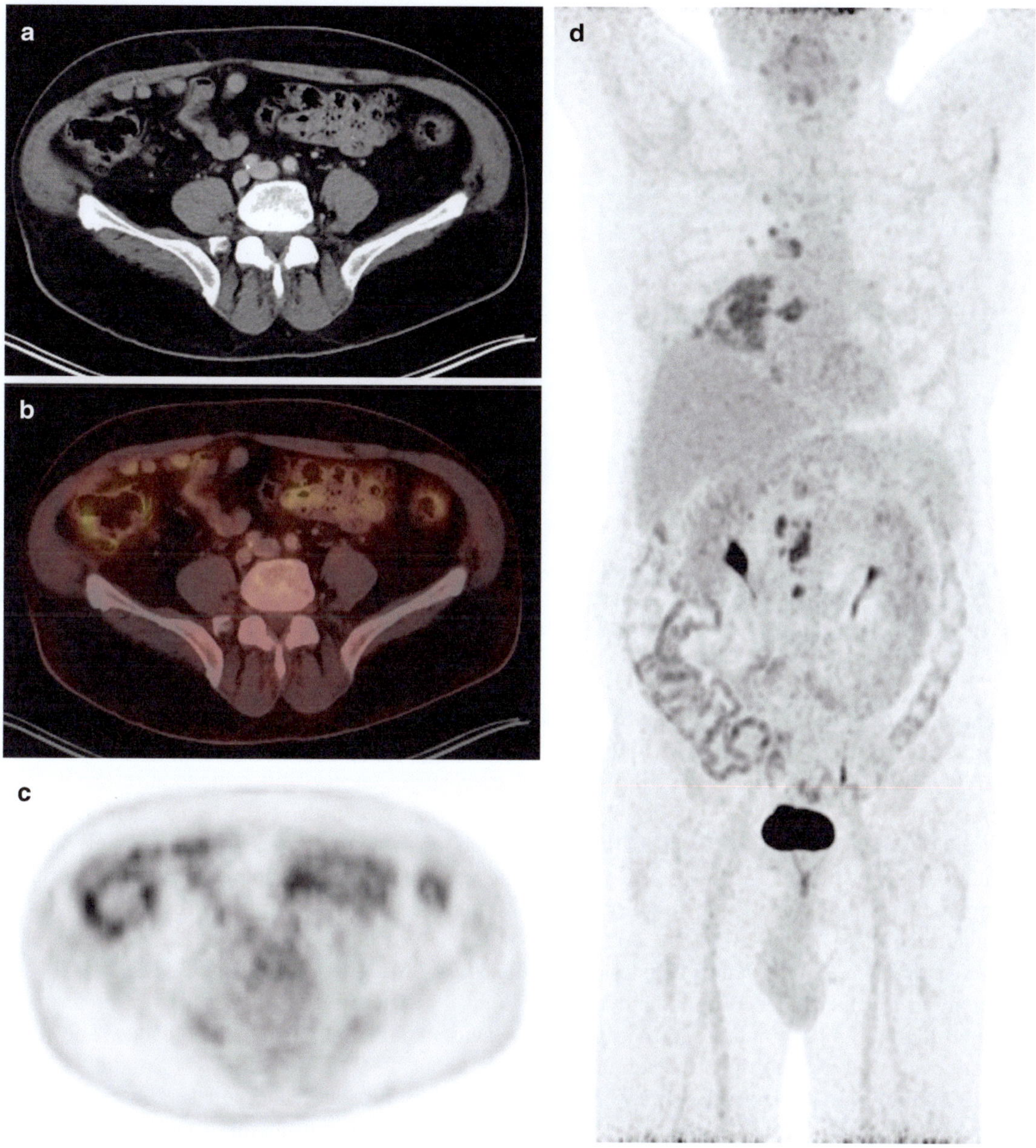

Fig. 8 63 year old male patient suffering diabetes type 2 who underwent hybrid imaging for whole-body lung cancer staging. Morphological CT (**a**), fused PET/CT (**b**) and PET images (**c**) as well as a PET maximum intensity projection image (**d**) are displayed. Due to treatment with metformin, an intense tracer uptake can be observed in the colonic wall

2.4 Small Pelvis

2.4.1 Female Patients: Uterus and Ovaries

In premenopausal female patients, physiological uptake in the uterus and the ovaries is highly dependent on the menstrual cycle. Especially in the ovulatory phase, a markedly increased ^{18}F-FDG uptake can be observed in the ovaries and the endometrium. Additionally, a strong tracer uptake can be observed in the endometrium during early menstrual flow (see Fig. 9), while no

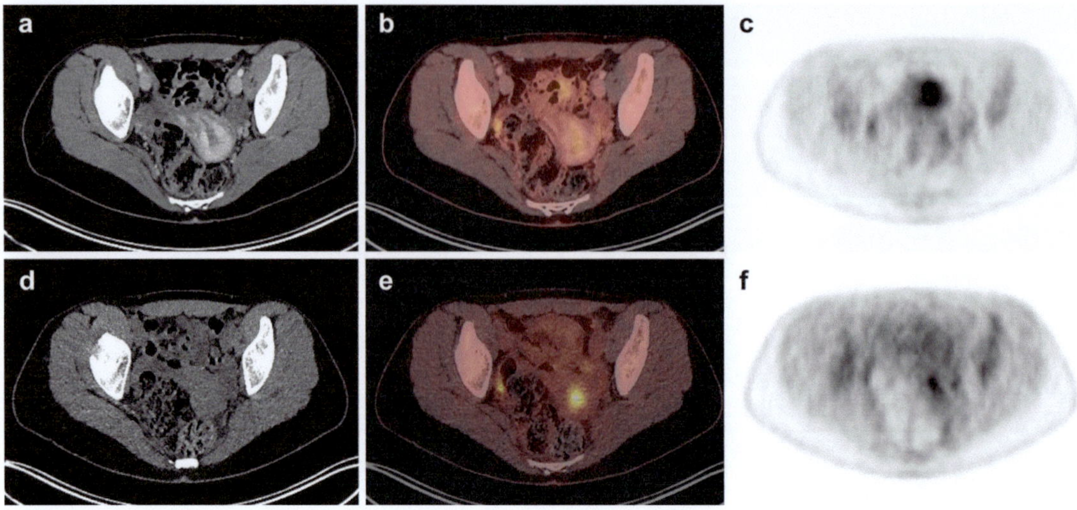

Fig. 9 28 year old female patient suffering from paraganglioma undergoing repeated PET/CT due to increased tracer uptake in disseminated brown adipose tissue. Morphological CT, fused PET/CT and PET images are displayed during the proliferative phase (**a–c**) and during menstrual flow (**d–f**). While no tracer uptake in the endometrium can be detected during the proliferative phase, a markedly increased tracer uptake in the endometrium can be observed during mentrual flow

increased tracer uptake is noted in the ovaries at this time. Therefore, it might be advisable to perform ^{18}F-FDG a week before or shortly after menses to exclude physiological tracer uptake if a gynecological malignancy is suspected (Lerman et al. 2004; Nishizawa et al. 2004).

In patients with cervical cancer, an increased endometrial tracer uptake can be observed. However, this is not an indicator of endometrial invasion but is rather induced by local cytokines excreted by the tumor or increased uterine fluid collections caused by a consecutive cervical stenosis. Therefore, PET does not seem to improve the detection of endometrial invasion (Lerman et al. 2004).

In postmenopausal women, physiological tracer uptake in the uterus and the ovaries is rarely observed. In contrast to the glandular tissue in the breast, hormone replacement therapy does not seem to lead to an increased tracer uptake in the ovaries or in the endometrium. Hence, especially increased tracer uptake in the ovaries in postmenopausal women can indicate a malignant process and deserves further investigation (Lerman et al. 2004; Rosenbaum et al. 2006). Despite the high overall sensitivity of ^{18}F-FDG PET for ovarian cancer, only a moderate tracer uptake can be frequently observed in premalignant lesions or early stage cancers. Still, a moderate tracer uptake in the ovaries can also be caused by benign lesions such as endometriomas (Fenchel et al. 2002). Therefore, a close comparison with the morphological images is warranted here.

2.4.2 Male Patients: Prostate and Testes

Incidental tracer uptake in the prostate is detected in about 2 % of all PET/CT studies and is caused by prostate cancer in 17 %. Lesion localization in the peripheral zone and increased patient age seem to be predictors of malignancy, while an association with increased SUVmax is questionable (Bertagna et al. 2015). Still, the positive predictive value for incidental prostate uptake is low as tracer uptake in benign prostatic disease such as prostatitis or benign prostate hyperplasia is common. As the mortality of prostate cancer is low, discretion should be advised when applying invasive techniques to investigate incidental prostatic uptake, especially in oncological patients with a limited life expectancy (Reesink et al. 2015, see Fig. 10).

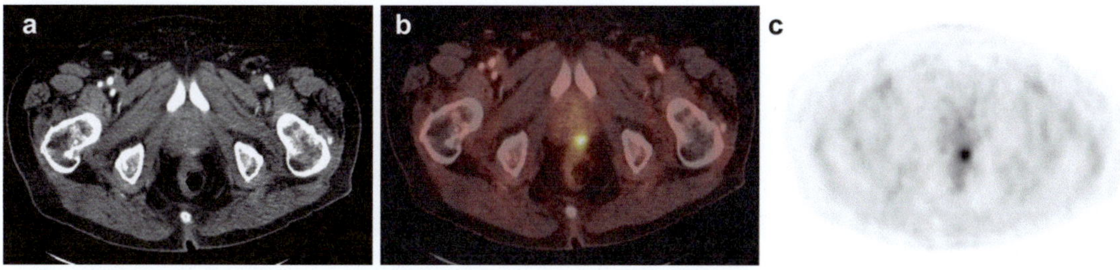

Fig. 10 A 90-year-old male patient suffering from Merkel cell carcinoma undergoing PET/CT for metastases detection. Contrast-enhanced CT (**a**), fused PET/CT (**b**), and PET images (**c**) are displayed. A strong tracer uptake (SUVmax 10.7) in the prostate indicated prostate cancer, which was confirmed by histopathology

^{18}F-FDG accumulation of the testes is age dependent. While a positive correlation between tracer uptake and patient age can be observed in pediatric patients, glucose metabolism decreases in aging male patients (Kitajima et al. 2007; Goethals et al. 2009). Asymmetrical tracer uptake, however, demands further evaluation as solitary metastases to the testes, or extranodal involvement in lymphoma patients have been reported (Weng and Schöder 2004; Sidhu et al. 2014).

2.5 Bone

In adult patients, hematopoietic bone marrow is replaced by fat. Therefore, the bone marrow normally shows a faint tracer uptake in adults, but in certain cases, this process can be reversed. Due to bone marrow activation after chemotherapy, an increased tracer uptake can be noted in adults. Additionally, intense tracer accumulation in the bone marrow can be observed after recent treatment with granulocyte colony-stimulating factor (Hollinger et al. 1998; Ulaner and Lyall 2013, see Fig. 11).

During the healing process, ^{18}F-FDG tracer uptake can be increased in recent fractures for up to 3 months. Therefore, CT images have to be analyzed carefully to detect acute fractures, postoperative fractures (such as fractures of the rips after thoracotomy for the resection of pulmonary tumors or metastases), and insufficiency fractures, for example, in the sacrum (Zhuang et al. 2003; Fayad et al. 2003). Furthermore, the precise depiction of osteolytic lesions by morphological CT images can be extraordinarily helpful to differentiate benign from malignant fractures.

In elderly patients with osteoarthritis, increased tracer uptake around the acromioclavicular joint, the glenohumeral joint, the hip, or the knee can be found. This uptake is considered to be caused by synovial proliferation in degeneratively changed joints and is rarely associated with symptoms (von Schulthess et al. 2001).

2.6 Inflammatory Lesions and Immunological Responses

Neutrophil granulocytes, monocytes, and macrophages are known to express the glucose transport protein GLUT1 as well as GLUT3 and show an increased hexokinase activity. If these cells are involved in an inflammatory reaction, the markedly increased glucose consumption can be visualized by ^{18}F-FDG PET/CT, leading to a growing number of indications for ^{18}F-FDG PET in inflammatory diseases (Jamar et al. 2013). In oncological ^{18}F-FDG PET imaging, however, it can be difficult to differentiate inflammatory processes from metastatic diseases, especially in patients with suspected lymph node metastases or in lymphoma patients.

Sarcoidosis is a chronic granulomatous disorder. Due to the ongoing inflammatory response, ^{18}F-FDG PET shows a markedly increased tracer accumulation in involved sites and can be therefore used to assess disease extent with a high sensitivity and specificity (Lewis and Salama 1994; Braun et al. 2008). In patients undergoing PET/CT for oncological indications, however, the differentiation between malignant and inflammatory

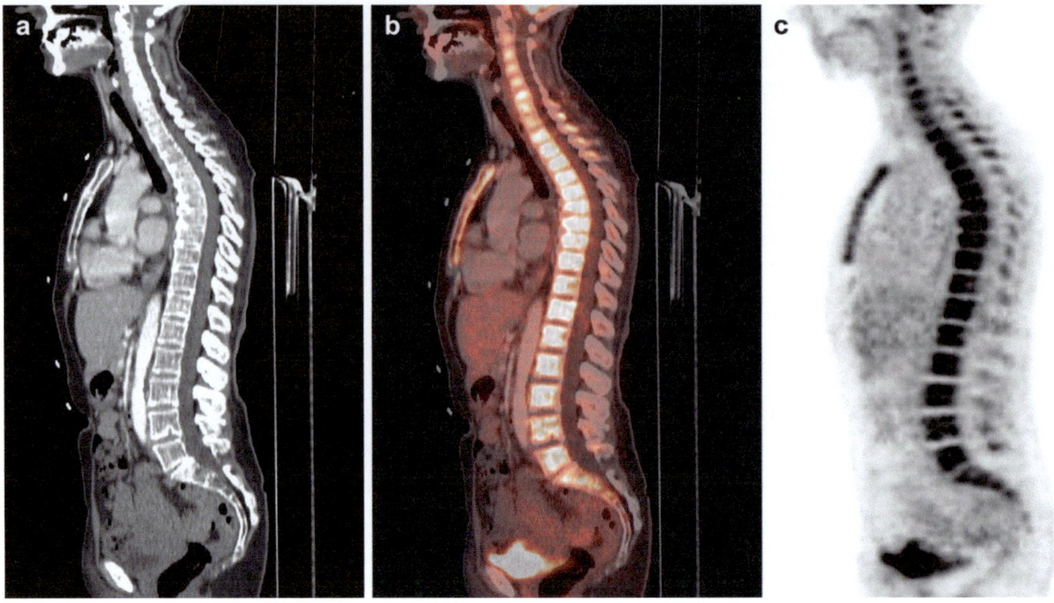

Fig. 11 A 64-year-old female patient suffering from acute myeloid leukemia and accompanying B-cell non-Hodgkin lymphoma with biopsy-proven bone marrow infiltration undergoing PET/CT after induction chemotherapy. Supportive therapy with granulocyte colony-stimulating factor (G-CSF) was performed until 2 days before the PET/CT examination. Contrast-enhanced CT (**a**), fused PET/CT (**b**), and PET images (**c**) are displayed. A markedly increased tracer uptake in the bone marrow was observed. As no malignant cells were observed in bone marrow biopsy, the tracer uptake in the bone marrow was most likely induced by G-CSF therapy

lesions can be challenging. Therefore, it is important not to rely on SUV measurements alone but to analyze the scans under consideration of usual metastatic patterns and suspect sarcoidosis as a possible explanation in the case of an unexpected metastatic spread (Cook et al. 1996, see Fig. 12).

Infectious diseases are another important pitfall in PET imaging. Especially in immunodeficient patients, opportunistic infectious diseases, such as fungal or mycobacterial infections, can mimic metastatic tumor spread due to disseminated disease (Sharma et al. 2014). As SUV measurements fail to correctly differentiate malignant from infectious lesions, the careful interpretation of the morphological images and ultimately biopsy might be necessary for a definite diagnosis (Rosenbaum et al. 2006).

Another cause for an inflammatory reaction with consecutive tracer uptake is vaccination. After injection, a faint muscular uptake at the vaccination site is frequently observed. Additionally, tracer uptake in the adjacent lymph nodes can be observed up to 1 month after this procedure (Thomassen et al. 2011; Shirone et al. 2012, see Fig. 13). Therefore, it is of utmost importance to identify patients that recently underwent vaccination to reduce the number of false-positive findings. In patients with potential axillary metastases, for example, breast cancer or melanoma patients, it might be advisory to postpone planned vaccination procedures to avoid this potential pitfall.

2.7 Miscellaneous

2.7.1 Skin and Subcutaneous Fat

Incidental increased tracer uptake in the skin is most frequently caused by inflammation. Especially focal inflammation, e.g., in infected atheroma or acne, can show an increased tracer uptake due to the increased presence of lymphatic cells. Apart from bacterial infections, viral infections such as an active herpes zoster infection can lead to an increased cutaneous tracer uptake that might even involve the associated lymph nodes (Wadih et al. 2015).

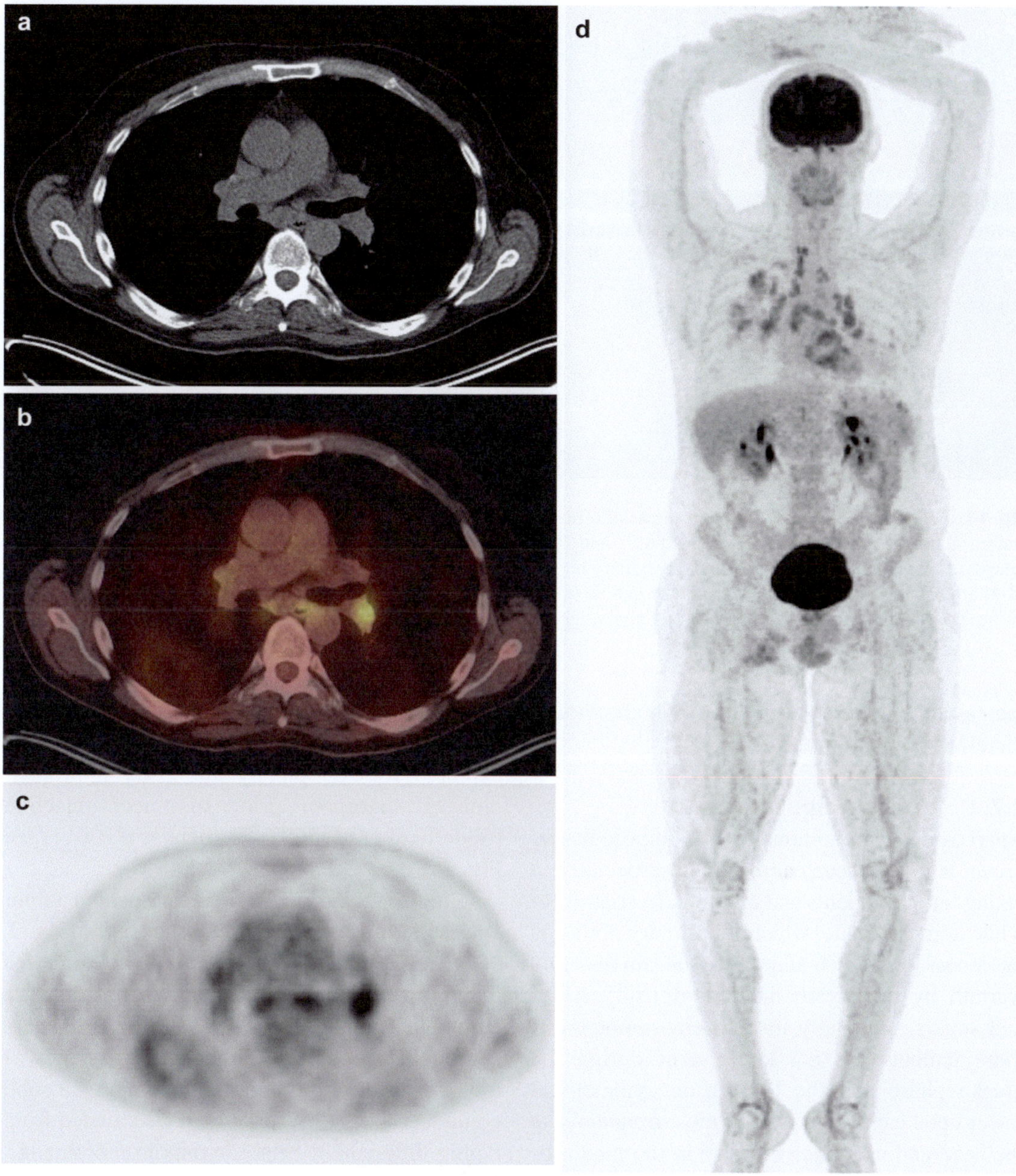

Fig. 12 41 year old male with newly detected mediastinal lympadenopathy. Morphological CT (**a**), fused PET/CT (**b**) and PET images (**c**) as well as a PET maximum intensity projection image (**d**) are displayed. Mild tracer uptake in mediastinal lymph nodes can be observed, but no primary was detected. Sarcoidosis was confirmed by histopathology after endobronchial ultrasound transbronchial needle aspiration

A rare inflammatory disease is hidradenitis suppurativa involving the hair follicles that can be predominantly found in the inguinal, perianal, and axillary region (see Fig. 14). Here, an intense tracer accumulation can be discovered involving the cutaneous tissue and the subcutaneous fat and can lead to fistulas and even osteomyelitis as well as malignant transformation (Simpson et al. 2011; Poh and Wong 2014). In most of the cases, diagnostic security can be

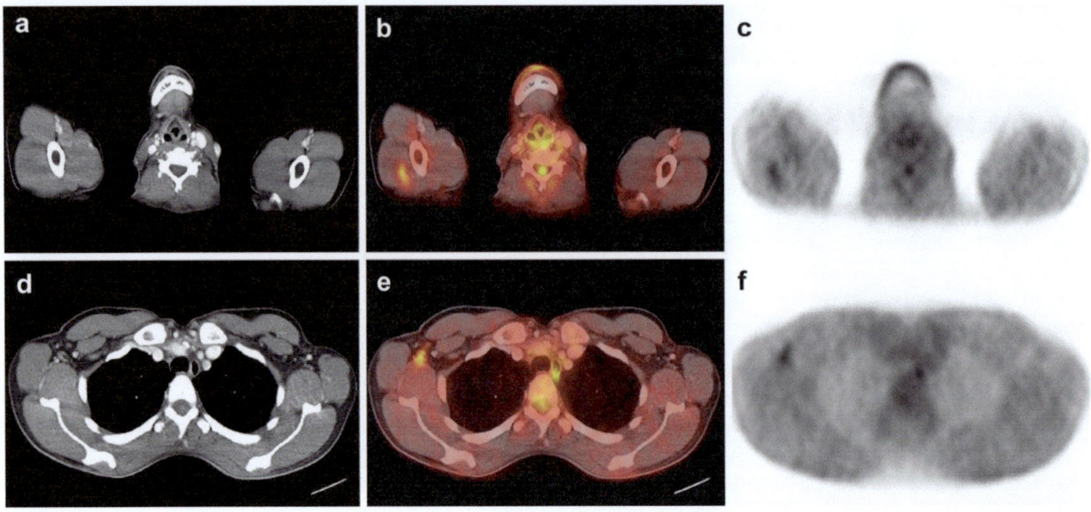

Fig. 13 Female patient suffering from metastatic breast cancer. Contrast-enhanced CT, fused PET/CT, and PET images of the right upper arm (**a–c**) and the axillary region (**d–f**) are displayed. Increased tracer uptake can be noted in the right deltoid muscle (**b–c**) and in the non-enlarged right axillary lymph nodes (**d-f**). This patient was vaccinated 14 days prior to [8]F-FDG PET/CT. In the follow-up examination 6 months later, no tracer uptake in the right deltoid muscle or the right axillary lymph nodes was observed

increased by mere inspection which should therefore not be omitted.

2.7.2 Brown Adipose Tissue

Apart from the predominant white adipose tissue, brown adipose tissue can be found especially in young female patients and children. In contrast to white adipose tissue, which its primary ability is fat deposition, brown adipose tissue can generate warmth by the metabolization of triglycerides and sugars, especially in cold environments. If these patients are not kept warm during the uptake phase and the PET scan, symmetrical tracer uptake can be observed most frequently in the head and neck area but also in the mediastinum and the perivertebral fatty tissue. Although brown adipose tissue can be correctly identified on fused PET/CT images by the pattern of distribution and identification of fat as morphological correlate of focal tracer uptake, small tracer avid lesions that are also situated in the fatty tissue, such as lymph node metastases, can be obscured. Therefore, it can be advisory to prepare patients with known high activity of brown adipose tissue by keeping the patients warm after ^{18}F-FDG injection (Boellaard et al. 2015). Furthermore, pharmacological means to decrease the glucose uptake in brown adipose tissue have been explored, for example, by administering propanolol or diazepam prior to tracer injection (Söderlund et al. 2007; Rakheja et al. 2011, see Fig. 15).

A rare variant is hibernoma, a benign tumor consisting of brown adipose tissue (Furlong et al. 2001, see Fig. 16). While the tumor mimics a lipoma in morphological imaging, it exhibits an extraordinary high tracer uptake in PET imaging. Although hibernomas neither do show signs of tumor invasion of the surrounding tissues nor solid components, it still cannot be differentiated from highly differentiated liposarcoma in morphological imaging. A possible tool of differentiation is a repeated PET imaging as strong SUV fluctuations of hibernomas have been observed in small cohorts (Smith et al. 2008). Still, histopathological correlation is necessary for a definite diagnosis.

2.7.3 Breast

Tracer uptake in the breast is observed in the glandular mammary tissue and can therefore be mainly observed in premenopausal women and postmenopausal women undergoing hormone

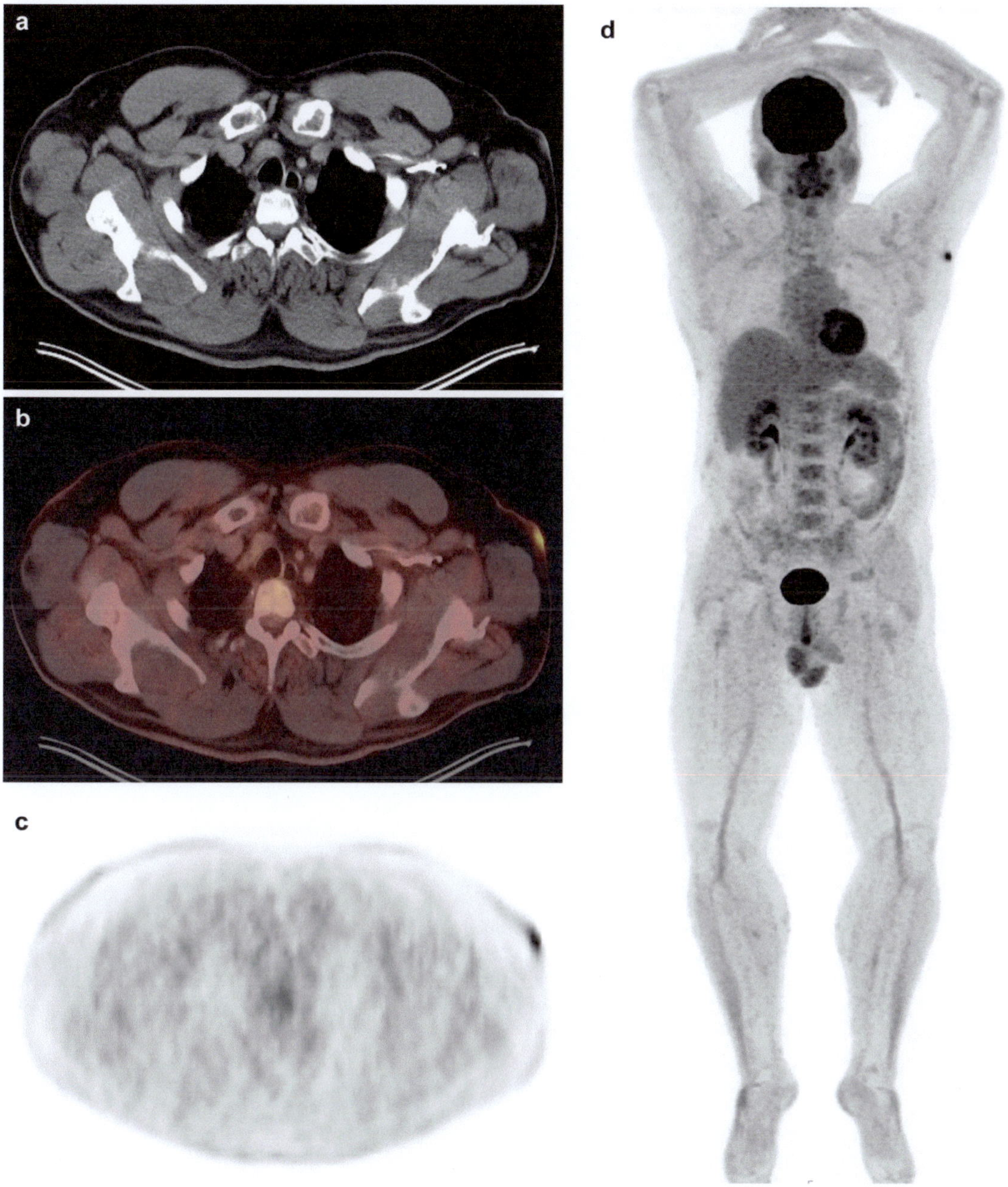

Fig. 14 51 year old male patient suffering from malignant melanoma who underwent hybrid imaging for whole-body staging. Morphological CT (**a**), fused PET/CT (**b**) and PET images (**c**) as well as a PET maximum intensity projection image (**d**) are displayed. Intense tracer uptake in the left axillary region with cutaneous thickening was suspicious of a second malignant melanoma. Local inspection showed a local inflammation in a patient with known hidradenitis suppurativa in the axillary region

replacement therapy. Intense tracer uptake of both breasts is frequently found in lactating women (see Fig. 17) but can also be asymmetrical if the child is predominantly fed from one side (Abhyankar et al. 2012). Therefore, especially small lesions can be obscured by the increased glandular uptake and can be difficult to detect in the PET dataset. Focal ^{18}F-FDG uptake

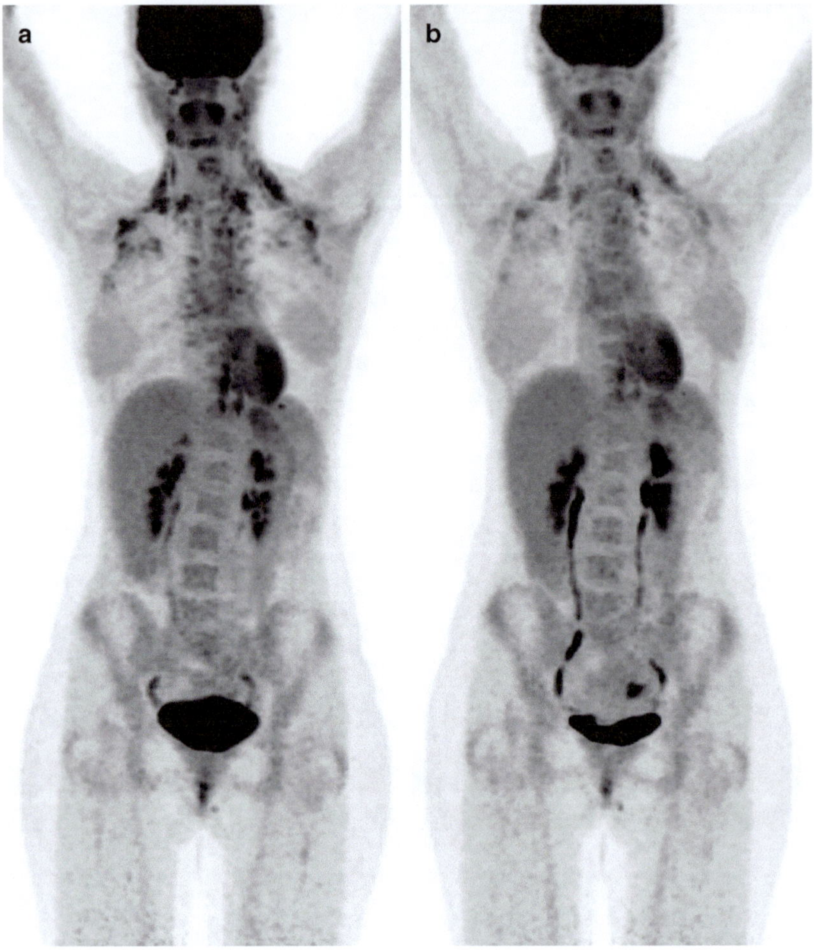

Fig. 15 28 year old female patient suffering from paraganglioma undergoing repeated PET/CT due to increased tracer uptake in disseminated brown adipose tissue. PET maximum intensity projection images are displayed. In the initial scan, a markedly increased tracer uptake can be observed in brown adipose tissue in the cervical and the mediastinal area (**a**). The second scan was performed after propanolol administration. Furthermore, the patient was kept warm during the tracer uptake phase, leading to a markedly reduced tracer accumulation in the brown adipose tissue (**b**)

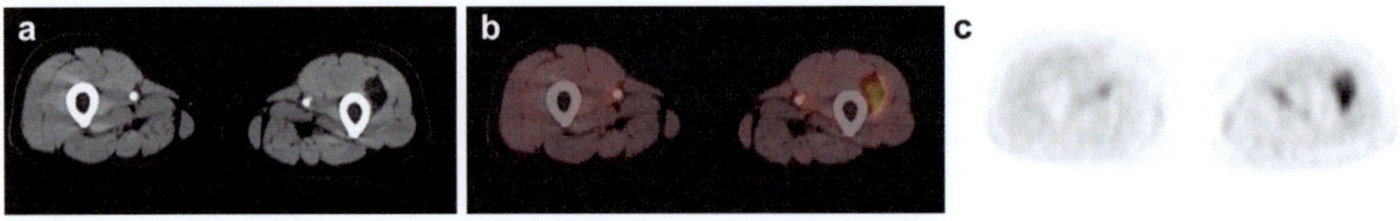

Fig. 16 A 72-year-old female patient suffering from a motoneuron disease of unknown origin undergoing PET/CT for tumor detection. Contrast-enhanced CT (**a**), fused PET/CT (**b**), and PET images (**c**) are displayed. A fatty lesion without local tumor invasion was detected in the left upper thigh with an increased tracer uptake without septae. In the histopathological examination of the resection specimen after tumor resection, the diagnosis of a hibernoma was confirmed

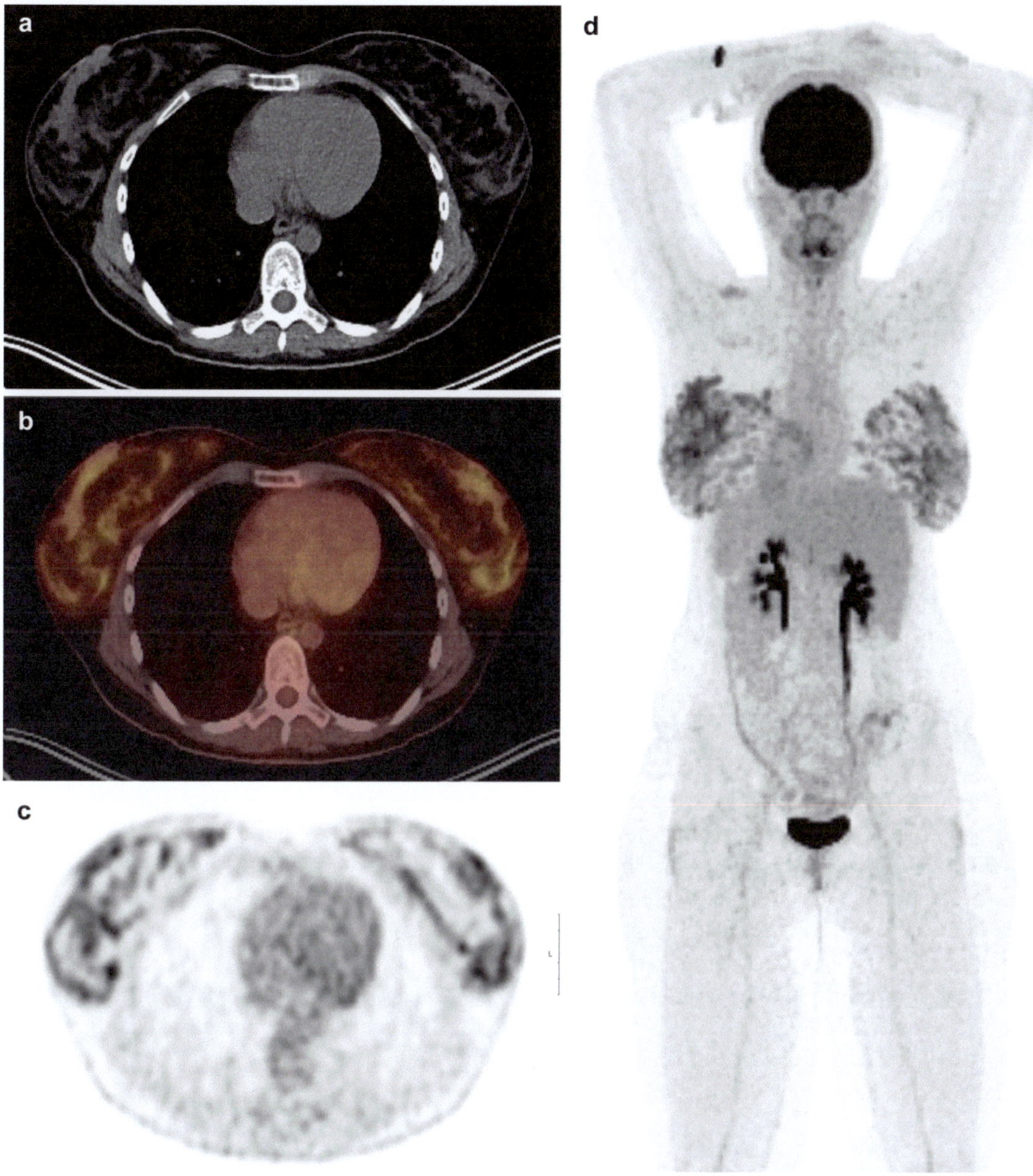

Fig. 17 27 year old female patient undergoing PET/CT after successful treatment of hodgkin lymphoma for tumor recurrence diagnostics. Morphological CT (**a**), fused PET/CT (**b**) and PET images (**c**) as well as a PET maximum intensity projection image (**d**) are displayed. A strong tracer uptake of the glandular mammary tissue can be observed in both breasts due to breastfeeding

in the breast, however, is a strong predictor of malignancy and demands further investigation (Bertagna et al. 2015).

3 Non-^{18}F-FDG Avid Incidental Findings in PET/CT

Incidental findings without tracer uptake are frequently discovered in PET/CT, both in CT examinations without contrast for attenuation correction and in diagnostic contrast-enhanced CT examinations (Bruzzi et al. 2006). Despite their frequency, these findings were considered of high clinical significance in up to 7 % of all patients (Osman et al. 2005; Schaaf et al. 2014). Although the immediate clinical impact of frequently encountered findings such as cystic kidney lesions, arteriosclerotic changes, or small pulmonary nodules might be low, the overall clinical significance should not be underestimated (Bruzzi et al. 2006). Therefore, it is important to review the available CT images with utmost care and mention non-^{18}F-FDG avid incidental findings in the final report, even if the CT scan was performed just for attenuation correction (Boellaard et al. 2015). However, there are some incidental findings frequently depicted in whole-body imaging where the additional PET information can be helpful or misleading and result in a significant change of interpretation. Therefore, the following paragraphs will cover frequent findings in morphological imaging that demand special attention in hybrid imaging.

3.1 Lung Nodules

Lung nodules are the most commonly encountered incidental finding in ^{18}F-FDG PET/CT (Bruzzi et al. 2006). Although PET has a high sensitivity for malignant pulmonary nodules, the low spatial resolution of the current generation detectors prohibit the adequate metabolic characterization of nodules that are smaller than 10 mm (Gould et al. 2001; Nomori et al. 2004). Here, the nonattenuation-corrected images can provide useful additional information on tracer uptake in small pulmonary nodules and should therefore be regularly reviewed to improve diagnostic accuracy (Reinhardt et al. 2005; Huang et al. 2010). Still, a considerate amount of small pulmonary nodules that are detectable on CT cannot be defined in a single PET/CT examination, even if the attenuation-corrected and the nonattenuation-corrected images are analyzed. In these cases, further follow-up examinations should be performed according to the "Guidelines for Management of Small Pulmonary Nodules Detected on CT Scans" published by the Fleischner Society in 2005 (MacMahon et al. 2005). In subsolid nodules, the "Recommendations for the Management of Subsolid Pulmonary Nodules Detected at CT" published by the Fleischner Society in 2013 should be adhered (Naidich et al. 2013). To reduce the number of follow-up examinations, all previously performed examinations should be used to detect changes in size and morphology. Lung nodules newly detected in follow-up examinations in oncological patients, however, are highly suspicious of malignancy and deserve special attention, short interval surveillance, or biopsy if relevant to therapeutic decisions.

3.2 Liver Lesions

Despite the significant improvement of sensitivity for liver metastases gained by the intravenous administration of iodine-based contrast agents in ^{18}F-FDG PET/CT, imaging of the liver can be troublesome in small lesions (Badiee et al. 2008; Niekel et al. 2010; Sacks et al. 2011). Liver lesions that are too small to characterize are encountered in up to 13 % of all oncological patients in CT and prove to be malignant in 11.7 % of all cases. Here ^{18}F-FDG PET fails to provide complimentary information to contrast-enhanced CT due to several reasons (Schwartz et al. 1999). First, the combination of the low spatial resolution of PET and the high background uptake of the liver parenchyma hinder the precise depiction and characterization of subcentimeter lesions (see Fig. 18). Additionally, liver movement during breathing causes blurring of

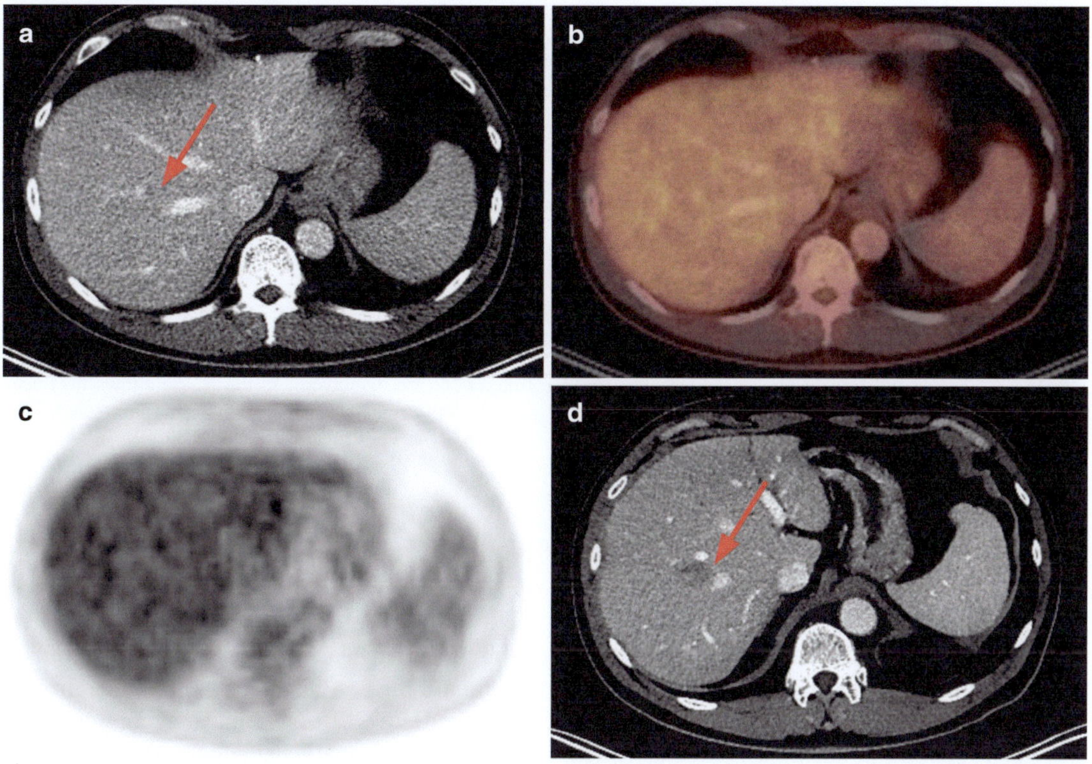

Fig. 18 53 year old male patient suffering from rectal cancer. Morphological CT (**a**), fused PET/CT (**b**) as well as attenuation corrected PET (**c**) and follow-up CT images (**d**) are displayed. A lesion that is too small to specify is detected in segment VII of the liver in CT (see *red arrow*, **a**) without a correlate in PET (**c**). In the follow-up examination, a liver metastasis is detected in the same location (see *red arrow*, **d**)

small lesions making them hard to detect even for experienced readers and preventing the diagnosis of early metastatic disease in some cases. Hence, liver lesions detected in 18F-FDG PET/CT that are too small to be adequately characterized as cysts should be referred to an additional contrast-enhanced MRI examination of the liver, especially if potential metastatic spread to the liver is of relevance for treatment decisions or preoperative imaging before liver metastasis resection is performed (Scharitzer et al. 2013).

3.3 Adrenal Lesions

Adrenal lesions, mostly attributable to adrenal adenomas, are detected with a frequency of up to 4.4 % in radiological patient cohorts. On the other hand, adrenal metastases are a common finding in patients with an extraadrenal tumor. Primary cancers of the adrenal gland, however, are exceedingly rare (Barzon et al. 2003; Bovio et al. 2006). Therefore, the correct characterization of adrenal lesions is crucial. While lipid-rich adenomas can be easily confirmed by low attenuation values on noncontrast-enhanced CT, lipid-poor adenomas are more challenging. Although delayed CT scans 15 min after the injection of iodine-based contrast agents can improve detection rates in these cases, it is difficult to adopt this strategy in the clinical imaging workflow, and moreover radiation exposure is increased by the additional scan (Park et al. 2007). Henceforth, chemical shift MR imaging is an alternative to differentiate adenomas from malignant lesions without additional radiation exposure (Haider et al. 2004; Park et al. 2007). ¹⁸F-FDG PET/CT, however, has an excellent sensitivity and specificity for malignant adrenal lesions. Yun et al. proposed to qualitatively evaluate adrenal masses

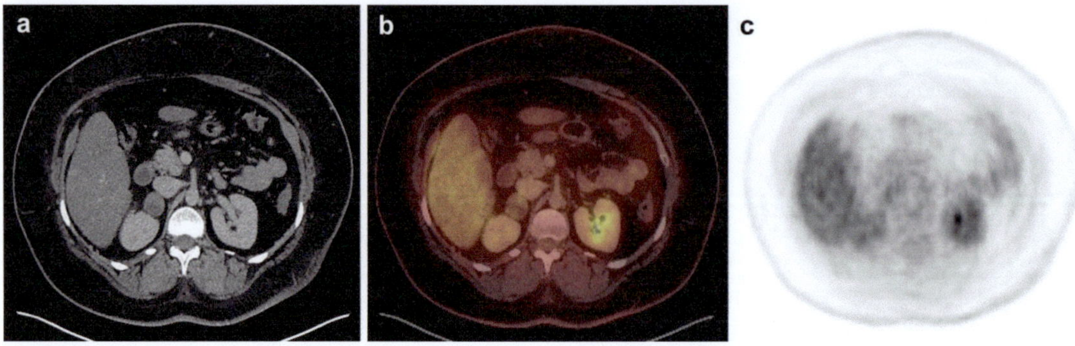

Fig. 19 A 28-year-old female patient undergoing PET/CT because of newly detected tumor of the right adrenal gland with a family history of adrenal carcinoma. Contrast-enhanced CT (**a**), fused PET/CT (**b**), and PET images (**c**) are displayed. As the lesion shows no tracer accumulation, an adrenal adenoma was suspected. The diagnosis was confirmed by histopathology

by comparing the tracer uptake of the adrenal mass to the liver uptake and found a sensitivity of 100 % and specificity of 94 %. Therefore, PET data can be used reliably for the differentiation of benign and adrenal masses (Yun et al. 2001, see Fig. 19). Still, increased tracer accumulation has also been reported in adenomas associated with Cushing's syndrome, posing a potential pitfall (Shimizu et al. 2003; Basu and Nair 2005).

4 Incidental Findings in PET/MR: Differences in Comparison to PET/CT

4.1 Introduction

Despite the success of PET/CT in clinical practice, it soon became obvious that the given limitations of CT, radiation exposure, and low soft tissue contrast are also inherent to PET/CT and cannot be overcome, even if intravenous iodine-based contrast agent is routinely administered. Due to the increased soft tissue contrast and the lack of ionizing radiation, the combination of MRI and PET is a promising perspective. However, the idea of integrating MRI and PET into one single modality is far more challenging than the combination of PET and CT. At first, standard photomultiplier tubes used in PET and PET/CT to read out the signal induced by gamma-radiation in scintillating crystals cannot operate in a strong magnetic field. Therefore, they had to be replaced by a new type of detector technology that is not disturbed by the high electromagnetic field strengths of the MR component, for example, by avalanche photo diodes or silicon photomultipliers (Quick 2014). Although two integrated PET/MR systems are commercially available, technical challenges still lie ahead. One prevailing problem is attenuation correction. While linear attenuation coefficients, which are necessary for attenuation correction of PET data, can be easily derived from the transmission data of the accompanying CT scan in PET/CT, a different approach has to be found in PET/MR, since the MR signal is not directly related to the radiodensity of the tissue but proton density. Therefore, T1-weighted images acquired in Dixon technique are used to determine the fat and water fraction of the tissue. Based on these results, the tissue is segmented into tissue groups (e.g., air, lung, fat, muscle). Standard attenuation coefficients are then used to create an attenuation map for correction of PET data in PET/MR (Martinez-Möller et al. 2009). To increase accuracy of quantification even further, PET in PET/MR is also corrected for attenuation caused by stationary coils and rigid MRI components. However, the gamma-quant attenuation of radiofrequency coils used for high-quality MR imaging has to be reduced to improve PET quality, a problem that can be only solved by the development of low-profile coil systems (Quick 2014).

Still, the inclusion of attenuation caused by bone and artifacts caused by metal implants remains problematic. While ultrashort echo time sequences can be used to image bone in MRI, the long acquisition time and the reduced field of view make its application in whole-body imaging problematic at the current time (Martinez-Möller and Nekolla 2012; Quick 2014).

Despite these limitations, PET/MR offers new opportunities in oncological imaging as the increased soft tissue contrast might be advantageous in the brain, head and neck, breast, heart and musculoskeletal imaging (Antoch and Bockisch 2009; Buchbender et al. 2012a, b; Nensa and Schlosser 2014). Furthermore, the combined acquisition of metabolic information derived from PET and functional MRI biomarkers such as diffusion-weighted imaging (DWI) could provide valuable additional information for tumor characterization and response assessment (Heusch et al. 2013; Gatidis et al. 2013). Still, this new modality holds some specific implications due to the MRI component. Therefore, this chapter will provide a brief overview of incidental findings in PET/MR and possible differences in comparison to PET/CT.

4.2 PET/MR Protocols: Basic Principles

A special challenge in clinical PET/MR imaging is protocol optimization. As a quick examination is necessary to increase patient comfort and economic profitability, the examiner is required to choose an appropriate set of pulse sequences that supplement information derived from PET without producing redundant information. Especially the combination of a dedicated MRI protocol of the primary, for example, of the breast in breast cancer patients or of the head and neck region in patient with squamous cell carcinoma, with a swift whole-body PET/MR promises "one-stop shop" examinations and is therefore highly advocated (Martinez-Möller et al. 2012; von Schulthess and Veit-Haibach 2014).

Initial studies tried to evaluate the possibilities of the T1-weighted Dixon images acquired for attenuation correction to perform fast whole-body examinations, but the quality of these images is low, especially in lung imaging (Appenzeller et al. 2013; Schaarschmidt et al. 2015a). As PET acquisition in PET/MR should be performed for at least 2 min per bed position to improve the quality of the PET images, this time can be used for additional pulse sequence acquisition in a whole-body protocol (Hartung-Knemeyer et al. 2013). Cystic lesions are frequently encountered in the abdomen; hence, a fast T2-weighted sequence might be advisory here (Martinez-Möller et al. 2012; von Schulthess and Veit-Haibach 2014; Schaarschmidt et al. 2015b). Additional T1-weighted, 3D gradient echo sequences allow a more accurate depiction of lung nodules and can be acquired rapidly (Biederer et al. 2001, 2003). If a gadolinium-based contrast agent is administered for local tumor staging, this sequence should be performed after contrast media injection for additional diagnostic security. Therefore, the combination of these two sequences allows a reliable diagnostic workup of most incidental findings and can be therefore used in clinical PET/MR protocols (Grueneisen et al. 2015).

4.3 Advantages of ^{18}F-FDG PET/MR in Comparison to PET/CT

4.3.1 Liver

As mentioned in Chapter 3.2, imaging of small liver lesions that are frequently malignant in oncological patients is challenging even in contrast-enhanced ^{18}F-FDG PET/CT (Schwartz et al. 1999). In these frequently encountered cases, additional MR imaging of the liver provides complementary information to contrast-enhanced PET/CT by allowing the precise characterization of small lesions (Antoch et al. 2003b; Kong et al. 2008; Scharitzer et al. 2013). Here, contrast-enhanced MRI is expected to supplement the information derived from PET if simultaneous PET and MR imaging is performed, leading to a markedly increase in staging accuracy. Therefore, the combination of PET and MRI in an integrated hybrid scanner is a thrilling perspective for liver imaging (Antoch and Bockisch 2009; Pichler et al. 2010). But apart

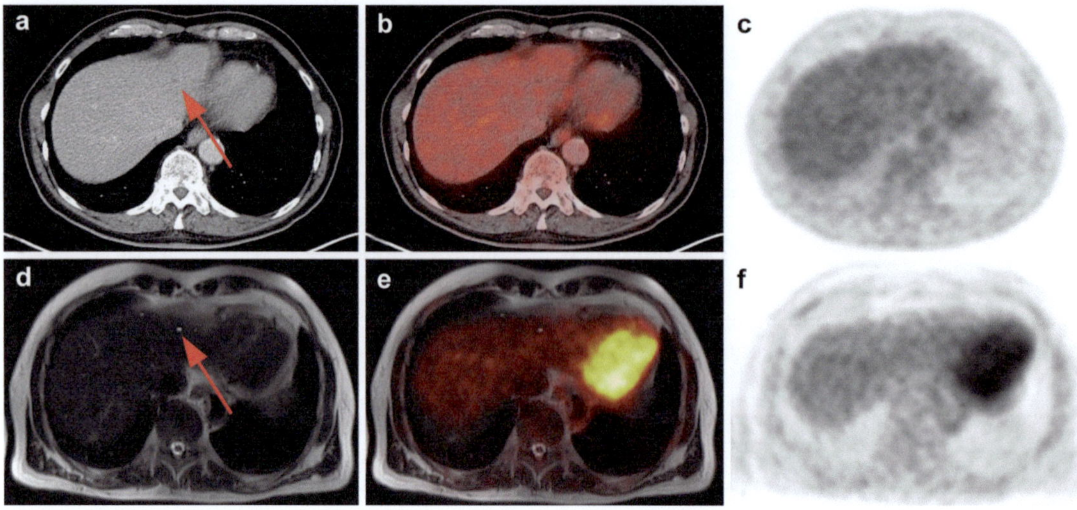

Fig. 20 50 year old male patient suffering from malignant melanoma. Morphological, fused and PET images are displayed for PET/CT (**a–c**) and PET/MR (**d–f**). A lesion that is too small to specify is detected in segment II of the liver in CT (see *red arrow*, **a**) without a correlate in PET (**c**), the high signal in T2-weighted imaging in PET/MR (see *red arrow*, **d**) indicates a benign liver cyst

from the improved sensitivity for liver metastases detection, the first studies also indicate an improved diagnostic confidence for PET/MR in the differentiation between benign and malignant liver lesions in contrast to PET/CT, thus leading to an increased diagnostic certainty (Beiderwellen et al. 2013; Schaarschmidt et al. 2015c, see Fig. 20). Therefore, the number of incidentally detected subcentimeter lesions that are too small to characterize in PET/CT could be reduced by in PET/MR. Still, the clinical and economic benefits of PET/MR in liver imaging in comparison to PET/CT have to be evaluated further for a definite recommendation.

4.3.2 Adrenal Gland

Adrenal lesions are frequently detected in morphological imaging, and their correct characterization is of utmost importance since adrenal metastases are frequently encountered in oncological patients. While the identification of lipid-rich adenomas is generally straightforward in CT, the discrimination between lipid-poor adenomas and malignant solid tumor or metastases poses a diagnostic challenge. Although an increased tracer uptake in the adrenal gland in comparison to liver parenchyma in ^{18}F-FDG PET/CT is a strong predictor of malignancy, an increased tracer uptake can be also observed in benign lesions (Yun et al. 2001). Therefore, additional CT scans such as the acquisition of a delayed phase might be necessary for a definite differentiation between benign and malignant lesions with an increased tracer uptake, disrupting clinical workflow and increasing radiation exposure (Park et al. 2007).

In MRI, the acquisition of in- and opposed-phase images allows the differentiation between benign and malignant adrenal lesions. As fat and water have different resonance frequencies, a marked signal drop in the opposed-phase images in comparison to the in-phase images can be found in fatty lesions, thus allowing the characterization of adrenal adenomas even in hyperattenuating adrenal lesions in CT (Haider et al. 2004). In standard protocols for integrated PET/MR, these exact images are acquired for attenuation correction and are therefore also at hand for diagnostic use, thus increasing diagnostic security (Schaarschmidt et al. 2015c). However, further research is needed to evaluate if additional in- and opposed-phase images in PET/MR increase the diagnostic accuracy in adrenal lesions in comparison to PET/CT.

4.4 Disadvantages of ¹⁸F-FDG PET/MR in Comparison to PET/ CT

4.4.1 Lung Nodules

3D gradient echo sequences have led to a dramatic increase in the sensitivity of MRI for lung nodule detection. Still, CT is preferred for lung imaging by most radiologists as CT is considered to be superior in lung nodule detection due to higher spatial resolution (Biederer et al. 2001, 2003; Schroeder et al. 2005; Sommer et al. 2014). Due to the lack of the CT component in integrated PET/MR scanners, the reduced sensitivity for pulmonary nodules is also inherent to PET/MR, even if dedicated lung imaging sequences have been included in the examination protocol (Sawicki et al. 2016b). Although 78.6 % of the missed lung nodules in the study of Sawicki et al. were benign, 21.4 % of the missed nodules turned out to be small lung metastases (Sawicki et al. 2016a, see Fig. 21). Apart from the risk of missing early metastatic disease, undetected lung nodules in PET/MR could be problematic if follow-up examinations are performed with a different modality such as CT. However, new pulse sequences such as ultrashort echo time sequences could further increase the sensitivity of MRI for small lung nodules and may lead to an improved performance of PET/MR in lung imaging in the future (Burris et al. 2015).

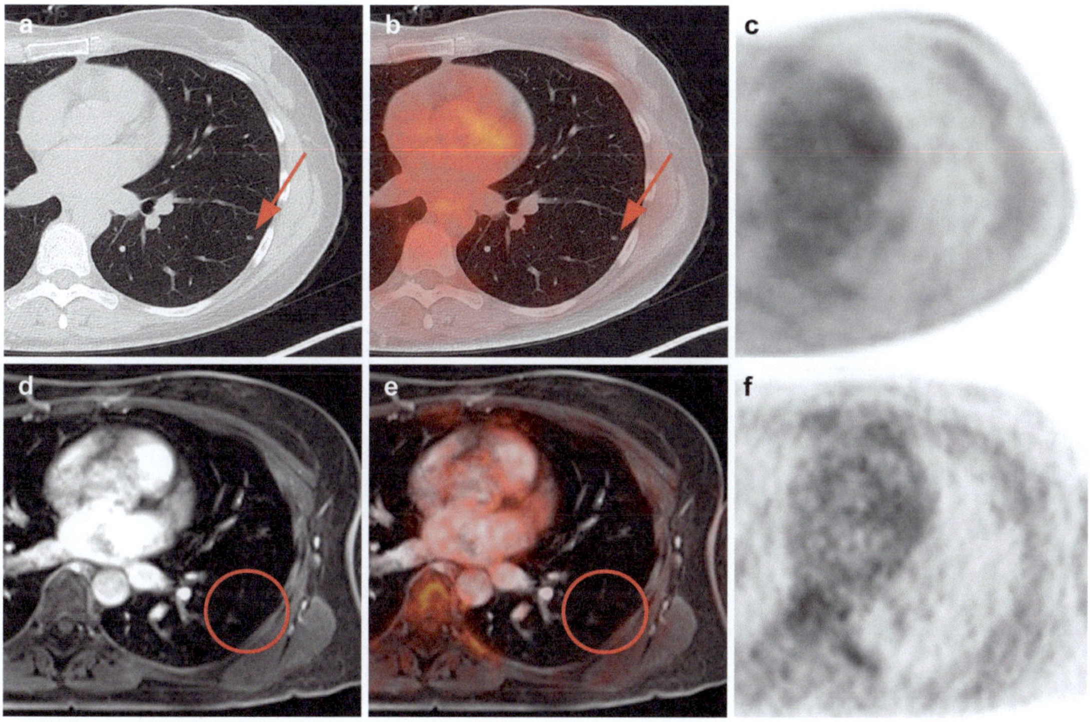

Fig. 21 41 year old female patient suffering from malignant melanoma. Morphological, fused and PET images are displayed for PET/CT (**a**–**c**) and PET/MR (**d**–**f**). While a small lung nodule without tracer uptake is detected by CT in the left lower lobe (see *red arrow*, **a** and **b**), no correlate is found by PET/MR (see *red circle*, **d** and **e**). No metastatic growth was detected during follow-up

References

Abhyankar A, Joshi J, Basu S (2012) FDG uptake in unilateral breast related to breastfeeding practice in a patient of pulmonary hydatid cyst. Clin Nucl Med 37:676–678

Abrams HL, Spiro R, Goldstein N (1950) Metastases in carcinoma. Analysis of 1000 autopsied cases. Cancer 3:74–85

Antoch G, Bockisch A (2009) Combined PET/MRI: a new dimension in whole-body oncology imaging? Eur J Nucl Med Mol Imaging 36:113–120

Antoch G, Stattaus J, Nemat AT, Marnitz S, Beyer T, Kuehl H, Bockisch A, Debatin JF, Freudenberg LS (2003a) Non–small cell lung cancer: dual-modality PET/CT in preoperative staging. Radiology 229:526–533

Antoch G, Vogt FM, Freudenberg LS, Nazaradeh F, Goehde SC, Barkhausen J, Dahmen G, Bockisch A, Debatin JF, Ruehm SG (2003b) Whole-body dual-modality PET/CT and whole-body MRI for tumor staging in oncology. JAMA 290:3199–3206

Appenzeller P, Mader C, Huellner MW, Schmidt D, Schmid D, Boss A, von Schulthess G, Veit-Haibach P (2013) PET/CT versus body coil PET/MRI: how low can you go? Insights Imaging 4:481–490

Avril N (2004) GLUT1 expression in tissue and 18F-FDG uptake. J Nucl Med 45:930–932

Badiee S, Franc BL, Webb EM, Chu B, Hawkins RA, Coakley F (2008) Role of IV iodinated contrast material in 18F-FDG PET/CT of liver, metastases. Am J Roentgenol 191:1436–1439

Bailey CJ (1995) Metformin and intestinal glucose handling. Diabetes Metab Rev 11:23–32

Barzon L, Sonino N, Fallo F, Palu G, Boscaro M (2003) Prevalence and natural history of adrenal incidentalomas. Eur J Endocrinol 149:273–285

Basu S, Nair N (2005) 18F-FDG uptake in bilateral adrenal hyperplasia causing Cushing's syndrome. Eur J Nucl Med Mol Imaging 32:384

Beiderwellen K, Gomez B, Buchbender C, Hartung V, Poeppel TD, Nensa F, Kuehl H, Bockisch A, Lauenstein TC (2013) Depiction and characterization of liver lesions in whole body [18F]-FDG PET/MRI. Eur J Radiol 82:669–675

Bertagna F, Evangelista L, Piccardo A, Bertoli M, Bosio G, Giubbini R, Orlando E, Treglia G (2015) Multicentric study on 18F-FDG-PET/CT breast incidental uptake in patients studied for non-breast malignant purposes. Rev Esp Med Nucl Imagen Mol 34:24–29

Biederer J, Graessner J, Heller M (2001) Magnetic resonance imaging of the lung with a volumetric interpolated 3D-Gradient echo sequence. Rofo Fortschr Dem Geb Rontgenstr Bildgeb Verfahr 173:883–887

Biederer J, Schoene A, Freitag S, Reuter M, Heller M (2003) Simulated pulmonary nodules implanted in a dedicated porcine chest phantom: sensitivity of MR imaging for detection. Radiology 227:475–483

Bockisch A, Beyer T, Antoch G, Veit P, Müller S, Pink R, Rosenbaum S, Kühl H (2004) Grundlagen und klinischer Nutzen von PET-CT. Radiologe 44: 1045–1054

Boeckmann J, Bartel T, Siegel E, Bodenner D, Stack BC (2012) Can the pathology of a thyroid nodule be determined by positron emission tomography uptake? Otolaryngol Head Neck Surg 146:906–912

Boellaard R, Delgado-Bolton R, Oyen WJ, Giammarile F, Tatsch K, Eschner W, Verzijlbergen FJ, Barrington SF, Pike LC, Weber WA, Stroobants S, Delbeke D, Donohoe KJ, Holbrook S, Graham MM, Testanera G, Hoekstra OS, Zijlstra J, Visser E, Hoekstra CJ, Pruim J, Willemsen A, Arends B, Kotzerke J, Bockisch A, Beyer T, Chiti A, Krause BJ (2015) FDG PET/CT: EANM procedure guidelines for tumour imaging: version 2.0. Eur J Nucl Med Mol Imaging 42:328–354

Börner AR, Voth E, Wienhard K, Wagner R, Schicha H (1998) F-18-FDG-PET der Schilddrüse bei Morbus Basedow. Nukl Nucl Med 37:227–233

Bovio S, Cataldi A, Reimondo G, Sperone P, Novello S, Berruti A, Borasio P, Fava C, Dogliotti L, Scagliotti GV, Angeli A, Terzolo M (2006) Prevalence of adrenal incidentaloma in a contemporary computerized tomography series. J Endocrinol Invest 29:298–302

Braun JJ, Kessler R, Constantinesco A, Imperiale A (2008) 18F-FDG PET/CT in sarcoidosis management: review and report of 20 cases. Eur J Nucl Med Mol Imaging 35:1537–1543

Brink I, Reinhardt MJ, Hoegerle S, Altehoefer C, Moser E, Nitzsche EU (2001) Increased metabolic activity in the thymus gland studied with 18F-FDG PET: age dependency and frequency after chemotherapy. J Nucl Med 42:591–595

Bruzzi JF, Truong MT, Marom EM, Mawlawi O, Podoloff DA, Macapinlac HA, Munden RF (2006) Incidental findings on integrated PET/CT that do not accumulate 18F-FDG. Am J Roentgenol 187:1116–1123

Buchbender C, Heusner TA, Lauenstein TC, Bockisch A, Antoch G (2012a) Oncologic PET/MRI, part 1: tumors of the brain, head and neck, chest, abdomen, and pelvis. J Nucl Med 53:928–938

Buchbender C, Heusner TA, Lauenstein TC, Bockisch A, Antoch G (2012b) Oncologic PET/MRI, part 2: bone tumors, soft-tissue tumors, melanoma, and lymphoma. J Nucl Med 53:1244–1252

Burris NS, Johnson KM, Larson PE, Hope MD, Nagle SK, Behr SC, Hope TA (2015) Detection of small pulmonary nodules with ultrashort echo time sequences in oncology patients by using a PET/MR system. Radiology 278:239–246

Cheson BD, Fisher RI, Barrington SF, Cavalli F, Schwartz LH, Zucca E, Lister TA (2014) Recommendations for initial evaluation, staging, and response assessment of Hodgkin and non-Hodgkin lymphoma: the Lugano classification. J Clin Oncol 32:3059–3067

Choi JY, Lee KS, Kim HJ, Shim YM, Kwon OJ, Park K, Baek CH, Chung JH, Lee KH, Kim BT (2006) Focal thyroid lesions incidentally identified by integrated

18F-FDG PET/CT: clinical significance and improved characterization. J Nucl Med 47:609–615

Chondrogiannis S, Marzola MC, Grassetto G, Zorzi A, Milan E, Rampin L, Rubello D, Colletti PM (2015) 18F-FDG PET/CT lung "focalities" without coregistered CT findings: an interpretative clinical dilemma. Nucl Med Commun 36:334–339

Cohen M, Hill C, Cangir A, Sullivan M (1980) Thymic rebound after treatment of childhood tumors. Am J Roentgenol 135:151–156

Cook GJ, Fogelman I, Maisey MN (1996) Normal physiological and benign pathological variants of 18-fluoro-2-deoxyglucose positron-emission tomography scanning: potential for error in interpretation. Semin Nucl Med 26:308–314

Dong A, Zhao T, Gong J, Zuo C (2014) Diffuse FDG uptake of the bilateral atrial walls in a patient with atrial fibrillation. Clin Nucl Med 39:167–169

Fan CM, Fischman AJ, Kwek BH, Abbara S, Aquino SL (2005) Lipomatous hypertrophy of the interatrial septum: increased uptake on FDG PET. Am J Roentgenol 184:339–342

Fayad LM, Cohade C, Wahl RL, Fishman EK (2003) Sacral fractures: a potential pitfall of FDG positron emission tomography. Am J Roentgenol 181:1239–1243

Fenchel S, Grab D, Nuessle K, Kotzerke J, Rieber A, Kreienberg R, Brambs HJ, Reske SN (2002) Asymptomatic adnexal masses: correlation of FDG PET and histopathologic findings. Radiology 223: 780–788

Furlong MA, Fanburg-Smith JC, Miettinen M (2001) The morphologic spectrum of hibernoma: a clinicopathologic study of 170 cases. Am J Surg Pathol 25:809–814

Gatidis S, Schmidt H, Claussen CD, Schwenzer NF (2013) Multiparametrische Bildgebung mittels simultaner MR/PET. Radiologe 53:669–675

Goethals I, De Vriendt C, Hoste P, Smeets P, Ham H (2009) Normal uptake of F-18 FDG in the testis as assessed by PET/CT in a pediatric study population. Ann Nucl Med 23:817–820

Gontier E, Fourme E, Wartski M, Blondet C, Bonardel G, Stanc EL, Mantzarides M, Foehrenbach H, Pecking AP, Alberini JL (2007) High and typical 18F-FDG bowel uptake in patients treated with metformin. Eur J Nucl Med Mol Imaging 35:95–99

Gould MK, Maclean CC, Kuschner WG, Rydzak CE, Owens DK (2001) Accuracy of positron emission tomography for diagnosis of pulmonary nodules and mass lesions: a meta-analysis. JAMA 285:914–924

Grueneisen J, Schaarschmidt BM, Heubner M, Suntharalingam S, Milk I, Kinner S, Heubner A, Forsting M, Lauenstein T, Ruhlmann V, Umutlu L (2015) Implementation of FAST-PET/MRI for whole-body staging of female patients with recurrent pelvic malignancies: a comparison to PET/CT. Eur J Radiol 84:2097–2102

Haber RS, Weiser KR, Pritsker A, Reder I, Burstein DE (1997) GLUT1 glucose transporter expression in benign and malignant thyroid nodules. Thyroid 7:363–367

Haider MA, Ghai S, Jhaveri K, Lockwood G (2004) Chemical shift MR imaging of hyperattenuating (>10 HU) adrenal masses: does it still have a role? Radiology 231:711–716

Hany TF, Heuberger J, von Schulthess GK (2003) Iatrogenic FDG foci in the lungs: a pitfall of PET image interpretation. Eur Radiol 13:2122–2127

Hartung-Knemeyer V, Beiderwellen KJ, Buchbender C, Kuehl H, Lauenstein TC, Bockisch A, Poeppel TD (2013) Optimizing positron emission tomography image acquisition protocols in integrated positron emission tomography/magnetic resonance imaging. Invest Radiol 48:290–294

Heusch P, Buchbender C, Köhler J, Nensa F, Beiderwellen K, Kühl H, Lanzman R, Wittsack H, Gomez B, Gauler T, Schuler M, Forsting M, Bockisch A, Antoch G, Heusner T (2013) Correlation of the apparent diffusion coefficient (ADC) with the standardized uptake value (SUV) in hybrid 18F-FDG PET/MRI in non-small cell lung cancer (NSCLC) lesions: initial results. Rofo Fortschr Dem Geb Rontgenstr Bildgeb Verfahr 185:1056–1062

Heusner TA, Hahn S, Hamami ME, Kim UH, Baumeister R, Forsting M, Stahl A, Bockisch A, Antoch G (2009) Gastrointestinal 18F-FDG accumulation on PET without a corresponding CT abnormality is not an early indicator of cancer development. Eur Radiol 19: 2171–2179

Heyer CM, Kagel T, Lemburg SP, Bauer TT, Nicolas V (2003) Lipomatous hypertrophy of the interatrial septum: a prospective study of incidence, imaging findings, and clinical symptoms. Chest 124:2068–2073

Hoang JK, Langer JE, Middleton WD, Wu CC, Hammers LW, Cronan JJ, Tessler FN, Grant EG, Berland LL (2015) Managing incidental thyroid nodules detected on imaging: white paper of the ACR Incidental Thyroid Findings Committee. J Am Coll Radiol 12: 143–150

Hollinger EF, Alibazoglu H, Ali A, Green A, Lamonica G (1998) Hematopoietic cytokine-mediated FDG uptake simulates the appearance of diffuse metastatic disease on whole-body PET imaging. Clin Nucl Med 23: 93–98

Horiuchi M, Yasuda S, Shohtsu A, Ide M (1998) Four cases of Warthin's tumor of the parotid gland detected with FDG PET. Ann Nucl Med 12:47–50

Horiuchi C, Tsukuda M, Taguchi T, Ishiguro Y, Okudera K, Inoue T (2008) Correlation between FDG-PET findings and GLUT1 expression in salivary gland pleomorphic adenomas. Ann Nucl Med 22:693–698

Huang YE, Pu YL, Huang YJ, Chen CF, Pu QH, Konda SD, Appelbaum DE (2010) The utility of the nonattenuation corrected 18F-FDG PET images in the characterization of solitary pulmonary lesions. Nucl Med Commun 31:945–951

Israel O, Yefremov N, Bar-Shalom R, Kagana O, Frenkel A, Keidar Z, Fischer D (2005) PET/CT detection of unexpected gastrointestinal foci of 18F-FDG uptake: incidence, localization patterns, and clinical significance. J Nucl Med 46:758–762

Jamar F, Buscombe J, Chiti A, Christian PE, Delbeke D, Donohoe KJ, Israel O, Martin-Comin J, Signore A (2013) EANM/SNMMI guideline for 18F-FDG use in inflammation and infection. J Nucl Med 54:647–658

James OG, Christensen JD, Wong TZ, Borges-Neto S, Koweek LM (2011) Utility of FDG PET/CT in inflammatory cardiovascular disease. Radiographics 31:1271–1286

Jeon TJ, Lee YS, Lee JH, Chang HS, Ryu YH (2014) Rebound thymic hyperplasia detected by 18F-FDG PET/CT after radioactive iodine ablation therapy for thyroid cancer. Thyroid 24:1636–1641

Kamel EM, Thumshirn M, Truninger K, Schiesser M, Fried M, Padberg B, Schneiter D, Stoeckli SJ, von Schulthess GK, Stumpe KD (2004) Significance of incidental 18F-FDG accumulations in the gastrointestinal tract in PET/CT: correlation with endoscopic and histopathologic results. J Nucl Med 45:1804–1810

Keyzer C, Dhaene B, Blocklet D, De Maertelaer V, Goldman S, Gevenois PA (2015) Colonoscopic findings in patients with incidental colonic focal FDG uptake. Am J Roentgenol 204:586–591

Kitajima K, Nakamoto Y, Senda M, Onishi Y, Okizuka H, Sugimura K (2007) Normal uptake of 18F-FDG in the testis: an assessment by PET/CT. Ann Nucl Med 21:405–410

Kong G, Jackson C, Koh DM, Lewington V, Sharma B, Brown G, Cunningham D, Cook GJ (2008) The use of 18F-FDG PET/CT in colorectal liver metastases–comparison with CT and liver MRI. Eur J Nucl Med Mol Imaging 35:1323–1329

Kostakoglu L, Wong JC, Barrington SF, Cronin BF, Dynes AM, Maisey MN (1996) Speech-related visualization of laryngeal muscles with Fluorine-18-FDG. J Nucl Med 37:1771–1773

Kuester LB, Fischman AJ, Fan CM, Halpern EF, Aquino SL (2005) Lipomatous hypertrophy of the interatrial septum: prevalence and features on fusion 18F fluorodeoxyglucose positron emission tomography/ CT. Chest 128:3888–3893

Lerman H, Metser U, Grisaru D, Fishman A, Lievshitz G, Even-Sapir E (2004) Normal and abnormal 18F-FDG endometrial and ovarian uptake in pre- and postmenopausal patients: assessment by PET/CT. J Nucl Med 45:266–271

Lewis PJ, Salama A (1994) Uptake of fluorine-18-fluorodeoxyglucose in sarcoidosis. J Nucl Med 35:1647–1649

Leyn PD, Lardinois D, Schil PEV, Rami-Porta R, Passlick B, Zielinski M, Waller DA, Lerut T, Weder W (2007) ESTS guidelines for preoperative lymph node staging for non-small cell lung cancer. Eur J Cardiothorac Surg 32:1–8

MacMahon H, Austin JH, Gamsu G, Herold CJ, Jett JR, Naidich DP, Patz EF Jr, Swensen SJ; Fleischner Society (2005) Guidelines for management of small pulmonary nodules detected on CT scans: a statement from the Fleischner Society. Radiology 237:395–400

Mäki M, Luotolahti M, Nuutila P, Iida H, Voipio-Pulkki LM, Ruotsalainen U, Haaparanta M, Solin O, Hartiala J, Härkönen R, Knuuti J (1996) Glucose uptake in the chronically dysfunctional but viable myocardium. Circulation 93:1658–1666

Martinez-Möller A, Nekolla SG (2012) Attenuation correction for PET/MR: problems, novel approaches and practical solutions. Z Med Phys 22:299–310

Martinez-Möller A, Souvatzoglou M, Delso G, Bundschuh RA, Chefd'hotel C, Ziegler SI, Navab N, Schwaiger M, Nekolla SG (2009) Tissue classification as a potential approach for attenuation correction in whole-body PET/MRI: evaluation with PET/CT data. J Nucl Med 50:520–526

Martinez-Möller A, Eiber M, Nekolla SG, Souvatzoglou M, Drzezga A, Ziegler S, Rummeny EJ, Schwaiger M, Beer AJ (2012) Workflow and scan protocol considerations for integrated whole-body PET/MRI in oncology. J Nucl Med 53:1415–1426

Maurer AH, Burshteyn M, Adler LP, Steiner RM (2011) How to differentiate benign versus malignant cardiac and paracardiac 18F FDG uptake at oncologic PET/ CT. Radiographics 31:1287–1305

Naidich DP, Bankier AA, MacMahon H, Schaefer-Prokop CM, Pistolesi M, Goo JM, Macchiarini P, Crapo JD, Herold CJ, Austin JH, Travis WD (2013) Recommendations for the management of subsolid pulmonary nodules detected at CT: a statement from the Fleischner society. Radiology 266:304–317

Nakahara T, Fujii H, Ide M, Nishiumi N, Takahashi W, Yasuda S, Shohtsu A, Kubo A (2001) FDG uptake in the morphologically normal thymus: comparison of FDG positron emission tomography andCT. Br J Radiol 74:821–824

Nakamoto Y, Tatsumi M, Hammoud D, Cohade C, Osman MM, Wahl RL (2005) Normal FDG distribution patterns in the head and neck: PET/CT evaluation. Radiology 234:879–885

Nensa F, Schlosser T (2014) Cardiovascular hybrid imaging using PET/MRI. Rofo Fortschr Dem Geb Rontgenstr Bildgeb Verfahr 186(12):1094–1101

Nensa F, Tezgah E, Poeppel TD, Jensen CJ, Schelhorn J, Köhler J, Heusch P, Bruder O, Schlosser T, Nassenstein K (2015) Integrated 18F-FDG PET/MR imaging in the assessment of cardiac masses: a pilot study. J Nucl Med 56:255–260

Niekel MC, Bipat S, Stoker J (2010) Diagnostic imaging of colorectal liver metastases with CT, MR imaging, FDG PET, and/or FDG PET/CT: a meta-analysis of prospective studies including patients who have not previously undergone treatment. Radiology 257:674–684

Nishizawa S, Inubushi M, Okada H (2004) Physiological 18F-FDG uptake in the ovaries and uterus of healthy female volunteers. Eur J Nucl Med Mol Imaging 32:549–556

Nomori H, Watanabe K, Ohtsuka T, Naruke T, Suemasu K, Uno K (2004) Evaluation of F-18 fluorodeoxyglucose (FDG) PET scanning for pulmonary nodules less than 3 cm in diameter, with special reference to the CT images. Lung Cancer 45:19–27

Oh JR, Song HC, Chong A, Ha JM, Jeong SY, Min JJ, Bom HS (2010) Impact of medication discontinuation on increased intestinal FDG accumulation in diabetic patients treated with metformin. Am J Roentgenol 195:1404–1410

Okamura T, Kawabe J, Koyama K, Ochi H, Yamada R, Sakamoto H, Matsuda M, Ohashi Y, Nakai Y (1998) Fluorine-18 fluorodeoxyglucose positron emission tomography imaging of parotid mass lesions. Acta Otolaryngol Suppl 538:209–213

Osman MM, Cohade C, Fishman EK, Wahl RL (2005) Clinically significant incidental findings on the unenhanced CT portion of PET/CT studies: frequency in 250 patients. J Nucl Med 46:1352–1355

Özülker T, Özülker F, Mert M, Özpaçacı T (2010) Clearance of the high intestinal 18F-FDG uptake associated with metformin after stopping the drug. Eur J Nucl Med Mol Imaging 37:1011–1017

Park BK, Kim CK, Kim B, Lee JH (2007) Comparison of delayed enhanced CT and chemical shift MR for evaluating hyperattenuating incidental adrenal masses. Radiology 243:760–765

Pichler BJ, Kolb A, Nägele T, Schlemmer HP (2010) PET/MRI: paving the way for the next generation of clinical multimodality imaging applications. J Nucl Med 51:333–336

Poh F, Wong SK (2014) Imaging of Hidradenitis Suppurativa and its complications. Case Rep Radiol 2014:294753

Purohit BS, Ailianou A, Dulguerov N, Becker CD, Ratib O, Becker M (2014) FDG-PET/CT pitfalls in oncological head and neck imaging. Insights Imaging 5:585–602

Quick HH (2014) Integrated PET/MR. J Magn Reson Imaging 39:243–258

Rakheja R, Ciarallo A, Alabed YZ, Hickeson M (2011) Intravenous administration of diazepam significantly reduces brown fat activity on 18F-FDG PET/CT. Am J Nucl Med Mol Imaging 1:29–35

Reesink DJ, Fransen van de Putte EE, Vegt E, De Jong J, van Werkhoven E, Mertens LS, Bex A, van der Poel HG, van Rhijn BW, Horenblas S, Meijer RP (2015) Clinical relevance of incidental prostatic lesions on FDG-PET/CT Scan. J Urol. Advance online publication

Reinhardt MJ, Wiethoelter N, Matthies A, Joe AY, Strunk H, Jaeger U, Biersack HJ (2005) PET recognition of pulmonary metastases on PET/CT imaging: impact of attenuation-corrected and non-attenuation-corrected PET images. Eur J Nucl Med Mol Imaging 33:134–139

Rosenbaum SJ, Lind T, Antoch G, Bockisch A (2006) False-positive FDG PET uptake – the role of PET/CT. Eur Radiol 16:1054–1065

Sacks A, Peller PJ, Surasi DS, Chatburn L, Mercier G, Subramaniam RM (2011) Value of PET/CT in the management of liver metastases, part 1. Am J Roentgenol 197:256–259

Sawicki LM, Grueneisen J, Buchbender C, Schaarschmidt BM, Gomez B, Ruhlmann V, Umutlu L, Antoch G, Heusch P (2016a) Evaluation of the outcome of lung nodules missed on 18F-FDG PET/MRI compared with 18F-FDG PET/CT in patients with known malignancies. J Nucl Med 57:15–20

Sawicki LM, Grueneisen J, Buchbender C, Schaarschmidt BM, Gomez B, Ruhlmann V, Wetter A, Umutlu L, Antoch G, Heusch P (2016b) Comparative performance of 18F-FDG PET/MRI and 18F-FDG PET/CT regarding detection and characterization of pulmonary lesions in 121 oncologic patients. J Nucl Med. Advance online publication

Schaaf WE, Patel Z, Retrouvey M, Cunningham TD, Johnson LS (2014) Frequency and clinical relevance of PET/CT incidentalomas. Abdom Imaging 39:657–662

Schaarschmidt B, Buchbender C, Gomez B, Rubbert C, Hild F, Köhler J, Grueneisen J, Reis H, Ruhlmann V, Wetter A, Quick HH, Antoch G, Heusch P (2015a) Thoracic staging of non-small-cell lung cancer using integrated 18F-FDG PET/MR imaging: diagnostic value of different MR sequences. Eur J Nucl Med Mol Imaging 42:1257–1267

Schaarschmidt BM, Grueneisen J, Heusch P, Gomez B, Beiderwellen K, Ruhlmann V, Umutlu L, Quick HH, Antoch G, Buchbender C (2015b) Oncological whole-body staging in integrated 18F-FDG PET/MR: value of different MR sequences for simultaneous PET and MR reading. Eur J Radiol 84:1285–1292

Schaarschmidt BM, Grueneisen J, Heusch P, Gomez B, Umutlu L, Ruhlmann V, Rosenbaum-Krumme S, Antoch G, Buchbender C (2015c) Does 18F-FDG PET/MRI reduce the number of indeterminate abdominal incidentalomas compared with 18F-FDG PET/CT? Nucl Med Commun 36:588–595

Scharitzer M, Ba-Ssalamah A, Ringl H, Kölblinger C, Grünberger T, Weber M, Schima W (2013) Preoperative evaluation of colorectal liver metastases: comparison between gadoxetic acid-enhanced 3.0-T MRI and contrast-enhanced MDCT with histopathological correlation. Eur Radiol 23:2187–2196

Schroeder T, Ruehm SG, Debatin JF, Ladd ME, Barkhausen J, Goehde SC (2005) Detection of pulmonary nodules using a 2D HASTE MR sequence: comparison with MDCT. Am J Roentgenol 185:979–984

Schwartz LH, Gandras EJ, Colangelo SM, Ercolani MC, Panicek DM (1999) Prevalence and importance of small hepatic lesions found at CT in patients with cancer. Radiology 210:71–74

Seo YL, Yoon DY, Baek S, Lim KJ, Yun EJ, Cho YK, Bae WJ, Chung EJ, Kwon KH (2015) Incidental focal FDG uptake in the parotid glands on PET/CT in patients with head and neck malignancy. Eur Radiol 25:171–177

Sharma P, Mukherjee A, Karunanithi S, Bal C, Kumar R (2014) Potential role of 18F-FDG PET/CT in patients with fungal infections. Am J Roentgenol 203:180–189

Shim JH, JH O, Oh SI, Yoo HM, Jeon HM, Park CH, Kim SH, Song KY (2012) Clinical significance of incidental colonic 18F-FDG uptake on PET/CT images in patients with gastric adenocarcinoma. J Gastrointest Surg 16:1847–1853

Shimaoka K, Sokal JE, Pickren JW (1962) Metastatic neoplasms in the thyroid gland. Pathological and clinical findings. Cancer 15:557–565

Shimizu A, Oriuchi N, Tsushima Y, Higuchi T, Aoki J, Endo K (2003) High [18F] 2-fluoro-2-deoxy-D-glucose

(FDG) uptake of adrenocortical adenoma showing subclinical Cushing's syndrome. Ann Nucl Med 17:403–406
Shirone N, Shinkai T, Yamane T, Uto F, Yoshimura H, Tamai H, Imai T, Inoue M, Kitano S, Kichikawa K, Hasegawa M (2012) Axillary lymph node accumulation on FDG-PET/CT after influenza vaccination. Ann Nucl Med 26:248–252
Sidhu P, Lin P, Son H, Rosenfeld D, Lin M (2014) Testicular fluorine-18 fludeoxyglucose uptake on positron emission tomography CT in patients with lymphoma: clinical significance and management impact. Br J Radiol 87:20140472
Simpson RC, Dyer MJ, Entwisle J, Harman KE (2011) Positron emission tomography features of hidradenitis suppurativa. Br J Radiol 84:164–165
Skolnik EM, Friedman M, Becker S, Sisson GA, Keyes GR (1977) Tumors of the major salivary glands. Laryngoscope 87:843–861
Smith CS, Teruya-Feldstein J, Caravelli JF, Yeung HW (2008) False-positive findings on 18F-FDG PET/CT: differentiation of hibernoma and malignant fatty tumor on the basis of fluctuating standardized uptake values. Am J Roentgenol 190:1091–1096
Söderlund V, Larsson SA, Jacobsson H (2007) Reduction of FDG uptake in brown adipose tissue in clinical patients by a single dose of propranolol. Eur J Nucl Med Mol Imaging 34:1018–1022
Soelberg KK, Bonnema SJ, Brix TH, Hegedüs L (2012) Risk of malignancy in thyroid incidentalomas detected by 18F-fluorodeoxyglucose positron emission tomography: a systematic review. Thyroid 22:918–925
Sommer G, Tremper J, Koenigkam-Santos M, Delorme S, Becker N, Biederer J, Kauczor HU, Heussel CP, Schlemmer HP, Puderbach M (2014) Lung nodule detection in a high-risk population: comparison of magnetic resonance imaging and low-dose computed tomography. Eur J Radiol 83:600–605
Stagg J, Farukhi I, Lazaga F, Thompson C, Bradshaw L, Kaif M, Gould-Simon A, Schmidt R (2014) Significance of 18F-fluorodeoxyglucose uptake at the gastroesophageal junction: comparison of PET to esophagogastroduodenoscopy. Dig Dis Sci 60:1335–1342
Stahl A, Dzewas B, Schwaiger M, Weber WA (2002) Excretion of FDG into saliva and its significance for PET imaging. Nukl Nucl Med 41:214–216
Thie JA (2004) Understanding the standardized uptake value, its methods, and implications for usage. J Nucl Med 45:1431–1434
Thomassen A, Lerberg Nielsen A, Gerke O, Johansen A, Petersen H (2011) Duration of 18F-FDG avidity in lymph nodes after pandemic H1N1v and seasonal influenza vaccination. Eur J Nucl Med Mol Imaging 38:894–898
Ulaner GA, Lyall A (2013) Identifying and distinguishing treatment effects and complications from malignancy at FDG PET/CT. Radiographics 33:1817–1834
von Schulthess GK, Veit-Haibach P (2014) Workflow considerations in PET/MR imaging. J Nucl Med 55:19–24
von Schulthess GK, Meier N, Stumpe KD (2001) Joint accumulations of FDG in whole body PET scans. Nukl Nucl Med 40:193–197
Wadih A, Rehm PK, Deng C, Douvas M (2015) Active herpes zoster infection with cutaneous manifestation and adenopathy on FDG PET/CT. Radiol Case Rep 10:27–29
Warburg O (1956) On the origin of cancer cells. Science 123:309–314
Weng L-J, Schöder H (2004) Melanoma metastasis to the testis demonstrated with FDG PET/CT. Clin Nucl Med 29:811–812
Wong WL, Gibson D, Sanghera B, Goodchild K, Saunders M (2007) Evaluation of normal FDG uptake in palatine tonsil and its potential value for detecting occult head and neck cancers: a PET CT study. Nucl Med Commun 28:675–680
Wu X, Pertovaara H, Korkola P, Dastidar P, Järvenpää R, Eskola H, Kellokumpu-Lehtinen PL (2014) Correlations between functional imaging markers derived from PET/CT and diffusion-weighted MRI in diffuse large B-cell lymphoma and follicular lymphoma. PLoS One 9:84999
Yasuda S, Shohtsu A, Ide M, Takagi S, Takahashi W, Suzuki Y, Horiuchi M (1998) Chronic thyroiditis: diffuse uptake of FDG at PET. Radiology 207:775–778
Yun M, Kim W, Alnafisi N, Lacorte L, Jang S, Alavi A (2001) 18F-FDG PET in characterizing adrenal lesions detected on CT or MRI. J Nucl Med 42:1795–1799
Zhuang H, Sam JW, Chacko TK, Duarte PS, Hickeson M, Feng Q, Nakhoda KZ, Guan L, Reich P, Altimari SM, Alavi A (2003) Rapid normalization of osseous FDG uptake following traumatic or surgical fractures. Eur J Nucl Med Mol Imaging 30:1096–1103

Incidental Findings in Ultrasound

J. Rübenthaler and D.-A. Clevert

Contents

1 **Preliminary Remarks** 197

2 **Abdominal Aortic Aneurysm** 198

3 **Hemangiomas and Liver Cysts** 198
3.1 Hemangiomas 198
3.2 Liver Cysts 199

4 **Cholelithiasis** 200

5 **Renal Cysts and Renal Cell Carcinoma** 201
5.1 Renal Cysts 201
5.2 Renal Cell Carcinoma 201

References 202

Abstract

This chapter describes the most common incidental findings in abdominal ultrasound and gives an overview about their etiologies, imaging features and treatment options. Being aware of unexpected incidental findings in ultrasound and their implications for patient management is a necessity for every sonographer and will assist the physician in clinical decision management. This chapter provides information about abdominal aortic aneurysms, hemangiomas, liver cysts, cholelithiasis, renal cysts and renal cell carcinoma.

1 Preliminary Remarks

Since the introduction of ultrasound into the clinical routine and the broad availability of ultrasound systems in modern hospitals, ultrasound has become the standard initial diagnostic tool for the initial work-up of unclear abdominal pathologies. Standard abdominal ultrasound includes native B-mode sonography and color-Doppler sonography. With the introduction of contrast-enhanced-ultrasound (CEUS) into modern ultrasound systems, it is now possible to add additional useful information for the final diagnosis without the need of using other imaging modalities.

The standard use of ultrasound for the diagnostic work up of all different kinds of abdominal pathologies results in a respectable amount of incidental findings originally not associated with

J. Rübenthaler • D.-A. Clevert (✉)
Department of Clinical Radiology, Interdisciplinary Ultrasound Center, Ludwig-Maximilians-University of Munich-Grosshadern Campus,
Marchioninistr. 15, Munich 81377, Germany
e-mail: dirk.clevert@med.uni-muenchen.de

Med Radiol Diagn Imaging (2016)
DOI 10.1007/174_2016_68, © Springer International Publishing Switzerland
Published Online: 20 Aug 2016

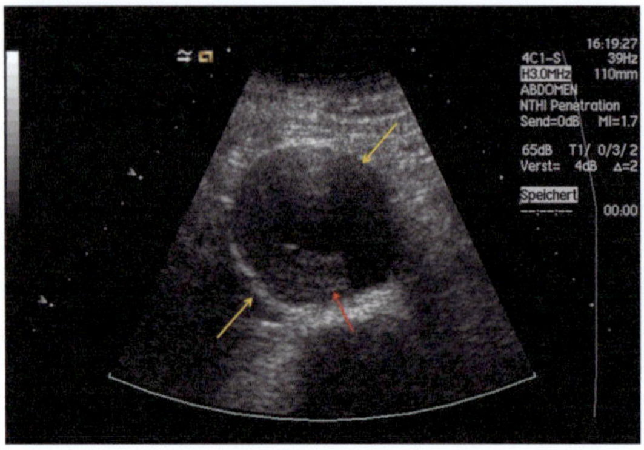

Fig. 1 An abdominal aortic aneurysm (*yellow arrows*) with intraluminal thrombotic material (*red arrow*)

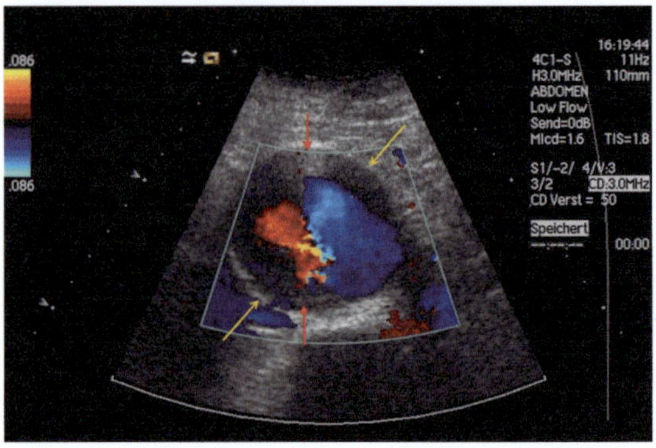

Fig. 2 Same patient as in Fig. 1. Color Doppler shows the blood flow in the abdominal aortic aneurysm (*yellow arrows*), with no detectable blood flow in the thrombotic areas of the aneurysm (*red arrows*)

the initial clinical question of the referring physician. This chapter is dedicated to describe the most common findings in abdominal ultrasound.

2 Abdominal Aortic Aneurysm

Abdominal aortic aneurysm (AAAs) is a common pathology found during standard ultrasound examinations. With an incidence of 2–8 % in men above the age of 65 and a fourfold lower incidence in women, aortic aneurysms are most likely to be seen incidentally in male patients (Kent 2014). AAAs are defined as an enlargement of the aorta with a diameter greater than 3.0 cm or greater than 50 % of the normal size and are considered as the most common form of aneurysms of the aorta (Kent 2014). The prevalence of AAAs is age dependent, with the most diagnoses made at the age of 65–70 (Kent 2014). Mostly they are asymptomatic and do not cause any signs or symptoms. Predisposing risk factors include smoking, hypertension, and genetic predisposition (Schmitz-Rixen et al. 2016). Additionally, ethnicity seems to play a role in the prevalence of AAAs (Salem et al. 2009). About 85 % of all AAAs can be seen below the kidney vessels (Kent 2014). In some states, ultrasound screening for AAAs is recommended above a certain age with an estimated number needed to screen of 850 patients (LeFevre 2014; Cina and Devereaux 2005). A surgical intervention is normally recommended above an average diameter of the AAA of 5.5 cm in men and 5.0 cm in women (Kent 2014). The main risk of AAAs is a rupture with a risk of less than 1 % for aneurysms with a diameter of less than 5.5 cm, 10 % for aneurysms measuring between 5.5 and 7.0 cm, and 33 % for aneurysms measuring more than 7.0 cm (Kent 2014). A ruptured AAA shows a mortality rate of 85–90 % (Kent 2014). Management of incidentally found AAAs includes conservative treatment with ultrasound surveillance for asymptomatic AAAs with a diameter of less than 5.5 cm, as there is a higher risk of repair than of rupture and surgical repair for AAAs above that size (Figs. 1 and 2) (Filardo et al. 2015; Powell et al. 2007; Lederle et al. 2002).

3 Hemangiomas and Liver Cysts

3.1 Hemangiomas

Hemangiomas of the liver are one of the most common incidental finding found during standard examinations of the liver. Although hemangiomas can occur at every site of the human body, about 30 % of all hemangiomas can be found inside the liver. The incidence rate is about 0.4–20 % (Bajenaru et al. 2015). Hemangiomas can be found four to five times more often in women as in men, which might be explained by estrogen as a stimulus (Kleinman et al. 2007; Dockerty et al. 1956). Hemangiomas are benign tumors which usually do not show a malignancy and do normally not

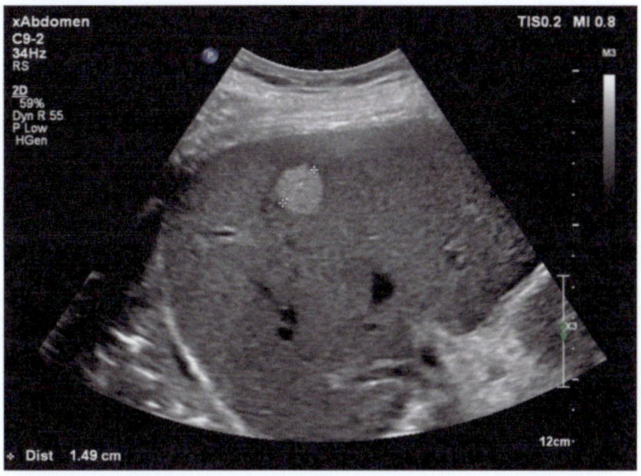

Fig. 3 Classical hemangioma in B-mode ultrasound. A solitary hyperechoic lesion can be seen with sharp margins, subcapsular located in the right liver lobe

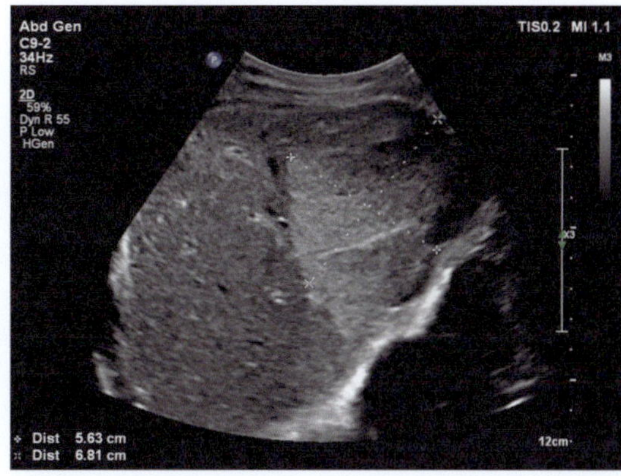

Fig. 4 Asymmetrically shaped hyperechoic lesion with sharp margins suggestive of a hemangioma, although not fulfilling the typical criteria for a hemangioma. An additional contrast-enhanced ultrasound was recommended for further diagnosis

cause any signs or symptoms (Bajenaru et al. 2015). Sonographic features include a hyperechoic lesion with sharp margins, posterior acoustic enhancement, and no visible perfusion in color Doppler due to the slow perfusion of the hemangiomas. Mostly, they are solitary and located subcapsular in the right lobe of the liver, although multilocular hemangiomas are possible, and show various sizes from a few millimeters up to 40 cm (Bajenaru et al. 2015; Koszka et al. 2010; Nakanuma 1995). Ultrasound surveillance should be performed on a regular basis, because about 10 % of all hemangiomas show a growth in size over time and bigger hemangiomas might cause symptoms, e.g., compression of adjacent structures (Bajenaru et al. 2015). CEUS can be used to verify the diagnosis, as hemangiomas show a specific contrast enhancement pattern after contrast agent injection with a peripheral nodular contrast enhancement and consecutive centripetal filling (Bajenaru et al. 2015). Normal hemangiomas do not require any treatment as long as they do not cause secondary problems. Ultrasound surveillance should also been carried out during pregnancy or in women using contraceptives, as estrogen can induce a size growth. Surgical therapy is only needed in cases of abnormal rapid size growth or risk for secondary problems and includes enucleation, segmental resection, or lobectomy (Figs. 3, 4, and 5) (Bajenaru et al. 2015).

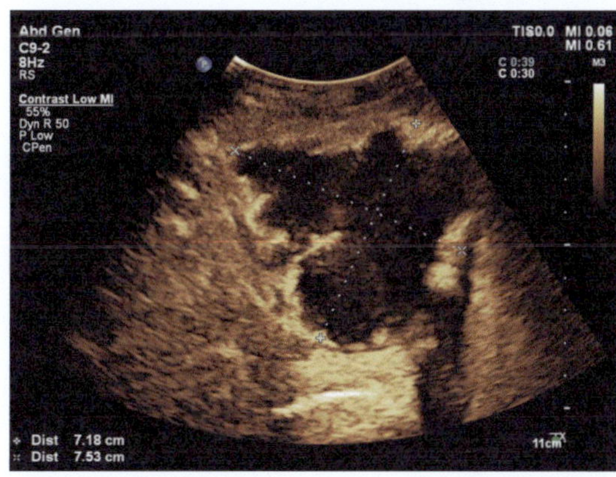

Fig. 5 Same patient as in Fig. 4. Contrast-enhanced ultrasound confirms the finding of a hemangioma with a classical nodular contrast enhancement pattern of the lesion

3.2 Liver Cysts

Liver cysts are a common incidental findings found during standard examinations of the liver. Liver cysts are benign fluid-filled cysts inside the liver parenchyma and are not considered as malignant. Normally they are anechoic and round to ovally shaped and show a characteristic posterior acoustic enhancement in B-mode ultrasound. They occur in about 2.5 % of the population with an age-dependent increasing incidence (Gaines and Sampson 1989). Comparable to the hemangiomas described earlier, they occur more commonly in women and

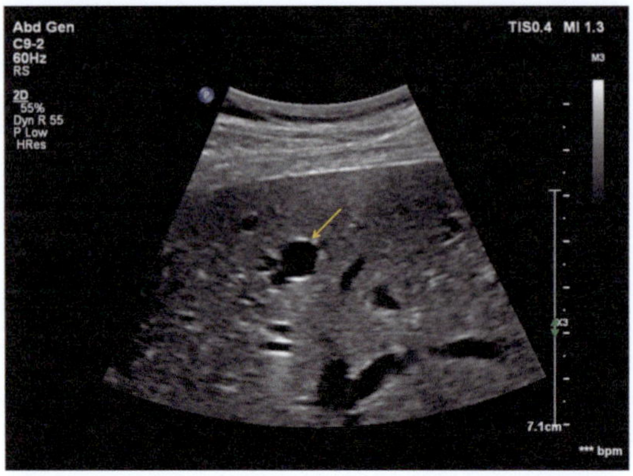

Fig. 6 A simple liver cyst (*yellow arrow*) of the right liver lobe in native B-mode ultrasound. The cyst shows the classical findings in B-mode ultrasound with a round shape, sharp margins, and posterior acoustic enhancement

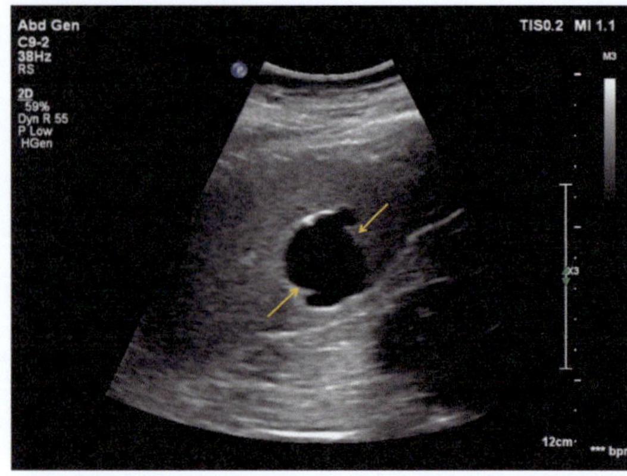

Fig. 8 Liver cyst (*yellow arrows*) with slightly lobulated walls still showing characteristics of a simple benign liver cyst, being anechoic in native B-mode ultrasound and characteristic posterior acoustic enhancement

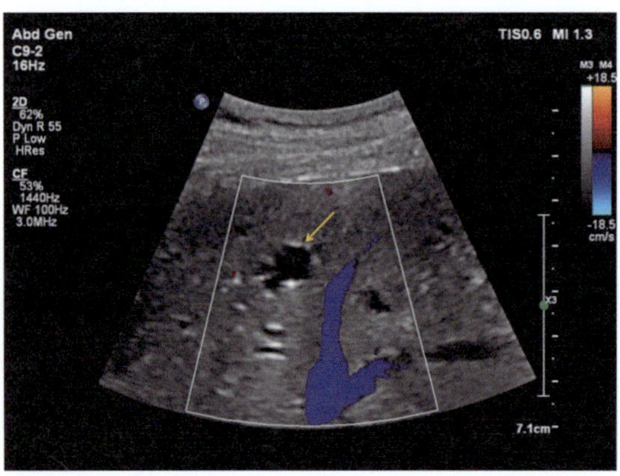

Fig. 7 Same patient as in Fig. 6. Color Doppler confirms the diagnosis of the native B-mode ultrasound with no detectable blood flow inside the cyst (*yellow arrow*)

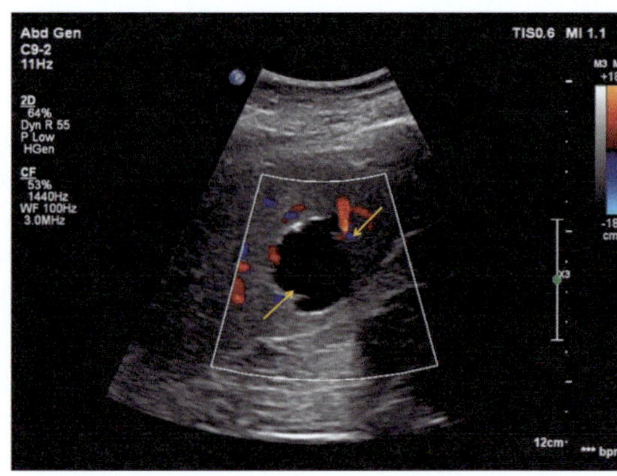

Fig. 9 Same patient as in Fig. 8. Color Doppler confirms the diagnosis of the native B-mode ultrasound with no detectable blood flow inside the cyst (*yellow arrows*)

are more often found solitary in the right liver lobe, although multiple liver cysts can also be found (Gaines and Sampson 1989). The etiology of most liver cysts is not known; they can occur at birth or can occur later on. Normal liver cysts do not require any further treatment as long as they do not cause any secondary problems (Figs. 6, 7, 8, and 9).

4 Cholelithiasis

Gallstones in the gallbladder are one of the most common findings in the ultrasound examination of the gallbladder in adolescents. They are mostly incidentally found in asymptomatic patients and do not require any treatment in asymptomatic patients regardless of size and number (Acalovschi et al. 2003). About 10–15 % of all adolescents are considered to have gallstones and they can be found about two times more often in women compared to men (Shaffer 2006). Common predisposing risk factors include, for example, genetic risk factors, obesity, hypercholesterolemia, pregnancy, and female sex (Shaffer 2006; Buch et al. 2007). About 25 % of all gallstones get symptomatic with a typical abdominal pain in the upper-right side. Typical sonographic features include an echoic focus inside the gallbladder that cast a dorsal acoustic shadow. The most common complication of gallstones is the obstruction of the common bile duct, which might result in acute cholecystitis, ascending cholangitis, or pancreatitis. Therapeutical options

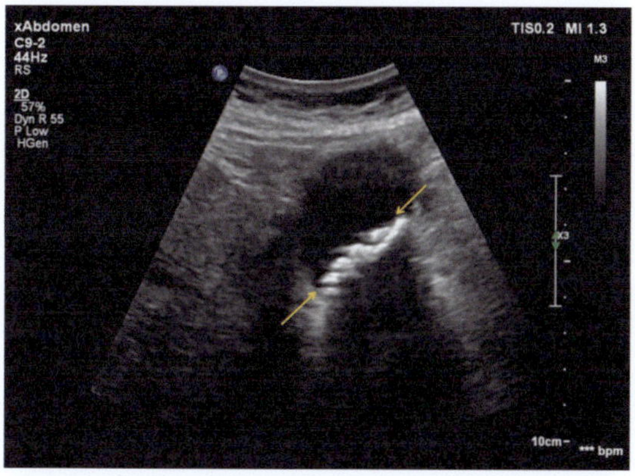

Fig. 10 Multiple hyperechoic foci (*yellow arrows*) inside the gallbladder that cast an acoustic dorsal shadow in line with the classical native B-mode findings of gallstones

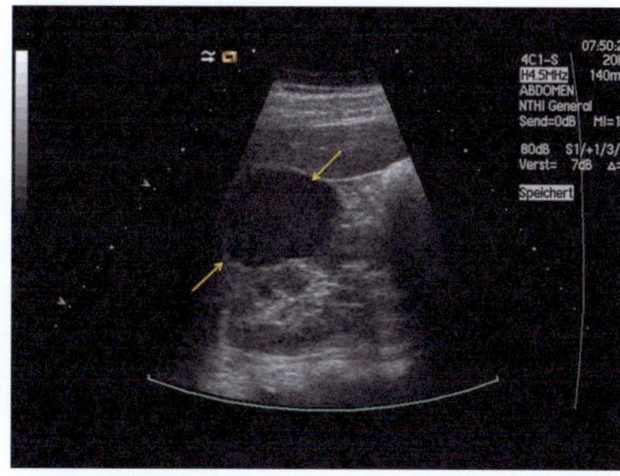

Fig. 12 Benign renal cyst that shows thin walls without any septae or calcifications and a characteristic posterior acoustic enhancement

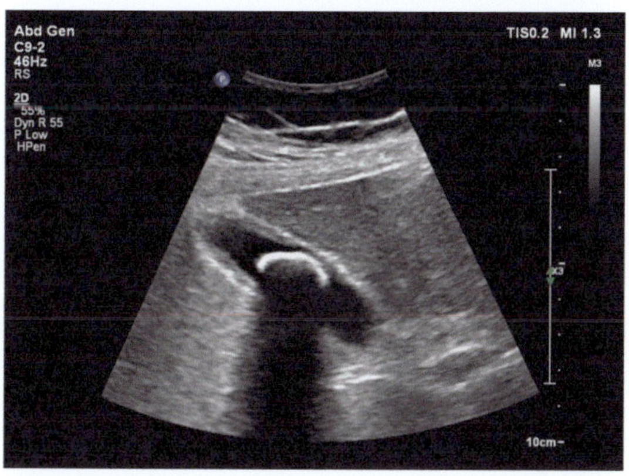

Fig. 11 A big single gallstone inside the gallbladder showing the classical sonographic features of gallstones with an hyperechoic focus and a dorsal acoustic shadow

include cholecystectomy, endoscopic retrograde cholangiopancreatography (ERCP), or extracorporeal shock wave lithotripsy (Figs. 10 and 11).

5 Renal Cysts and Renal Cell Carcinoma

5.1 Renal Cysts

Focal benign renal cysts are one of the most common incidental finding in the sonography of the kidneys. Renal cysts show an age-dependent increasing incidence with more renal cysts found in older patients. 20 % of all 50 years old show benign renal cysts, and in 50 % of all patients, renal cysts can be found after necropsy. They additionally show a gender-dependent distribution with a ratio of 2:1 in favor of women (Ravine et al. 1993). In native B-mode ultrasound, benign renal cysts show characteristic features: thin walls without septa or calcifications, an anechoic water-equal density, and a posterior acoustic enhancement (Radermacher 2003). Normally they do not cause any signs or symptoms and no intervention is usually needed, except in cases they cause secondary problems, e.g., due to their size causing hydronephrosis or abdominal pain. If they cause any symptoms, therapeutic options include, for example, laparoscopic decortication (Fig. 12) (Shiraishi et al. 2006).

5.2 Renal Cell Carcinoma

The most important differential diagnosis for renal lesions is the renal cell carcinoma with an incidence rate of 3 %. Of all malignant neoplasms, it is most commonly found in patients between an age of 60–70 and with a ratio of 3:2 in favor of women (Hock et al. 2002; Chow et al. 1999; Decastro and McKiernan 2008; Landis et al. 1999; Wallen et al. 2007; Woldrich et al. 2008). Predisposing risk factors for renal cell carcinoma include hypertension, smoking, genetics, and obesity (Haggstrom et al. 2013; Lipworth et al. 2009). The classical clinical triad for patients referred for diagnosis consists of hematuria, flank pain, and an abdominal mass, but they can only be found in about 10–15 % of all patients

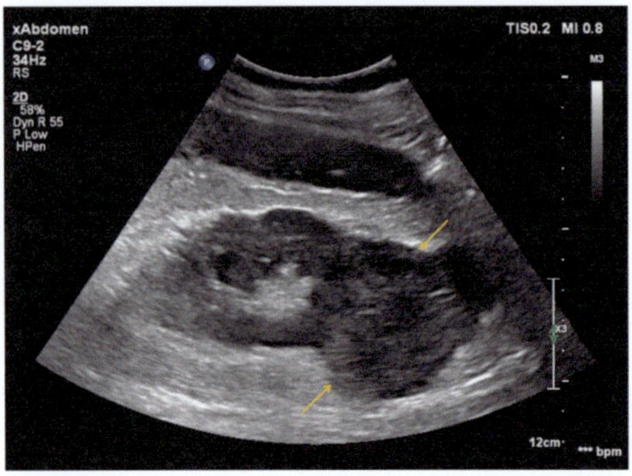

Fig. 13 Hypoechoic solid soft tissue renal lesion of the kidney (*yellow arrows*) suggestive of a renal cell carcinoma

(Cohen and McGovern 2005). Mostly, renal cell carcinomas are incidentally found in asymptomatic patients (Motzer et al. 2007). Typical sonographic features include hypoechoic soft tissue components adjacent to the kidney with visible vascularization in color Doppler (Jubelirer and Rubin 1993). Treatment options include radical nephrectomy as the treatment option of choice or, if possible, nephron-sparing tumor surgery (Fig. 13) (Tannir 2014).

Literature

Acalovschi M, Blendea D, Feier C, Letia AI, Ratiu N, Dumitrascu DL et al (2003) Risk factors for symptomatic gallstones in patients with liver cirrhosis: a case–control study. Am J Gastroenterol 98(8):1856–1860

Bajenaru N, Balaban V, Savulescu F, Campeanu I, Patrascu T (2015) Hepatic hemangioma -review. J Med Life 8(Spec Issue):4–11

Buch S, Schafmayer C, Volzke H, Becker C, Franke A, von Eller-Eberstein H et al (2007) A genome-wide association scan identifies the hepatic cholesterol transporter ABCG8 as a susceptibility factor for human gallstone disease. Nat Genet 39(8):995–999

Chow WH, Devesa SS, Warren JL, Fraumeni JF Jr (1999) Rising incidence of renal cell cancer in the United States. JAMA 281(17):1628–1631

Cina CS, Devereaux PJ (2005) Review: population-based screening for abdominal aortic aneurysm reduces cause-specific mortality in older men. ACP J Club 143(1):11

Cohen HT, McGovern FJ (2005) Renal-cell carcinoma. N Engl J Med 353(23):2477–2490

Decastro GJ, McKiernan JM (2008) Epidemiology, clinical staging, and presentation of renal cell carcinoma. Urol Clin North Am 35(4):581–592; vi

Dockerty MB, Gray HK, Henson SW Jr (1956) Benign tumors of the liver. II. Hemangiomas. Surg Gynecol Obstet 103(3):327–331

Filardo G, Powell JT, Martinez MA, Ballard DJ (2015) Surgery for small asymptomatic abdominal aortic aneurysms. Cochrane Database Syst Rev 2:CD001835

Gaines PA, Sampson MA (1989) The prevalence and characterization of simple hepatic cysts by ultrasound examination. Br J Radiol 62(736):335–337

Haggstrom C, Rapp K, Stocks T, Manjer J, Bjorge T, Ulmer H et al (2013) Metabolic factors associated with risk of renal cell carcinoma. PLoS One 8(2):e57475

Hock LM, Lynch J, Balaji KC (2002) Increasing incidence of all stages of kidney cancer in the last 2 decades in the United States: an analysis of surveillance, epidemiology and end results program data. J Urol 167(1):57–60

Jubelirer SJ, Rubin M (1993) The use of modern radiologic methods in identifying incidental renal cell carcinoma. W V Med J 89(1):21–23

Kent KC (2014) Clinical practice. Abdominal aortic aneurysms. N Engl J Med 371(22):2101–2108

Kleinman ME, Greives MR, Churgin SS, Blechman KM, Chang EI, Ceradini DJ et al (2007) Hypoxia-induced mediators of stem/progenitor cell trafficking are increased in children with hemangioma. Arterioscler Thromb Vasc Biol 27(12):2664–2670

Koszka AJ, Ferreira FG, de Aquino CG, Ribeiro MA, Gallo AS, Aranzana EM et al (2010) Resection of a rapid-growing 40-cm giant liver hemangioma. World J Hepatol 2(7):292–294

Landis SH, Murray T, Bolden S, Wingo PA (1999) Cancer statistics, 1999. CA Cancer J Clin 49(1):8–31, 1

Lederle FA, Wilson SE, Johnson GR, Reinke DB, Littooy FN, Acher CW et al (2002) Immediate repair compared with surveillance of small abdominal aortic aneurysms. N Engl J Med 346(19):1437–1444

LeFevre ML (2014) Force USPST. Screening for abdominal aortic aneurysm: U.S. Preventive Services Task Force recommendation statement. Ann Intern Med 161(4):281–290

Lipworth L, Tarone RE, Lund L, McLaughlin JK (2009) Epidemiologic characteristics and risk factors for renal cell cancer. Clin Epidemiol 1:33–43

Motzer RJ, Hutson TE, Tomczak P, Michaelson MD, Bukowski RM, Rixe O et al (2007) Sunitinib versus interferon alfa in metastatic renal-cell carcinoma. N Engl J Med 356(2):115–124

Nakanuma Y (1995) Non-neoplastic nodular lesions in the liver. Pathol Int 45(10):703–714

Powell JT, Brown LC, Forbes JF, Fowkes FG, Greenhalgh RM, Ruckley CV et al (2007) Final 12-year follow-up of surgery versus surveillance in the UK Small Aneurysm Trial. Br J Surg 94(6):702–708

Radermacher J (2003) Ultrasound of the kidney and renal vessels. I: normal findings, congenital diseases,

diseases of the kidney parenchyma. Internist 44(10):1283–1297; quiz 98–9

Ravine D, Gibson RN, Donlan J, Sheffield LJ (1993) An ultrasound renal cyst prevalence survey: specificity data for inherited renal cystic diseases. Am J Kidney Dis 22(6):803–807

Salem MK, Rayt HS, Hussey G, Rafelt S, Nelson CP, Sayers RD et al (2009) Should Asian men be included in abdominal aortic aneurysm screening programmes? Eur J Vasc Endovasc Surg 38(6):748–749

Schmitz-Rixen T, Keese M, Hakimi M, Peters A, Bockler D, Nelson K et al (2016) Ruptured abdominal aortic aneurysm-epidemiology, predisposing factors, and biology. Langenbecks Arch Surg/Deutsche Gesellschaft fur Chirurgie 401(3):275–288

Shaffer EA (2006) Gallstone disease: epidemiology of gallbladder stone disease. Best Pract Res Clin Gastroenterol 20(6):981–996

Shiraishi K, Eguchi S, Mohri J, Kamiryo Y (2006) Laparoscopic decortication of symptomatic simple renal cysts: 10-year experience from one institution. BJU Int 98(2):405–408

Tannir NM (2014) Renal cell carcinoma. Oxford University Press, Oxford; pp 1–187

Wallen EM, Pruthi RS, Joyce GF, Wise M (2007) Urologic diseases in America P. Kidney cancer. J Urol 177(6):2006–2018; discussion 18–9

Woldrich JM, Mallin K, Ritchey J, Carroll PR, Kane CJ (2008) Sex differences in renal cell cancer presentation and survival: an analysis of the National Cancer Database, 1993–2004. J Urol 179(5):1709–1713; discussion 13

Index

A
Abdomen
  ^{18}F-FDG PET/CT
    stomach and bowel, 176
    urinary tract, 176–177
  IF (*see also* Incidental findings (IFs))
    adnexal findings, 109–110
    adrenal mass, 108–109
    cystic renal masses, 107–108
    liver mass, 108
Abdominal aortic aneurysm (AAA), 155–156, 198
Adnexal cysts, 110
Adnexal lesions, 156–157
  cysts and teratomas, 157–159
  uterus, 159–160
Adrenal gland, 121
Adrenal lesions, non-^{18}F-FDG PET/CT, 187–188, 190–191
Adrenal mass
  CT characteristics, 143–144
  extra-adrenal malignancy, 146
  frequency, 143
  IF, 108–109
  management, 145
  shape and size, 145
  young patients with, 146
Appendix, 155

B
Biliary tree, 150–151
Body imaging, 117–118
Bone, ^{18}F-FDG PET/CT, 179
Brain imaging, 115–117
Breast, ^{18}F-FDG PET/CT, 182–186
Brown adipose tissue, ^{18}F-FDG PET/CT, 182

C
Carotid Doppler ultrasound image, 74
Cholelithiasis, 200–201
Colonography, 129–131
Computed tomography (CT)
  characteristics, adrenal mass, 143–144
  incidentalomas, 26
  population-based imaging, 39
  SCAPIS, 93–94
Coronary Artery Calcium Score (CACS), 94
Coronary artery disease (CAD), 174
Coronary artery stenosis (CAS)
  challenges with calcifications, 97
  guidelines, 96–97
  handling, 97–98
Coronary CT angiography (CCTA), 94
Cystic renal masses, 107–108

D
Diffusion-weighted imaging (DWI), 189
Disclosure
  design, 14
  false-negative results, 11, 12
  plans, 18–20
  positive outcomes, 12
Dual-energy X-ray absorptiometry (DXA), 74

E
e-Medicine, potential impact of, 164
Esophagus, ^{18}F-FDG PET/CT, 175–176

F
Female reproductive system, ^{18}F-FDG PET/CT, 177–178
^{18}F-FDG PET/CT
  abdomen
    stomach and bowel, 176
    urinary tract, 176–177
  bone, 179
  breast, 182–186
  brown adipose tissue, 182
  head and neck, 170
    larynx, 173
    salivary glands, 171
    thyroid, 171–173
    Waldeyer's ring, 171
  immunological responses, 179–180
  inflammatory lesions, 179–180
  nonattenuation-corrected images, 186

DOI 10.1007/174_2016, © Springer International Publishing Switzerland

^{18}F-FDG PET/CT (*cont.*)
  and PET/MR
    advantages, 189–191
    disadvantages, 191
  skin and subcutaneous fat, 180–182
  small pelvis
    prostate and testes, 178–179
    uterus and ovaries, 177–178
  thorax
    esophagus, 175–176
    gastroesophageal junction, 175–176
    heart, 174–175
    lung, 173
    thymus, 173–174
^{18}F-FDG PET/MR, and PET/CT, 188
  advantages, 189–191
  disadvantages, 191

G
Gallbladder, 150–151
Gallstones, 200–201
Gastroesophageal junction, ^{18}F-FDG PET/CT, 175–176
Gastrointestinal tract
  appendix, 155
  IF, 153–154
  large bowel, 154–155
  small bowel, 154
  stomach, 154
G-CSF. *See* Granulocyte colony-stimulating factor (G-CSF)
German National Cohort (GNC)
  design of MRI study within, 59
  goal, 58
  IF
    clinically relevant, 62–65
    clinical work-up outside, 62
    concept, 68–69
    ethical framework, 60
    false positives, disproportionate increase of, 61–62
    limited clinical context, 61
    problems, 60–62
    quality assurance, 67–68
    radiologists, training and certification of, 67
    reliability, reproducibility, and consistency, 62
    scientific imaging sequences, 61
    technical translation, 65–67
  imaging, 58
  MR sequences within, 58
Granulocyte colony-stimulating factor (G-CSF), 179, 180

H
Head and neck, ^{18}F-FDG PET/CT, 170
  larynx, 173
  salivary glands, 171
  thyroid, 171–173
  Waldeyer's ring, 171
Healing process, ^{18}F-FDG tracer uptake, 179
Heart, ^{18}F-FDG PET/CT, 174–175
Hemangiomas, 198–199
Hibernoma, 182, 184
Hidradenitis suppurativa, 181, 183
Hormone replacement therapy, 178, 182–183

I
IFs. *See* Incidental findings (IFs)
Imaging-derived phenotypes (IDP), 73
Imaging modalities
  CT, 39
  MRI, 38–39
  properties, 38
  US, 39–40
Immune response, ^{18}F-FDG PET/CT, 179–180
Incidental findings (IFs)
  abdominal CT
    adnexal findings, 109–110
    adnexal and uterine lesions, 156–160
    adrenal masses, 108–109, 143–146
    in clinical work, 161–162
    colonography, 129–131
    cystic renal masses, 107–108
    description, 128–129
    detection, 131
    e-Medicine, potential impact of, 164
    examinations, 128
    gallbladder and biliary tree, 150–151
    gastrointestinal tract, 153–155
    kidneys, 132–141
    liver, 146–150
    liver mass, 108
    lymph nodes, 151
    pancreas, 152–153
    patients need, 162–163
    prostate, 160–161
    radiologists report, 162
    refer physician, 163–164
    retrospective study, 129
    skeletal lesions, 161
    spleen, 151
    technical factors affecting, 131–132
    urinary bladder and upper urinary tract tumors, 141–143
    vascular structures, 155–156
  in broad sense, 4–5
  characteristics, 5
  classification
    clinical setting, 118–124
    research setting, 114–118
  clinical studies, 7
  concept, 4
  diagnostic findings, 4
  ethical aspects
    challenges, 9–10
    classification, 19
    disclosure algorithms, 18
    disclosure and non-disclosure, 12–13, 18–21
    discovery findings, 10
    frequency of occurrence, 10–11
    inform, 21

medical practice and research, 22–23
positive and negative effects, 13–14
possible consequences, 14
potential outcome, 11
prerequisites, 14–17
principles, 14–17
recommendations, 17–22
study protocol design, 21–22
typical fields, 11
whole-body scans, 10
GNC
clinical work-up outside, 62
concept, 68–69
ethical framework, 60, 62–68
false positives, disproportionate increase of, 61–62
limited clinical context, 61
problems, 60–62
quality assurance, 67–68
radiologists, training and certification of, 67
reliability, reproducibility, and consistency, 62
scientific imaging sequences, 61
technical translation, 65–67
indicative dignity, 6
medical fundamental research, 7
MESA
aortic valve calcification, 88
CAC, 87–88
electron-beam CT, 88
four-detector row CT, 88
pericardial effusion, 88, 89
pleural thickening, 88, 89
prevalence, 88
pulmonary nodule, 88, 89
significant alerts, 89–90
in narrow sense, 5
neuroscientific fundamental research, 7
occurrence, 6–7
PFN, 107
population-based screening study, 113
Rotterdam study
on brain MRI, 85
detection and management protocol, 81–82
feedback, 85
frequency, 82–85
participants' expectations and experience, 85–86
review of scans, 82
SCAPIS
aim, 92–93
asymptomatic coronary artery stenosis, 96–98
CT, 93–94
ethics, 98–99
imaging, 92
information collect, 92, 93
pulmonary nodules, 94–96
SHIP
assessment and handling, 49–51
distribution, 51–52
impact, 52–53
signal abnormality, 5–6
small pulmonary nodules, 106
subsolid pulmonary nodules, 106–107
UK Biobank
consent processes, 74–75
development, 74
evaluating participants, 75–76
feedback, 75
identification, 75
ongoing evaluation, 76–77
qualitative work, 76
with radiologists, 76
ultrasound
AAA, 198
cholelithiasis, 200–201
hemangiomas, 198–199
liver cysts, 199–200
preliminary remarks, 197–198
renal cell carcinoma, 201–202
renal cysts, 201
Incidentalomas
author's advice, 32
CT, 26
definition, 26
incidence, 27
radiologists, 31–32
Informed consent
SHIP, 46–49
types, 31
Interatrial septum, lipomatous hypertrophy, 175

K
Kidney, 120
benign renal lesions, 135–136
Bosniak classification, 139
complex cysts, 138–139
cystic renal lesions, 137
false-positive renal masses, 140
hydronephrosis, 141
normal variants and malformations, 141
renal calcifications, 140
renal size, 140
simple cysts, 137–138
small lesions, 136–137
solid renal tumors, 132–135

L
Larynx, ^{18}F-FDG PET/CT, 173
Lipomatous hypertrophy, interatrial septum, 175
Liver, 189–190
ACR recommendations, 122
CT colonography, 146
cystic lesions, 146–147
cysts, ultrasound, 199–200
hemangioma, 147–148
incidental liver mass detected, 149–150
mass, 108
non-cystic benign liver lesions, 148–149
non-^{18}F-FDG PET/CT, 186–187
steatosis, 150

Lung, 119–120, 173
Lung nodules, 186, 191
Lymph nodes, 151

M
Magnetic resonance imaging (MRI)
population-based imaging, 38–39
Rotterdam study, 85
Male reproductive system, ^{18}F-FDG PET/CT, 178–179
Medicolegal aspects
duty of researchers, 30
exposure to radiation, 30–31
frequency engenders dilemma, 26–27
incidentaloma, in American courtroom, 29–30
incidentalomas
author's advice, 32
CT, 26
definition, 26
incidence, 27
radiologists, 31–32
informed consent (*see* Informed consent)
radiology literature, 26
standard of care, 27–29
unnecessary imaging, 30–31
Metformin, 176
Multiethnic Study of Atherosclerosis (MESA) Study
aortic valve calcification, 88
CAC, 87–88
electron-beam CT, 88
four-detector row CT, 88
pericardial effusion, 88, 89
pleural thickening, 88, 89
prevalence, 88
pulmonary nodule, 88, 89
significant alerts, 89–90

N
Non-^{18}F-FDG PET/CT
adrenal lesions, 187–188
liver lesions, 186–187
lung nodules, 186

O
Ovary, ^{18}F-FDG PET/CT, 177–178

P
Pancreas
cystic lesions, 152–153
solid tumors, 152
Papillary muscles, focal tracer uptake in, 174
Pelvis, ^{18}F-FDG PET/CT
prostate and testes, 178–179
uterus and ovaries, 177–178
Population-based imaging
data
post-processing and analysis, 40–41
storage and distribution, 40
general requirements, 37–38
imaging modalities
CT, 39
MRI, 38–39
properties, 38
US, 39–40
Positron emission tomography/computed tomography (PET/CT), 169–170
^{18}F-FDG (*see* ^{18}F-FDG PET/CT)
and PET/MR, 188–191
squamous cell carcinoma, 175
Positron emission tomography/magnetic resonance (PET/MR), 170
and PET/CT, 188–191
protocols, 189
Presidential Commission for Study of Bioethical Issues, 10
Prostate, 160–161, 178–179
Pulmonary nodules
guidelines, 94–95
handle
in main trial, 96
in pilot trial, 95–96
Pulmonary perifissural nodules (PFN), 107

R
Radiofrequency coils, gamma-quant attenuation, 188
Renal cell carcinoma, 201–202
Renal cysts, 201
Rotterdam study
hardware and imaging protocol, 80–81
IF
on brain MRI, 85
detection and management protocol, 81–82
feedback, 85
frequency, 82–85
participants' expectations and experience, 85–86
review of scans, 82
neuroimaging, 80
setup, 79–80

S
Salivary glands, ^{18}F-FDG PET/CT, 171
Sarcoidosis, 179–181
SCAPIS. *See* Swedish CArdioPulmonary bioImage Study (SCAPIS)
SHIP. *See* Study of Health in Pomerania (SHIP)
Signal abnormality, 5–6
Skeletal lesions, 161
Skin, ^{18}F-FDG PET/CT, 180–182
Small pulmonary nodules, 106
Spine, 122–124
Spleen, 151
Squamous cell carcinoma, PET/CT, 175
Standardized uptake value (SUV), 170, 180, 182
Standard of care (SOC), 27–29
Study of Health in Pomerania (SHIP)
cohort study, 45
comprehensive examination programs, 45

incidental findings
assessment and handling, 49–51
distribution, 51–52
impact, 52–53
informed consent, 46–49
perception of study, 46–49
WB-MRI, 46
Subcutaneous fat, ^{18}F-FDG PET/CT, 180–182
Subsolid pulmonary nodules, 106–107
SUV. *See* Standardized uptake value (SUV)
Swedish CArdioPulmonary bioImage Study (SCAPIS)
aim, 92–93
asymptomatic coronary artery stenosis, 96–98
CT, 93–94
ethics, 98–99
imaging, 92
information collect, 92, 93
pulmonary nodules, 94–96

T

Testes, ^{18}F-FDG PET/CT, 178–179
Thorax, ^{18}F-FDG PET/CT
esophagus, 175–176
gastroesophageal junction, 175–176
heart, 174–175
lung, 173
thymus, 173–174
3D gradient echo sequences, 189, 191
Thymus, ^{18}F-FDG PET/CT, 173–174
Thyroid, ^{18}F-FDG PET/CT, 171–173

U

UK Biobank
carotid Doppler ultrasound, 74
DXA, 74
generates IDP, 73
IF protocol
consent processes, 74–75
development, 74
evaluating participants, 75–76
feedback, 75
identification, 75
ongoing evaluation, 76–77
qualitative work, 76
with radiologists, 76
imaging study, 72–74
non-contrast cardiac MRI, 73
research imaging, 72
Ultrasound
AAA, 198
cholelithiasis, 200–201
hemangiomas, 198–199
liver cysts, 199–200
population-based imaging, 39–40
preliminary remarks, 197–198
renal cell carcinoma, 201–202
renal cysts, 201
Upper urinary tract tumors, 141–143
Urinary bladder, 141–143
Urinary tract, ^{18}F-FDG PET/CT, 176–177
Uterine lesions, 156–157
cysts and teratomas, 157–159
uterus, 159–160
Uterus, ^{18}F-FDG PET/CT, 177–178

W

Waldeyer's ring, ^{18}F-FDG PET/CT, 171
Warburg effect, 170
White adipose tissue, 182
Whole body-MRI (WB-MRI), 15, 41, 46

MIX
Papier aus verantwortungsvollen Quellen
Paper from responsible sources
FSC® C105338

If you have any concerns about our products,
you can contact us on
ProductSafety@springernature.com

In case Publisher is established outside the EU,
the EU authorized representative is:
Springer Nature Customer Service Center GmbH
Europaplatz 3, 69115 Heidelberg, Germany

Printed by Libri Plureos GmbH
in Hamburg, Germany